Ultrasonography of Musculoskeletal Pain

Ke-Vin Chang
Editor

Ultrasonography of Musculoskeletal Pain

Insights into the Upper Extremity

Springer

Editor
Ke-Vin Chang, MD, PhD, CIPS, RMSK, ASRA-PMUC, Professor
Bei-Hu Branch
National Taiwan University Hospital
Taipei, Taiwan

ISBN 978-981-96-6786-4 ISBN 978-981-96-6787-1 (eBook)
https://doi.org/10.1007/978-981-96-6787-1

This Springer imprint is published by the registered company Springer Nature Singapore Pte Ltd.
The registered company address is: 152 Beach Road, #21-01/04 Gateway East, Singapore 189721, Singapore

Foreword by Levent Özçakar

After the *Blue* [1], *Black* [2], and *Red* [3] *books*, I am now very much pleased/flattered to contribute to *Ke-Vin's book*. Our collaboration with him has already surpassed a decade during which we tried our best to work as "1 + 1 + ... + 1 = 1 1 ... 1." In this sense, we also hope to have added our "cents" to the "renaissance" of musculoskeletal medicine, i.e., ultrasonography [4]. It is again our great pleasure to also witness the new (post-ultrasound) era where we are now discussing its "haute couture" use in our daily practice [5]. Yet, while all musculoskeletal physicians need ultrasound; depending on their patient spectrum, working place, or available infrastructure, the actual utility might vary. In this book, those who are dealing with painful conditions and (in the same time) who would like to intervene are rather zeroed in on. Further, the individual scenarios are discussed more with emphasis on the coupling of ultrasound imaging and guidance. In other words, ultrasound guidance refers not only to precise targeting during the intervention but also to its impact on the whole process including the (pre-procedural) diagnostic stage and the (post-procedural) follow-up. After reading this first volume and having substantial insight into better understanding the optimal interventional approach to common painful conditions, I strongly believe that colleagues will start looking forward to the incoming volumes, which are all planned as "sugarcoated" and "spoon-fed."

Levent Özçakar, MD, Professor

Department of Physical
and Rehabilitation Medicine
Hacettepe University Medical School
Ankara, Turkey

Vice President, ISPRM, Istanbul, Turkey

References

1. Özçakar L, De Muynck M, Eds. Musculoskeletal ultrasound in Physical and Rehabilitation Medicine. Edi.Ermes, Milan, 2014.
2. Özçakar L, Ed. Sonographic atlas for common musculoskeletal pathologies. Edi.Ermes, Milan, 2017.
3. Özçakar L, Ed. Ultrasound imaging and guidance for musculoskeletal interventions in Physical and Rehabilitation Medicine. Edi.Ermes, Milan, 2020.
4. Özçakar L. AI (as an Ally) for musculoskeletal ultrasound in PRM - Haute couture after renaissance. Am J Phys Med Rehabil 2024;103:967–9.
5. Özçakar L. Advances in musculoskeletal ultrasound – Chronicle of a 25-year live witness. PM R (in press).

Foreword by Der-Sheng Han

Musculoskeletal ultrasonography has revolutionized the diagnostic and therapeutic approach for pain physicians, particularly in the management of musculoskeletal disorders. The dynamic, noninvasive nature of ultrasound imaging has become an indispensable tool for identifying structural abnormalities and guiding interventions with precision. *Ultrasonography of Musculoskeletal Pain: Insights into the Upper Extremity* serves as a comprehensive resource, addressing the unique needs of practitioners who focus on diagnosing and treating painful syndromes of the upper extremity.

Unlike traditional texts that emphasize the normal sonoanatomy of musculoskeletal systems, this book adopts a clinically oriented perspective. It integrates detailed anatomical insights with real-world application, enabling pain physicians to bridge the gap between diagnosis and intervention. Each chapter has consistent organization, and is designed to address common clinical syndromes, offering step-by-step ultrasonographic evaluations, diagnostic criteria, and interventional techniques. High-resolution cadaveric and ultrasonographic images, along with dynamic illustrations, provide unparalleled clarity in visualizing complex anatomical structures.

From shoulder pathologies like adhesive capsulitis and sub-coracoid pain to intricate wrist conditions such as carpal tunnel syndrome and triangular fibrocartilage complex injuries, this book explores a spectrum of conditions. For each topic, emphasis is placed on understanding the sonoanatomy, recognizing pathologies, and mastering ultrasound-guided interventions. Pain physicians will find value in the actionable protocols, evidence-based approaches, and practical tips tailored for real-world application.

Authored by leading experts in the field—Drs. Ke-Vin Chang, Wei-Ting Wu, Yuan-Yuan Tsai, Shao-Yu Chi, Jia-Chi Wang, and Levent Özçakar—this book aspires to enhance the clinical skills and confidence of its readers. Whether you are a pain physician, orthopedist, physiatrist, neurologist, or physical therapist, I recommend this book as a vital companion in the evolving field of musculoskeletal ultrasonography. I hope it not only enriches your practice but also empowers you to improve patient outcomes through precision diagnostics and targeted therapies.

Let this journey through the upper extremity, guided by the probes of ultrasonography, deepen your expertise and refine your approach to managing musculoskeletal pain.

Department of Physical Medicine and Rehabilitation, College of Medicine
National Taiwan University
Taipei, Taiwan

Bei-Hu Branch, National Taiwan University Hospital
Taipei, Taiwan

Der-Sheng Han, MD, PhD, EMBA, Professor

Preface

Pain management demands a precise understanding of the intricate interplay between musculoskeletal and neural structures that contribute to pain. While numerous books systematically introduce musculoskeletal ultrasound imaging or detail ultrasound-guided injection techniques, few focus on specific body regions paired with strategic ultrasound approaches and selected intervention tips. Addressing this gap is the primary aim of the present book.

Designed for physicians and healthcare practitioners managing painful musculoskeletal conditions across all specialties, this book integrates diagnostic principles with guided interventions. Central to its philosophy is the concept of "diagnosis ahead of intervention," emphasizing that accurate diagnosis is paramount to effective treatments.

This book can also be viewed as an extension of *Ultrasound Imaging & Guidance for Musculoskeletal Interventions* (Levent Özçakar, *Editor*), where we had the initial privilege of coupling "imaging" and "guidance," i.e., the concept of "ultrasound guides the procedure." Additionally, the content has been enriched by insights gained through the USMSIT (Ultrasound Musculoskeletal Workshop in Taiwan) and NMUSIT (Neuro-muscular Ultrasound Workshop in Taiwan) courses, which annually blend classical principles with innovative approaches to musculoskeletal ultrasound education.

Authored and edited primarily by physiatrists from National Taiwan University Hospital, Bei-Hu branch—including myself, Wei-Ting Wu, Yuan-Yuan Tsai, and Shao-Yu Chi—this book features a unified writing style and consistently edited figures to minimize cognitive load for readers. We owe immense gratitude to the MSK ultrasound team at the main hospital for their unwavering support and to the teachings and writings of esteemed pioneers in the field. Images adapted from cadaveric images provided by the Visible Human Project® of the National Library of Medicine. Excerpts from the VH Dissector are included with permission from Touch of Life Technologies Inc., and we acknowledge their valuable contributions to this work.

As part of a series, this book focuses on the upper extremities, while future volumes will explore the lower extremities and the head, neck, and trunk. Guided by the belief that "perfection may be out of reach, but dedication unites us," this first edition may not be flawless, but it is imbued with our collective enthusiasm and commitment. We hope it resonates with all physicians managing painful musculoskeletal conditions and reflects the excitement we felt during its creation.

Personally, I find myself moved each time I revisit its chapters and wholeheartedly recommend it as an invaluable resource for your practice.

With gratitude and anticipation,

Taipei, Taiwan Ke-Vin Chang

Contents

Contributors

Ke-Vin Chang Bei-Hu Branch, National Taiwan University Hospital, Taipei, Taiwan

Shao-Yu Chi Bei-Hu Branch, National Taiwan University Hospital, Taipei, Taiwan

Levent Özçakar Department of Physical and Rehabilitation Medicine, Hacettepe University Medical School, Ankara, Turkey

Yuan-Yuan Tsai Bei-Hu Branch, National Taiwan University Hospital, Taipei, Taiwan

Jia-Chi Wang Arkship Rehabilitation Clinic, New Taipei City, Taiwan

Wei-Ting Wu Bei-Hu Branch, National Taiwan University Hospital, Taipei, Taiwan

Part I
Shoulder

Chapter 1
Targeting the Rotator Cuff and the Rotator Interval in Shoulder Pathologies

Ke-Vin Chang, Wei-Ting Wu, Yuan-Yuan Tsai, and Levent Özçakar

1.1 Introduction

The rotator interval is a triangular space between the subscapularis and supraspinatus tendons, often implicated in various shoulder conditions including adhesive capsulitis. The four tendons of the rotator cuff—supraspinatus, infraspinatus, teres minor, and subscapularis—work together to stabilize and facilitate shoulder movements. While the supraspinatus primarily assists in shoulder abduction, the infraspinatus and teres minor are responsible for external rotation. Meanwhile, the subscapularis enables internal rotation of the shoulder. The rotator cuff interval is anatomically connected to these tendons and helps to prevent excessive anterior translation of the humeral head, thereby maintaining joint stability during arm movements.

Ultrasound is a highly effective tool for evaluating rotator cuff tendon tears, with distinct advantages over magnetic resonance imaging (MRI) in various scenarios. Although MRI is often considered the gold standard for soft tissue assessment, ultrasound offers quick, cost-effective, dynamic, and real-time imaging that enables clinicians to assess tendon integrity and functionality. A meta-analysis by Farooqi et al. [1] reviewed 23 studies involving 2054 shoulders and demonstrated that ultrasound had high diagnostic accuracy for identifying rotator cuff tendon tears. Specifically, ultrasound showed a median accuracy of 0.83 for supraspinatus tendon tears and 0.93 for biceps tendon tears, with a notably higher accuracy for full-thickness (0.93) vs. partial-thickness (0.81) supraspinatus tendon tears.

K.-V. Chang (✉) · W.-T. Wu · Y.-Y. Tsai
Bei-Hu Branch, National Taiwan University Hospital, Taipei, Taiwan

L. Özçakar
Department of Physical and Rehabilitation Medicine, Hacettepe University Medical School, Ankara, Turkey

K.-V. Chang (ed.), *Ultrasonography of Musculoskeletal Pain*,
https://doi.org/10.1007/978-981-96-6787-1_1

Adhesive capsulitis, commonly known as frozen shoulder, affects between 3% and 5% of the general population [2]. It typically develops in people aged 40 to 59 years, but evidence shows that it can also occur in older age groups. A German study [3] reported a one-year prevalence of 0.4% and a lifetime prevalence of 2.4% among older adults. Arthroscopic examinations of shoulders affected by adhesive capsulitis reveal specific pathological features, including subacromial fibrosis, proliferative synovitis, and capsular thickening. These characteristics contribute to the limited range of motion and pain associated with frozen shoulder.

Several imaging studies have highlighted important findings in adhesive capsulitis. A meta-analysis by Suh et al. [4] identified common features such as coracohumeral ligament thickening, fat obliteration in the rotator interval, and enhanced visibility of the axillary joint capsule. Additionally, hyperintensity and thickening of the inferior glenohumeral ligament are frequently observed. Another meta-analysis by Wu et al. [5] focused on ultrasound imaging and noted similar results. They reported thickened coracohumeral ligament and axillary recess capsule in addition to rotator interval abnormalities as key diagnostic indicators for adhesive capsulitis.

Traditional treatment for adhesive capsulitis often involves corticosteroid injections into the posterior glenohumeral joint. However, a newer approach via the rotator interval has also shown comparable effectiveness [6] with a more targeted and less invasive treatment option. This chapter aims to elaborate on the sonoanatomy of the rotator cuff and rotator interval with special emphasis on the diagnosis/treatment of rotator cuff tendon tears as well as adhesive capsulitis.

1.2 Anatomy

The long head tendon of the biceps brachii lies within the rotator interval, where it stabilizes the shoulder joint by interacting closely with the surrounding tendons/ligaments. Its extra-articular portion, located in the bicipital groove between the lesser and greater tuberosities, is stabilized by the transverse humeral ligament (Fig. 1.1). Its intra-articular portion is stabilized by the biceps' reflection pulley at the medial aspect, which consists of the superior glenohumeral ligament and the medial bundle of the coracohumeral ligament (Fig. 1.1). The biceps brachii muscle is the flexor/supinator of the forearm at the elbow joint. It also contributes to arm flexion at the glenohumeral joint. Medially, the subscapularis muscle originates from the subscapular fossa and its tendon inserts onto the lesser tuberosity with four to five bundles. The transverse humeral ligament is considered a sling primarily formed by fibers of the subscapularis tendon [7], with additional support from the supraspinatus tendon and the coracohumeral ligament.

The residual three tendons of the rotator cuff all insert on the facets of the greater tuberosity (Fig. 1.2) [8]. The supraspinatus originates from the supraspinous fossa of the scapula and inserts onto the superior facet and the anterior portion of the middle facet of the greater tuberosity of the humerus. The infraspinatus originates from the infraspinous fossa of the scapula and inserts onto the middle facet of the

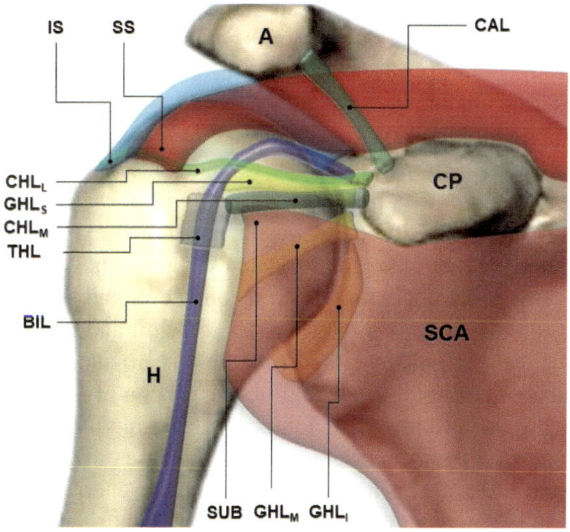

Fig. 1.1 The illustration depicts the rotator cuff interval. THL transverse humeral ligament; CHL$_L$ lateral bundle of the coracohumeral ligament; CHL$_M$ medial bundle of the coracohumeral ligament; GHL$_S$ superior glenohumeral ligament; GHL$_M$ middle glenohumeral ligament; GHL$_I$ inferior glenohumeral ligament; CAL coracoacromial ligament; BIL long head tendon of the biceps brachii; SUB subscapularis tendon; SS supraspinatus tendon; IS infraspinatus tendon; CP coracoid process; A acromion; SCA scapula; H humerus

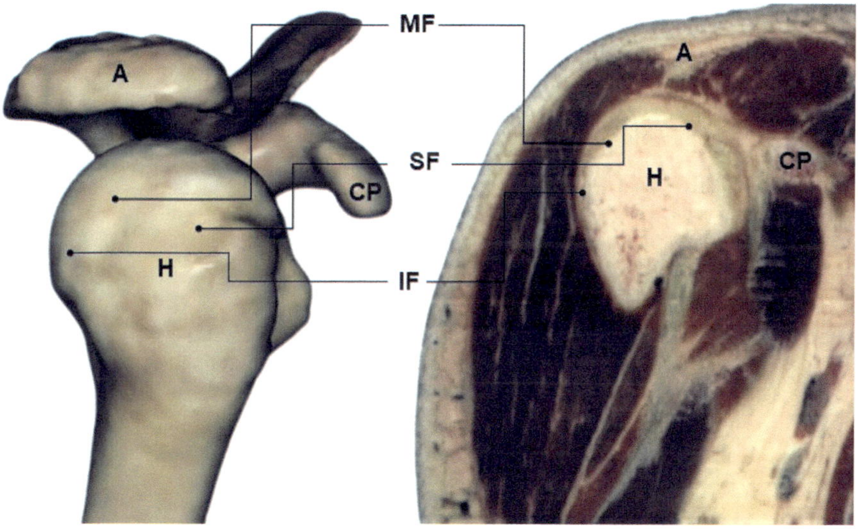

Fig. 1.2 The cadaveric images show the superior, middle, and inferior facets of the greater tuberosity of the humerus. SF superior facet; MF middle facet; IF inferior facet; CP coracoid process; A acromion; H humerus

greater tuberosity, overlapping the posterior aspect of the supraspinatus tendon (Fig. 1.3). The teres minor tendon originates from the posteroinferior surface of the scapula and inserts onto the inferior facet of the greater tuberosity (Fig. 1.3).

Soft tissues surrounding the rotator cuff include the bursae and labrum. The subacromial-subdeltoid bursa is located between the rotator cuff and the overlying deltoid muscle and the acromion, whereas the subcoracoid bursa is located anterior to the subscapularis and does not communicate with the glenohumeral joint. The glenoid labrum is a rim of fibrocartilage surrounding the glenoid edge, providing stabilization of the glenohumeral joint the area known as the rotator interval encompasses several structures, including the coracohumeral and superior glenohumeral ligaments, the long head tendon of the biceps brachii, and a thin layer of capsule (Fig. 1.4) [9]. Having originated either from the postero-superior labrum, the superior glenoid tubercle, or both, the intra-articular portion of the long head tendon of the biceps brachii passes through the joint capsule within this region [10].

The coracohumeral ligament originates from the base of the coracoid process and divides into two bundles [11]. One bundle inserts on the anterior edge of the supraspinatus tendon and the greater tuberosity, while the other attaches to the subscapularis tendon, transverse humeral ligament, and the lesser tuberosity. The medial bundle is of a smaller size; it wraps around the intra-articular portion of the long head tendon of the biceps brachii and attaches onto the lesser tuberosity, along with the cranial fibers of the subscapularis tendon and the superior glenohumeral joint. The larger lateral bundle surrounds the superolateral part of the intra-articular portion of the long

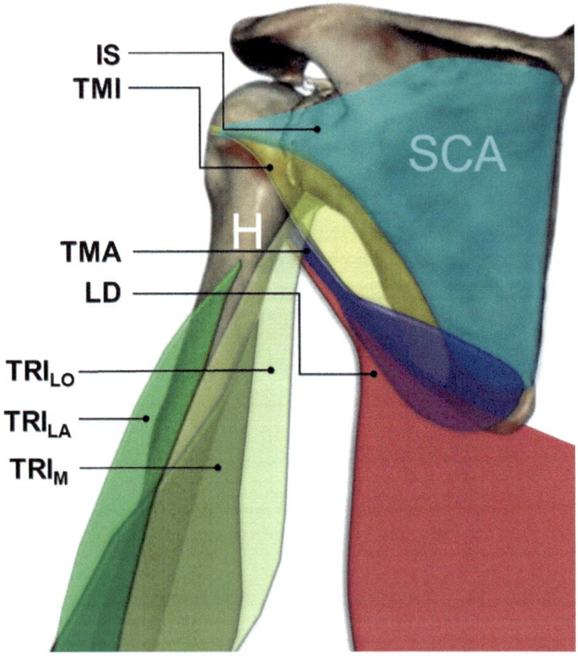

Fig. 1.3 The illustration shows the posterior aspect of the rotator cuff and associated muscles. IS infraspinatus; TMI teres minor; TMA teres major; LD latissimus dorsi; TRI_{LO} long head of the triceps brachii; TRI_{LA} lateral head of the triceps brachii; TRI_{M} medial head of the triceps brachii; SCA scapula; H humerus

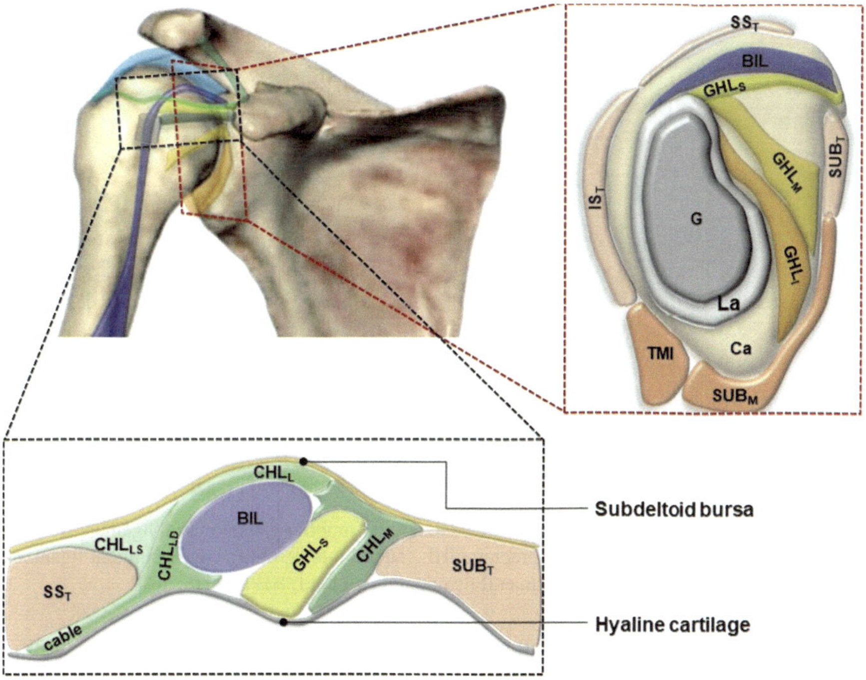

Fig. 1.4 Multi-planar illustration shows the rotator interval and associated structures, including the rotator cable. BIL long head tendon of the biceps brachii; SUB_T subscapularis tendon; SUB_M subscapularis muscle; SS_T supraspinatus tendon; IS_T infraspinatus tendon; CHL_L lateral bundle of the coracohumeral ligament; CHL_{LS} superficial band of the lateral bundle of the coracohumeral ligament; CHL_{LD} deep band of the lateral bundle of the coracohumeral ligament; CHL_M medial bundle of the coracohumeral ligament; GHL_S superior glenohumeral ligament; GHL_M middle glenohumeral ligament; GHL_I inferior glenohumeral ligament; TMI teres minor; G glenoid; La labrum; Ca capsule

head tendon of the biceps brachii, inserting at the greater tuberosity of the humerus and the anterior border of the supraspinatus tendon. This lateral part, also referred to as the rotator cable [12], extends from the coracohumeral ligament (Fig. 1.4), which plays a crucial role in preventing downward translation of the adducted arm. It is an extra-articular structure not visible during glenohumeral arthroscopy.

The superior glenohumeral ligament arises from the glenoid labrum near the supraglenoid tubercle (Fig. 1.5), crossing beneath the coracohumeral ligament within the rotator interval and attaching to the lesser tuberosity. The fibers of the superior glenohumeral ligament can be divided into two groups: the direct and oblique fibers. The former originates from the glenoid labrum, while the latter originates from the supraglenoid tubercle [13]. The long head tendon of the biceps brachii lies between the coracohumeral and superior glenohumeral ligaments. The superior glenohumeral ligament inserts near the lesser tuberosity and is an intra-articular capsular ligament visible during arthroscopy. It plays a crucial role in

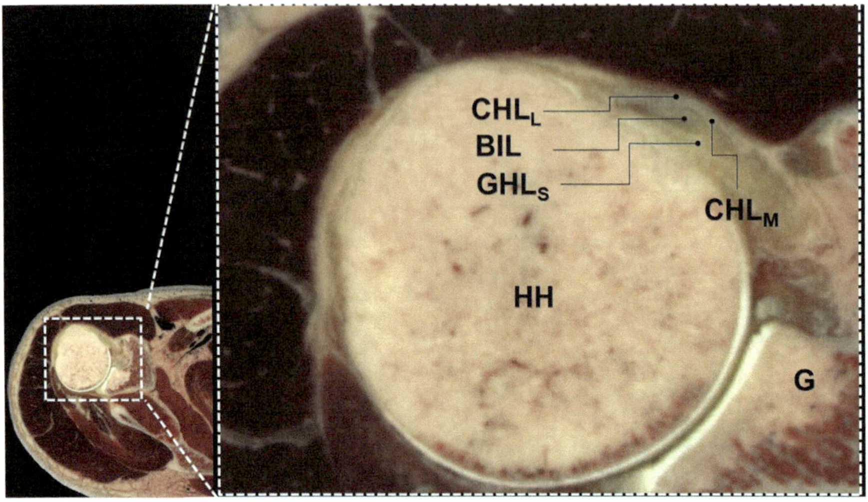

Fig. 1.5 The cadaveric dissection (axial view) shows the superior glenohumeral ligament (GHL_S). BIL long head tendon of the biceps brachii; CHL_L lateral bundle of the coracohumeral ligament; CHL_M medial bundle of the coracohumeral ligament; G glenoid; HH humeral head

resisting inferior translation of the shoulder. The capsule or synovial layer within this interval is exceptionally thin, measuring less than 0.1 mm in thickness. Despite its minimal thickness, this layer serves as a barrier and helps to maintain the joint's negative intra-articular pressure.

1.3 Sonoanatomy

Since the long head tendon of the biceps brachii is central to the rotator cuff interval, ultrasound examination typically starts for its axial imaging within the bicipital groove (Fig. 1.6a, c). To evaluate its intra-articular portion, the patient is instructed to assume the modified Crass position, which involves humeral internal rotation and extension. This position shifts the supraspinatus tendon away from the acromion, improving visualization. At the bicipital groove, the long head tendon of the biceps brachii is stabilized by the groove's shape and the transverse humeral ligament. Its fibrillar pattern is readily visible in the long-axis view (Fig. 1.6b, d). In this area, the tendon is encased in a synovial sheath which extends from the glenohumeral joint and continues about 3–4 cm beyond the distal end of the groove. The tendon sheath is connected to the glenohumeral joint, allowing communication in between.

To examine the proximal portion of the long head tendon of the biceps brachii, the ultrasound probe is placed over the superior aspect of the humerus. At this level, the coracohumeral and superior glenohumeral ligaments form a ring-like structure, encircling the tendon (Fig. 1.7a, b). The coracohumeral ligament can be further

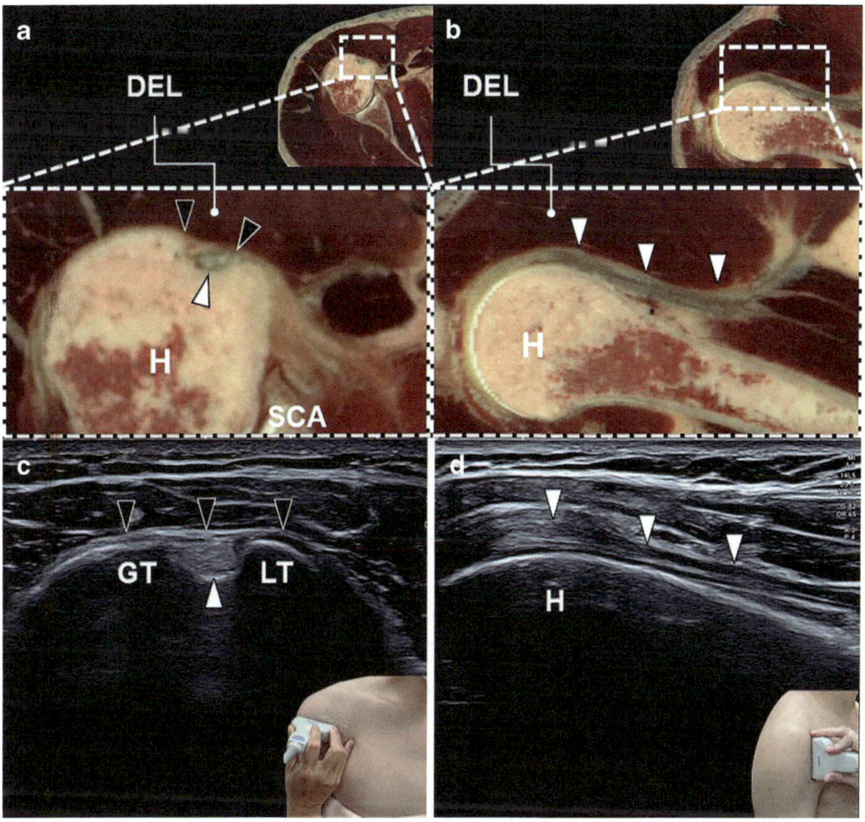

Fig. 1.6 The cadaveric and ultrasound images illustrate the long head tendon of the biceps brachii (white arrowheads) at the bicipital groove in the short-axis (**a**, **c**) and long-axis (**b**, **d**) views. Black arrowheads: transverse humeral ligament; DEL deltoid; SCA scapula; GT greater tuberosity; LT lesser tuberosity; H humerus

divided into lateral and medial bundles. The latter merges with the superior glenohumeral ligament, creating a medial boundary that prevents medial shift of the long head tendon of the biceps brachii. Conversely, the lateral bundle bifurcates into superficial and deep fibers. The superficial part courses over the anterior edge of the supraspinatus tendon, while the deep part passes beneath the anterior edge of the supraspinatus tendon and transitions into the rotator cable. Of note, during axial imaging, the shape of the long head tendon of the biceps brachii is oval near the humeral head but becomes more rounded proximally.

As the examiner tracks the long head tendon of the biceps brachii upward, it sharply changes direction, diving into the shoulder joint and attaching onto the supraglenoid tubercle (Fig. 1.8a). It is difficult to visualize this point from a standard axial view, so rotating the transducer along the long axis of the tendon is suggested to better identify its connection with the superior labrum (Fig. 1.8b).

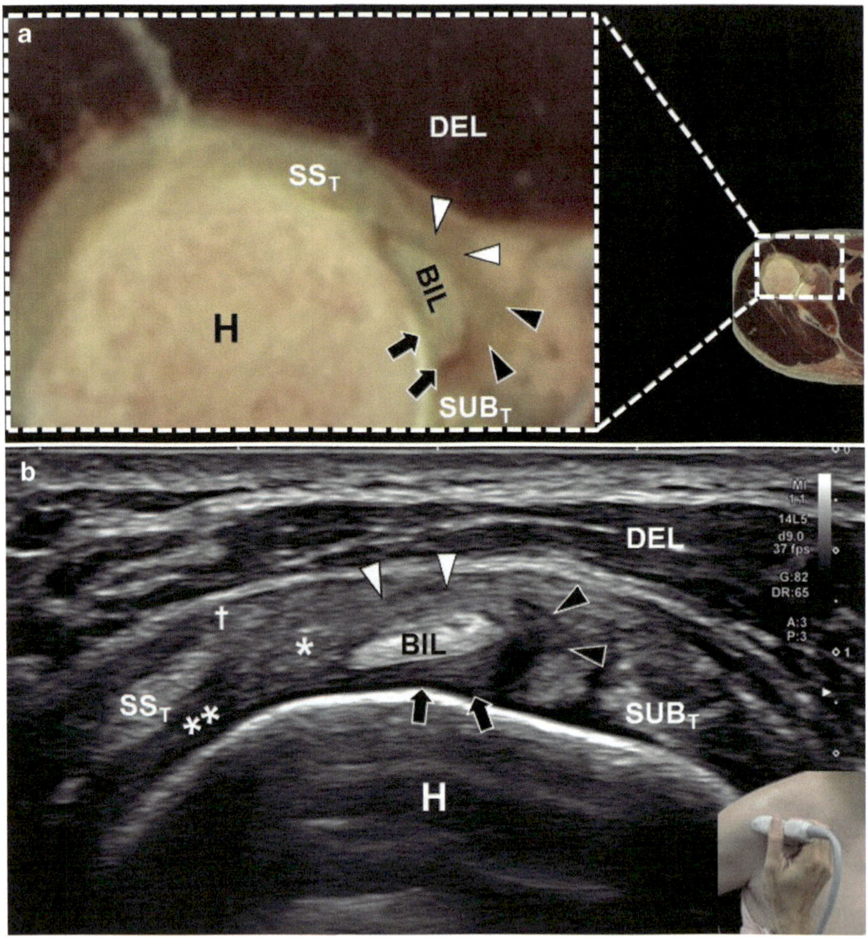

Fig. 1.7 The cadaveric (**a**) and ultrasound (**b**) images illustrate the tendons and ligaments at the rotator interval. White arrowheads: lateral bundle of the coracohumeral ligament; black arrowheads: medial bundle of the coracohumeral ligament; black arrows: superior glenohumeral ligament; asterisk: deep band of the lateral bundle of the coracohumeral ligament; dagger: superficial band of the lateral bundle of the coracohumeral ligament; double asterisks: rotator cable; SS_T supraspinatus tendon; BIL long head tendon of the biceps brachii; SUB_T subscapularis tendon; DEL deltoid; H humerus

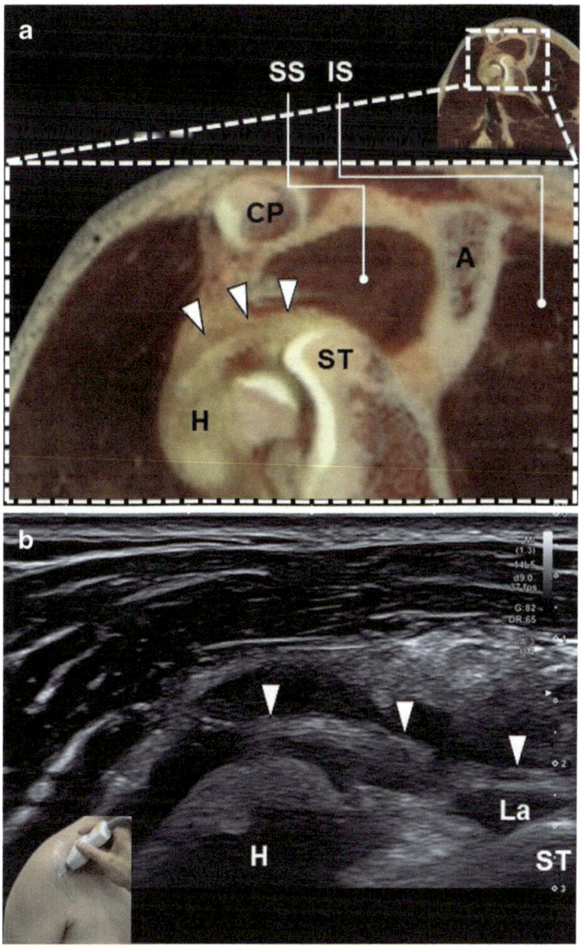

Fig. 1.8 The cadaveric (**a**) and sonographic (**b**) images illustrate the origin of the long head tendon of the biceps brachii (white arrowheads) at the supraglenoid tubercle. SS supraspinatus; IS infraspinatus; ST supraglenoid tubercle; CP coracoid process; La labrum; A acromion; H humerus

The supraspinatus tendon has a cylindrical bundle that runs anterior to its muscle belly [14]. Given the tendon's fibrillar pattern, the bundle is prone to anisotropy (similar to the long head tendon of the biceps brachii); therefore, scanning needs to be performed cautiously (Fig. 1.9a, c). The lateral bundle of the coracohumeral ligament extends outward and merges with the rotator cable, tapering posteriorly and infiltrating the underside of the cylindrical bundle. The rotator cable is a bright, fibrillar band that is a thin fibrous structure continuous with the deep band of the lateral bundle of the coracohumeral ligament [15]. It extends along the underside of the rotator cuff fibers and is positioned above the joint capsule. It can be located about 1.5 cm medial to the greater tuberosity. When scanning the supraspinatus tendon along its long axis, the rotator cable appears as a bright, transversely-oriented bundle of fibers running perpendicular to and beneath the supraspinatus tendon (Fig. 1.9b, d).

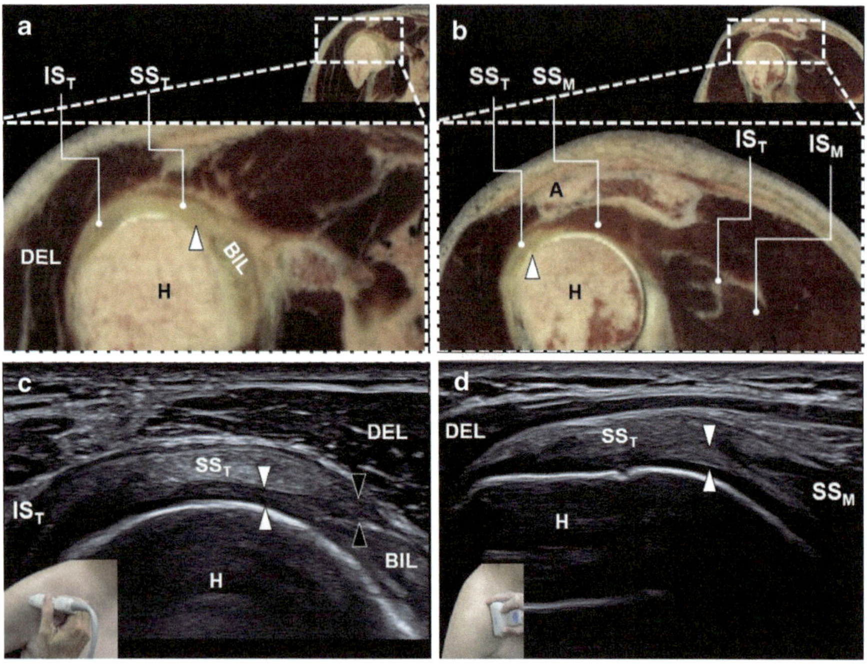

Fig. 1.9 The cadaveric and ultrasound images illustrate the rotator cable (white arrowheads) in the short-axis (**a**, **c**) and long-axis (**b**, **d**) views of the supraspinatus tendon. Black arrowheads: lateral bundle of the coracohumeral ligament; SS_T supraspinatus tendon; SS_M supraspinatus muscle; IS_T infraspinatus tendon; IS_M infraspinatus muscle; BIL long head tendon of the biceps brachii; DEL deltoid; A acromion; H humerus

The transducer is positioned between the lesser tuberosity of the humerus and the coracoid process to scan the subscapularis tendon in the long-axis view (Fig. 1.10a, c). Since the tendon comprises multiple bundles, the examination is performed from a cephalic to caudal direction. The transducer is then rotated 90 degrees to visualize the tendon in the short-axis view (Fig. 1.10b, d). Notably, the anterior glenohumeral capsule extends to the anatomic neck of the humerus, which appears as a groove situated between the greater tuberosity and the humeral head cartilage. Using high-resolution ultrasound, the lamination between the subscapularis tendon and the anterior glenohumeral capsule can be observed.

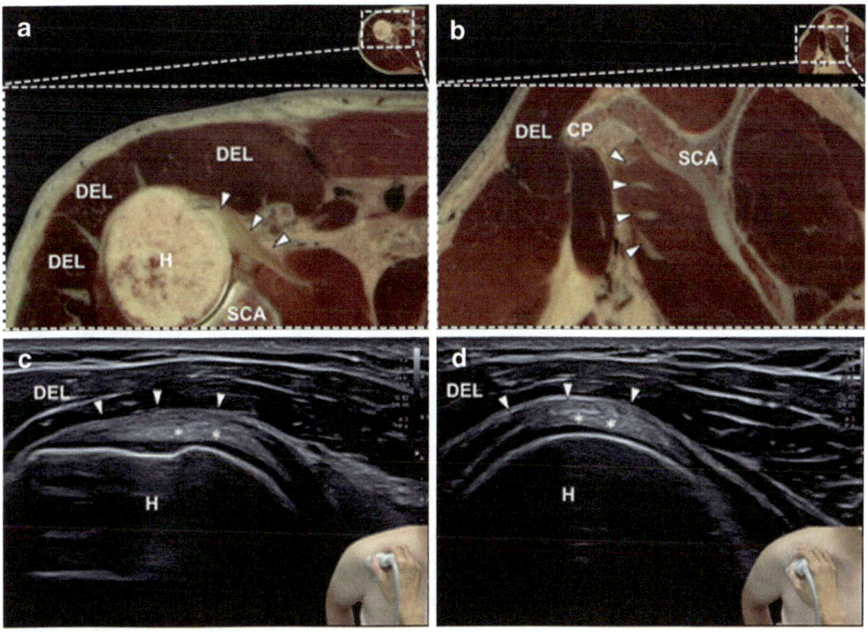

Fig. 1.10 Cadaveric and ultrasound images illustrate the subscapularis tendon (white arrowheads) in the long-axis (**a**, **c**) and short-axis (**b**, **d**) views. White asterisks: glenohumeral capsule; DEL deltoid muscle; CP coracoid process; SCA scapula; H humerus

To evaluate the infraspinatus and teres minor muscles and tendons (Fig. 1.11a), the transducer is positioned perpendicular to and just caudal to the scapular spine. In this view, the supraspinatus muscle is visualized in the suprascapular fossa, while the infraspinatus and teres minor muscles are seen caudally in their short-axis view (Fig. 1.11b). After identifying each hyperechoic intramuscular aponeurosis, the transducer is rotated 90 degrees and advanced toward each tendon's insertion point, allowing visualization of the infraspinatus (Fig. 1.12a, c) and teres minor (Fig. 1.12b, d) tendons in the long-axis view.

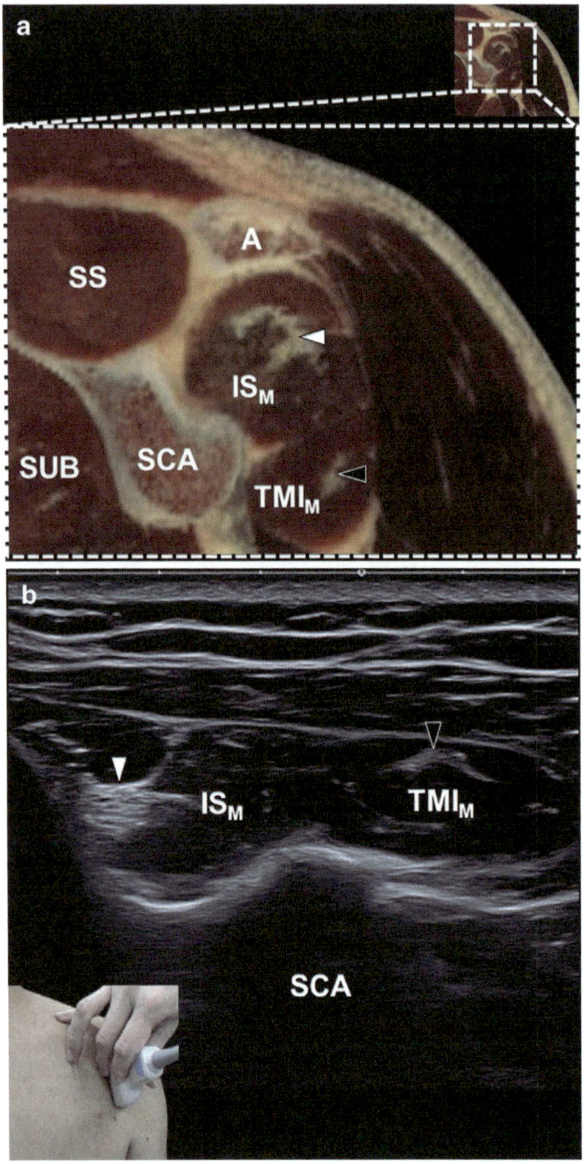

Fig. 1.11 The cadaveric images (**a**) and corresponding sonoanatomy (**b**) demonstrate infraspinatus and teres minor tendons at the musculotendinous junction in the short-axis views. White arrowheads: infraspinatus tendon; black arrowheads: teres minor tendon; SUB subscapularis; SS supraspinatus; IS_M infraspinatus muscle; TMI_M teres minor muscle; SCA scapula; A acromion

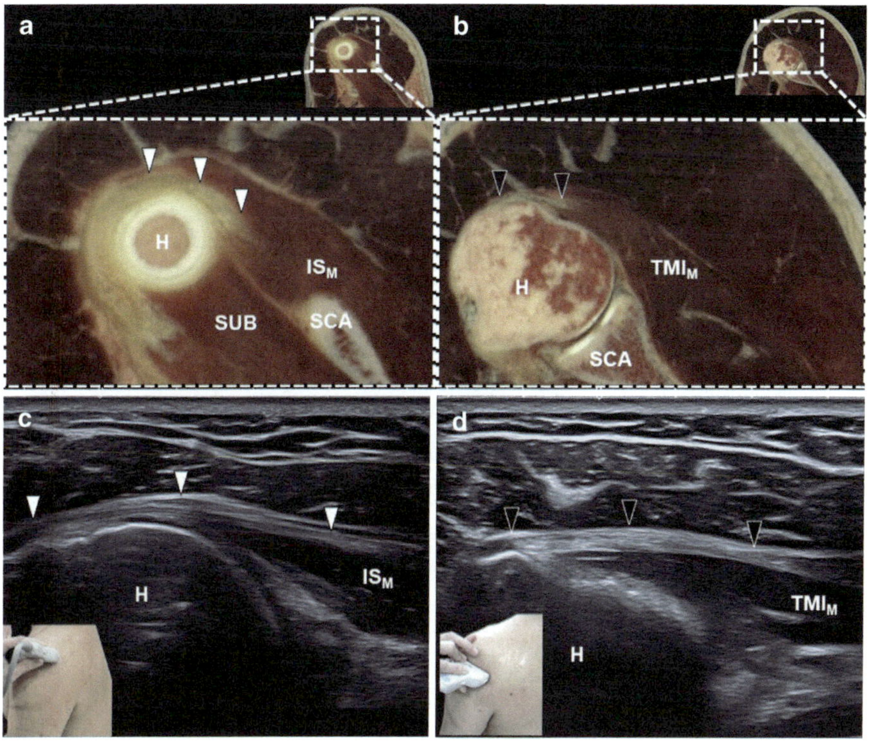

Fig. 1.12 The cadaveric and ultrasound images illustrate the infraspinatus (**a**, **c**) and teres minor (**b**, **d**) tendons in the long-axis views. White arrowheads: infraspinatus tendon; black arrowheads: teres minor tendon; SUB subscapularis; IS_M infraspinatus muscle; TMI_M teres minor muscle; SCA scapula; H humerus

1.4 Pathology

1.4.1 Rotator Cuff Tendon Tear

Although rotator cuff tendon tears are a common cause of anterior shoulder pain, peritendinous soft tissues, such as bursae or the underlying bone, may also be assessed with ultrasound. In addition to tears, the rotator cuff may also exhibit tendinosis, which is characterized by tendon thickening, loss of the fibrillar pattern, and often accompanied by calcification (Fig. 1.13a). Subdeltoid bursitis, presenting as bursal hypertrophy with or without fluid accumulation, may also be observed (Fig. 1.13b).

Rotator cuff tears most commonly affect the supraspinatus tendon. At the site of a tear, the hyperechoic interface between the area devoid of tendon fibers and the hyaline cartilage may become more conspicuous, a feature known as the cartilage interface sign. Supraspinatus tendon tears can occur at various sites, including the

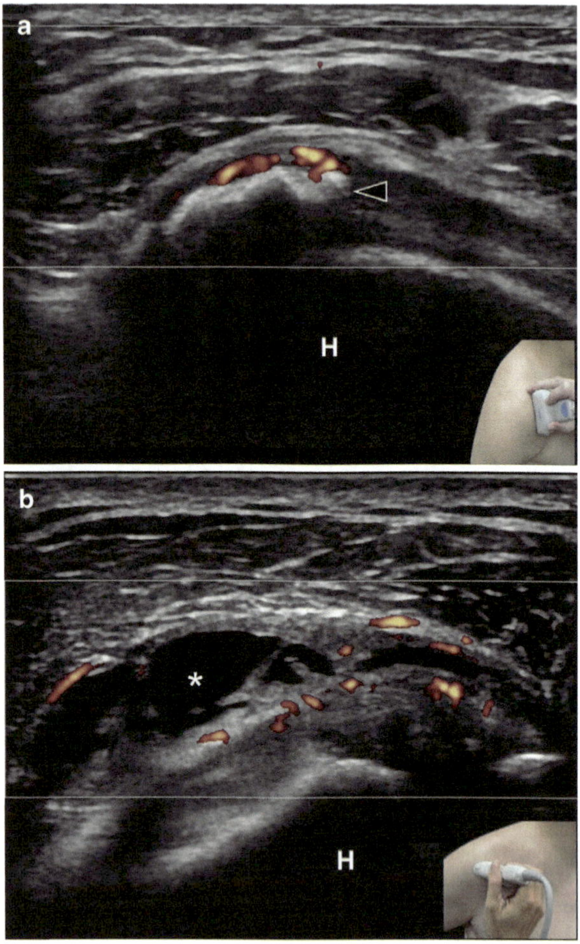

Fig. 1.13 The power Doppler ultrasound image demonstrates supraspinatus calcific tendinitis, that is, a well-defined hyperechoic deposit (black arrowhead) accompanied by acoustic shadowing and hyperemia (**a**). In another case, the ultrasound image reveals subacromial-subdeltoid bursitis (asterisk), that is, anechoic fluid accumulation and heterogeneous synovial hypertrophy (**b**). H humerus

insertion at the greater tubercle, the region near the rotator interval, the supraspinatus-infraspinatus junction, or the muscle-tendon junction. Partial-thickness tears are categorized as bursal-side (Fig. 1.14a), intrasubstance (Fig. 1.14b), or articular-side (Fig. 1.14c). A partial-thickness tear located on the far-distal articular side, specifically at the articular surface footprint where the tendon attaches to the greater tuberosity of the humerus, is referred to as a rim-rent tear or a PASTA (partial articular-side supraspinatus tendon avulsion) lesion [16] (Fig. 1.14d).

Full-thickness tears are categorized as focal (incomplete) or full-width (complete). An incomplete tear may present as a deficiency of tendon fibers across its entire thickness (Fig. 1.15a, b), with a cartilage interface sign visible between the accumulated fluid and the humeral head cartilage (Fig. 1.15c). Herniation of the deltoid muscle and the subacromial-subdeltoid bursa toward the humeral cortex, manifesting as flattening or concavity of the tendon surface can also be seen (Fig. 1.15d). In contrast, a complete tear extends across the entire tendon width

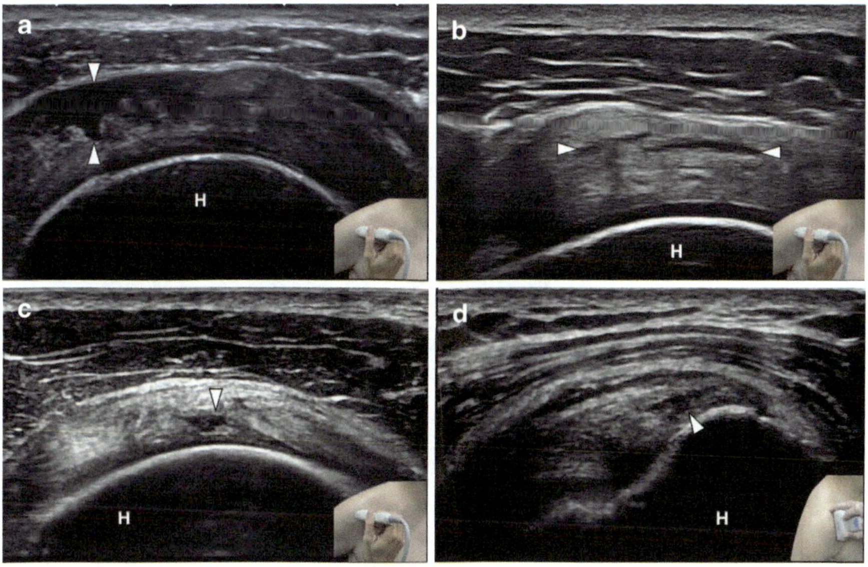

Fig. 1.14 The ultrasound images illustrate bursal-side (**a**), intrasubstance (**b**), and articular-side (**c**) partial-thickness supraspinatus tendon tears (white arrowheads) in the short-axis views and a rim-rent tear in the long-axis view (**d**). H humerus

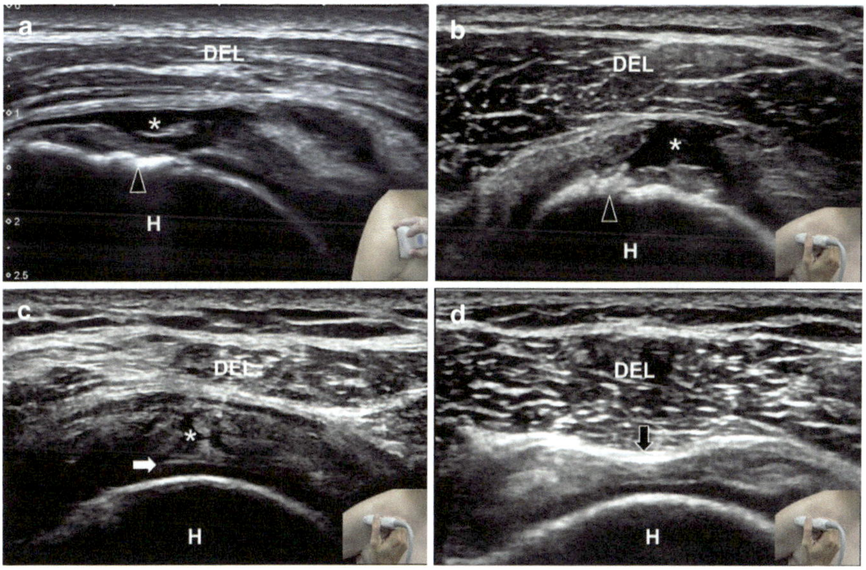

Fig. 1.15 The ultrasound images in the long-axis (**a**) and short-axis (**b**) views show an incomplete full-thickness tear of the supraspinatus tendon with absent fibers, effusion (asterisks) involving its entire thickness and cortical irregularities (black arrowheads). In a similar case, the cartilage interface sign (white arrow) is observed between the effusion and the humeral cartilage (**c**). In the third case, herniation of the deltoid muscle (black arrow) toward the humeral head is visible (**d**). DEL deltoid; H humerus

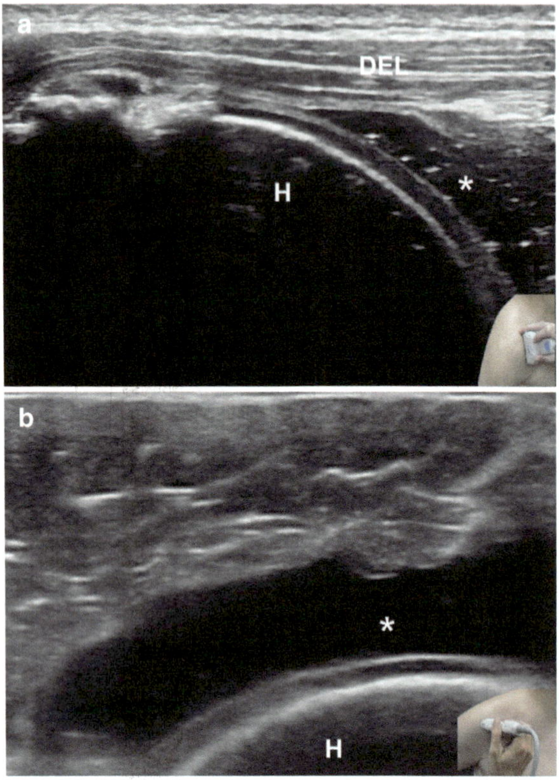

Fig. 1.16 The ultrasound images demonstrate a complete tear of the supraspinatus tendon, characterized by the absence of tendon fibers and fluid accumulation (asterisks) in the long-axis (**a**) and short-axis (**b**) views. DEL deltoid; H humerus

(long axis, Fig. 1.16a; short axis, Fig. 1.16b) and is often accompanied by tendon retraction or muscle atrophy.

In some cases, a supraspinatus tendon injury may involve the rotator cable (Fig. 1.17a) or ligaments within the rotator cuff interval, such as the coracohumeral ligament (Fig. 1.17b). A supraspinatus tendon tear can extend anteriorly through the rotator interval, either without (Fig. 1.18a) or with (Fig. 1.18b) tearing of the transverse humeral ligament, potentially leading to subluxation of the long head of the biceps brachii tendon. A partial (Fig. 1.18c) or complete (Fig. 1.18d) tear of the subscapularis tendon may also result in subluxation of the long head tendon of the biceps brachii.

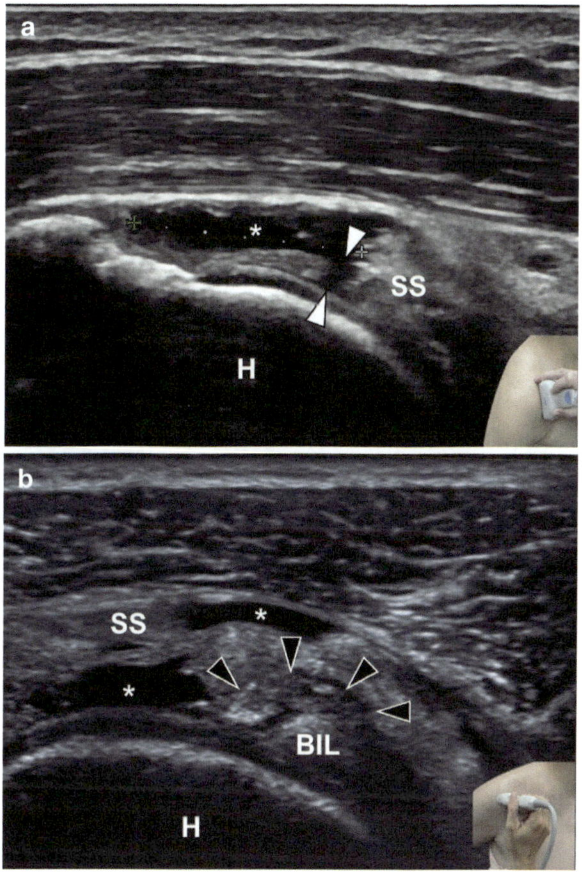

Fig. 1.17 The ultrasound imaging in the long-axis view (**a**) shows a supraspinatus tendon tear with effusion (asterisks) and injury of the rotator cable (white arrowheads). In the short-axis view (**b**), the lateral bundle of the coracohumeral ligament (black arrowheads) is also seen to be involved. BIL long head tendon of the biceps brachii; SS supraspinatus tendon; H humerus

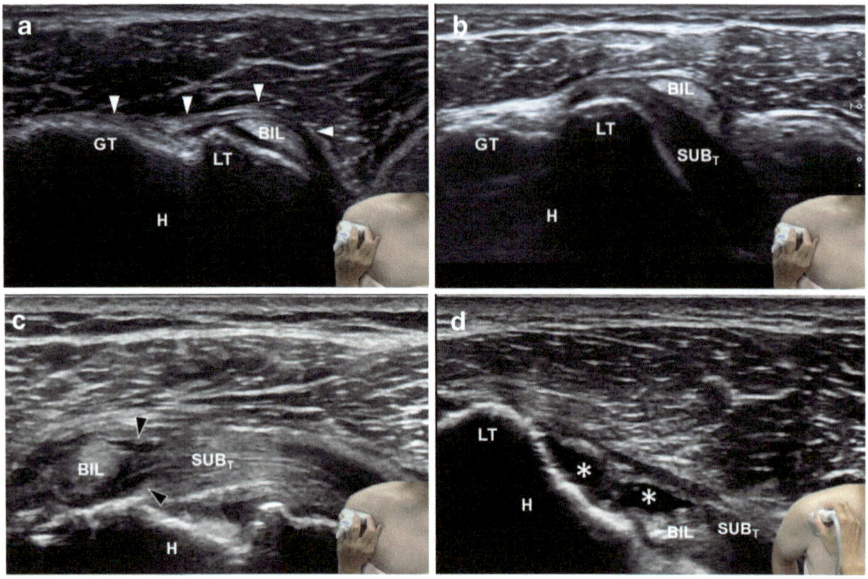

Fig. 1.18 The ultrasound images illustrate subluxation of the long head tendon of the biceps brachii (BIL) with intact transverse humeral ligament (white arrowheads) (**a**) and without (**b**). The subluxation may be associated with a partial tear of the subscapularis tendon (black arrowheads) (**c**) or a complete tear accompanied by effusion (asterisks) (**d**). SUB$_T$ subscapularis tendon; GT greater tuberosity; LT lesser tuberosity; H humerus

Incomplete subscapularis tendon tears are classified as partial-thickness (Fig. 1.19a, b) or full-thickness (Fig. 1.19c). Complete tears may result in proximal or distal retraction of the tendon stump (Fig. 1.20a), herniation of the pectoralis major muscle (Fig. 1.20b), or even complete loss of visible tendon fibers, exposing a naked humeral head (Fig. 1.20c).

Infraspinatus and teres minor tears, though less common than supraspinatus tears, may occur, often due to trauma. Infraspinatus injuries can manifest as tendinopathy (Fig. 1.21a), intra-substance partial tears (long axis, Fig. 1.21b; short axis, Fig. 1.21c), or complete tears with a retraction stump in both the short-axis (Fig. 1.22a) and long-axis (Fig. 1.22b) views. Teres minor tears may involve partial tearing at the myotendinous junction, demonstrated in both the short-axis (Fig. 1.23a) and long-axis (Fig. 1.23b) images. Furthermore, the long head tendon of the biceps brachii and myotendinous junctions may also be involved, with partial tears observed in both the short-axis (Fig. 1.24a) and long-axis (Fig. 1.24b) views, and complete tears presenting with a distal retraction stump (Fig. 1.24c).

In severe cases, rotator cuff surgery may be considered. However, fatty infiltration and atrophy of the supraspinatus (Fig. 1.25a) and infraspinatus (Fig. 1.25b) muscles are associated with poorer surgical outcomes. In post-surgical assessments, retears at the repaired insertion (Fig. 1.26a) or the myotendinous junction (Fig. 1.26b), screw loosening (Fig. 1.26c), and suture detachment (Fig. 1.26d) may be observed.

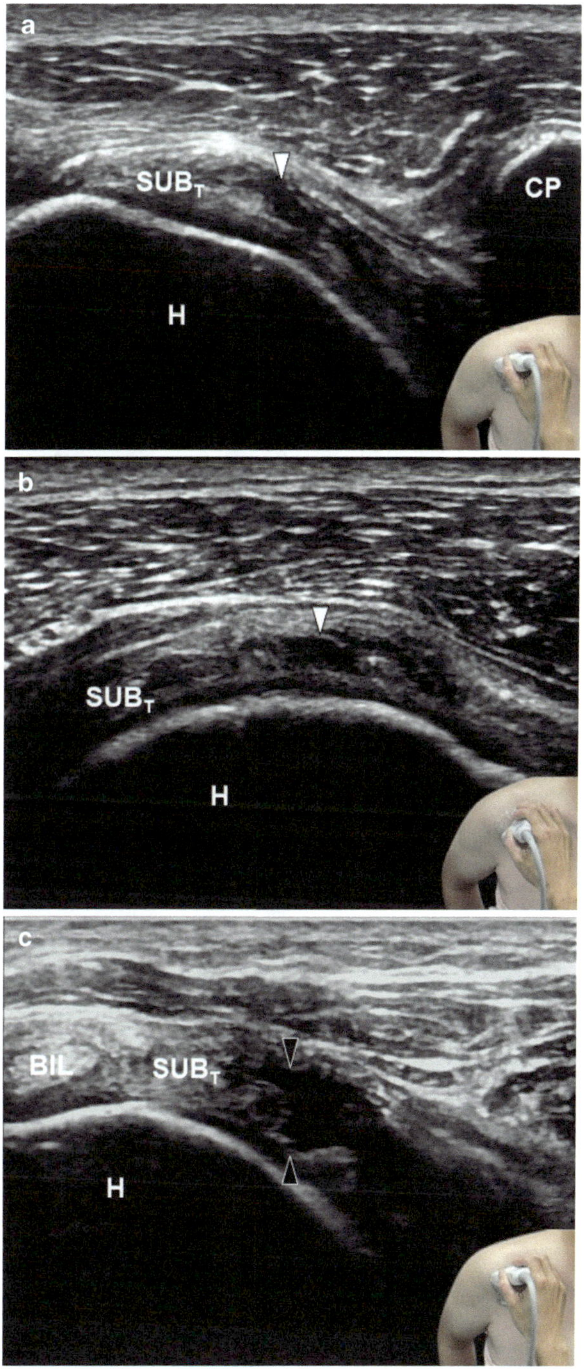

Fig. 1.19 The ultrasound images show a partial-thickness subscapularis tendon tear (white arrowheads) in the long- (**a**) and short-axis (**b**) views. In a different case, a full-thickness tear (black arrowheads) is visible in the short-axis view (**c**). BIL long head tendon of the biceps brachii; SUB_T subscapularis tendon; CP coracoid process; H humerus

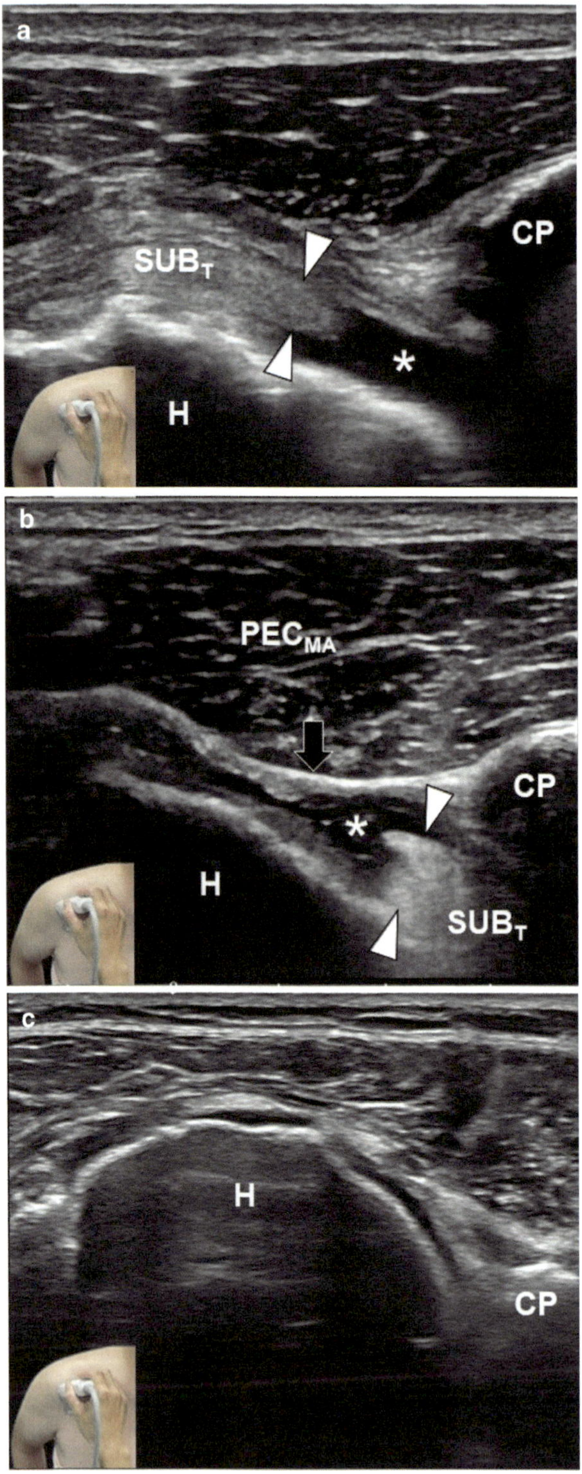

Fig. 1.20 The ultrasound images of the subscapularis tendon in the long-axis view illustrate complete tear with distal retraction stump (white arrowheads) and effusion (asterisks) (**a**) as well as proximal retraction stump with pectoralis major muscle herniation (black arrow) (**b**). In the short-axis view, there is the complete absence of the tendon (**c**). PEC_{MA} pectoralis major muscle; SUB_T subscapularis tendon; CP coracoid process; H humerus

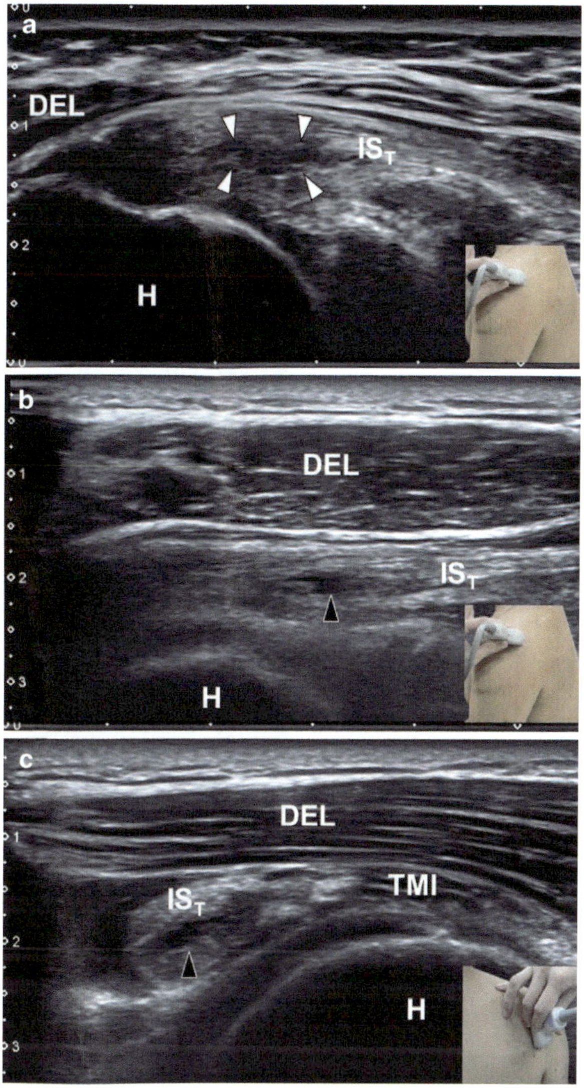

Fig. 1.21 The ultrasound images of the infraspinatus tendon show loss of the fibrillar pattern (white arrowheads), indicating tendinopathy (**a**), and a partial thickness intrasubstance tear (black arrowheads) at the myotendinous junction is visible in the long-axis (**b**) and short-axis (**c**) views. IS_T infraspinatus tendon; TMI teres minor; DEL deltoid; H humerus

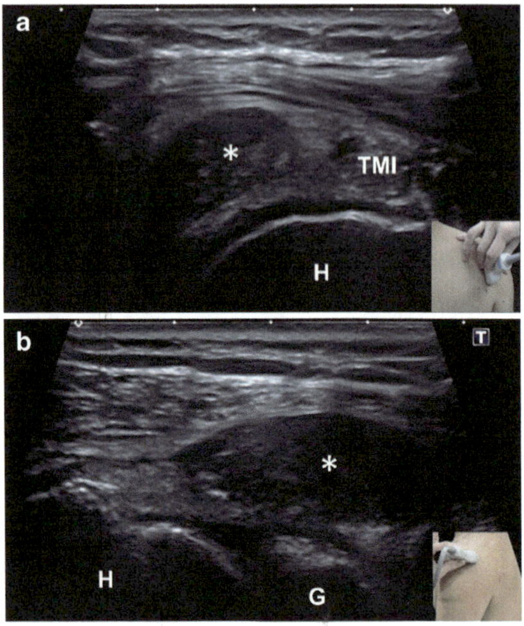

Fig. 1.22 Ultrasound images show complete infraspinatus tendon tear with a retracted stump (asterisks) in the short-axis (**a**) and long-axis (**b**) views. TMI teres minor; G glenoid; H humerus

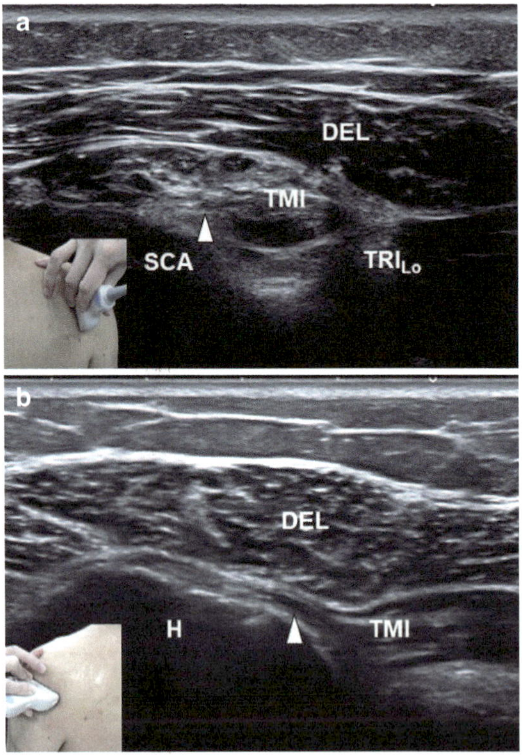

Fig. 1.23 The ultrasound images of the teres minor depict a partial-thickness tear (white arrowheads) in the short-axis (**a**) and long-axis (**b**) views. TMI teres minor; TRI_{LO} long head of the triceps brachii; DEL deltoid; SCA scapula; H humerus

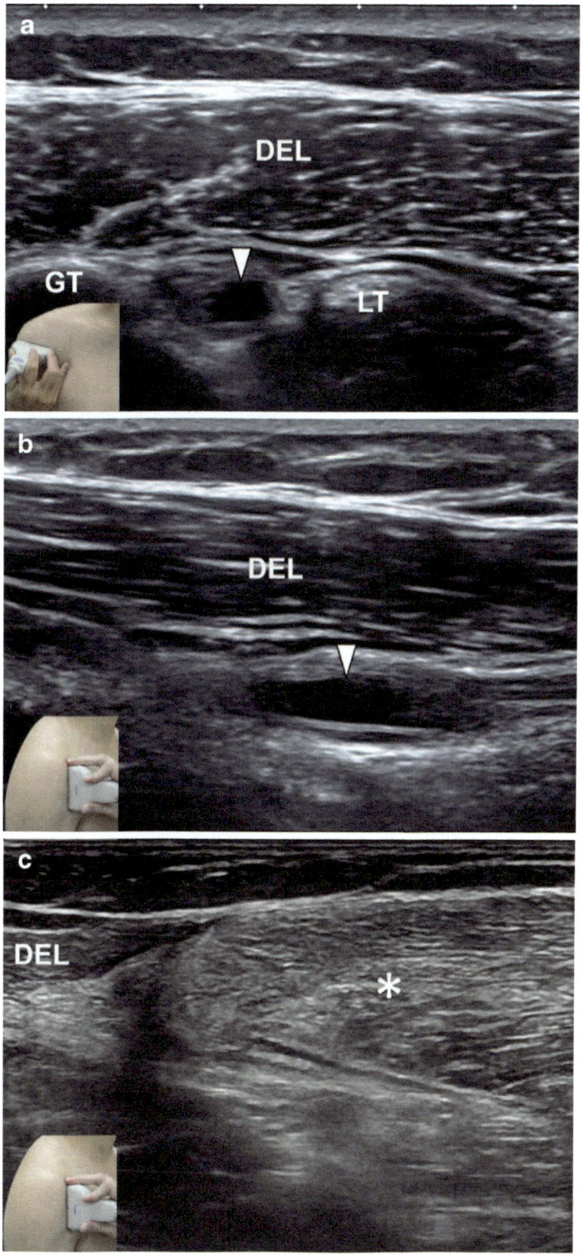

Fig. 1.24 The ultrasound images of the long head tendon of the biceps brachii show an intra-tendinous partial tear (white arrowheads) in the short-axis (**a**) and long-axis (**b**) views. In another case, the ultrasound image shows a complete tear with a distal retraction stump (asterisk) in the long-axis view (**c**). DEL deltoid; GT greater tuberosity of the humerus; LT lesser tuberosity of the humerus

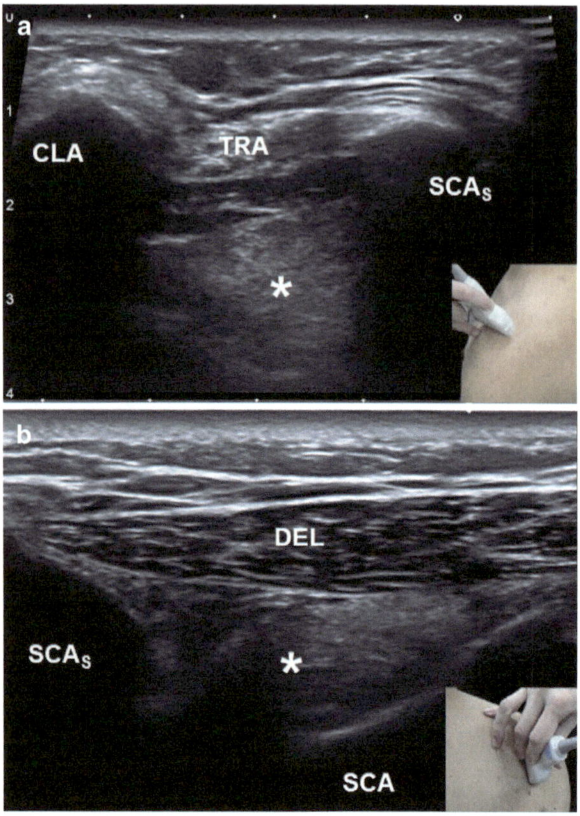

Fig. 1.25 The ultrasound images in the short-axis view depict fatty infiltration and muscle atrophy (asterisks) of the supraspinatus (**a**) and infraspinatus (**b**) muscles. DEL deltoid; TRA trapezius; CLA clavicle; SCA_S scapular spine; SCA scapula

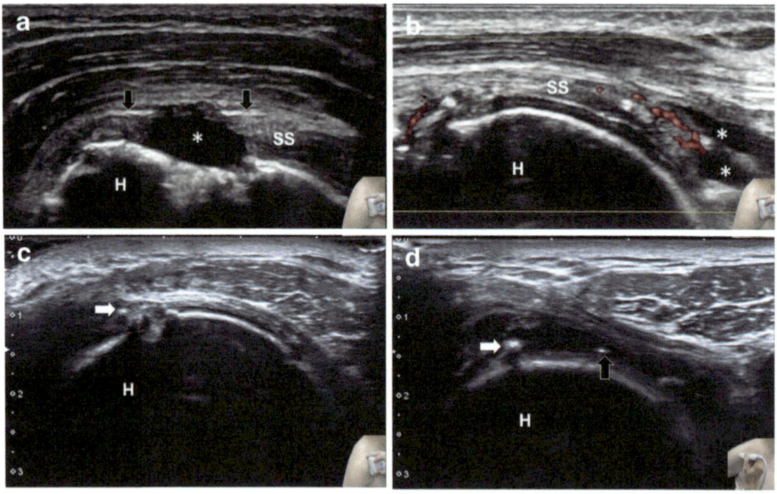

Fig. 1.26 The ultrasound images in the long-axis view depict suture rupture (black arrows) and retear (asterisks) at the distal insertion (**a**) and at the myotendinous junction (**b**). Complete retear with screw loosening (white arrows) and suture detachment are seen in the long-axis (**c**) and short-axis (**d**) views. SS supraspinatus; H humerus

1.4.2 Adhesive Capsulitis

Thickening of the coracohumeral ligament has been identified as a potential indicator of adhesive capsulitis. This is often accompanied by thickening (Fig. 1.27a) and periligamentous hypervascularity (Fig. 1.27b, c) of the coracohumeral ligament, as well as involvement of the superior glenohumeral ligament (Fig. 1.27d). In a study by Homsi et al. [17], ultrasound examinations were conducted on 498 shoulders from 306 participants, grouped into asymptomatic shoulders, painful shoulders, and shoulders with arthrographic evidence of adhesive capsulitis. The researchers compared the mean maximal thickness of the coracohumeral ligament among these three groups. The average thickness of the coracohumeral ligament in adhesive capsulitis was significantly greater (3 mm) compared to both the asymptomatic (1.34 mm) and painful (1.39 mm) shoulder groups.

In another study, Lee et al. [18] investigated the changes in ultrasound parameters and clinical symptoms in patients with adhesive capsulitis ($N = 56$). They had undergone ultrasound-guided intra-articular steroid injections (20 mg of triamcinolone with 5.5 mL of normal saline) using a posterior approach. Significant reduction in the thickness of the coracohumeral ligament was observed on the 1-month follow-up.

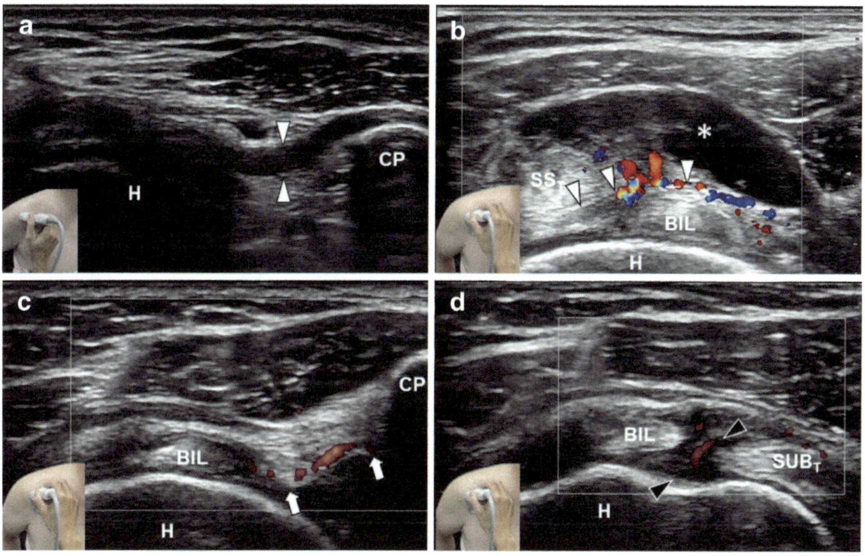

Fig. 1.27 The ultrasound image illustrates thickening of the lateral bundle of the coracohumeral ligament (white arrowheads) (**a**). In other cases, power Doppler ultrasound reveals hyperemia in the lateral bundle of the coracohumeral ligament (**b**), the medial bundle of the coracohumeral ligament (white arrows) (**c**), and the superior glenohumeral ligament (black arrowheads) (**d**). Asterisk: bursal effusion; SS_T supraspinatus tendon; BIL long head tendon of the biceps brachii; SUB_T subscapularis tendon; CP coracoid process; H humerus

Regarding the stiffness of the coracohumeral ligament, shear-wave elastography was studied in a group of healthy individuals (11 men and 19 women) vs. those suspected for adhesive capsulitis (9 men and 11 women) [19]. The median elastic modulus of the symptomatic shoulders (234.8 kPa) was notably higher than that of the unaffected shoulders (203.3 kPa) in neutral shoulder position ($p = 0.004$), but no significant difference was observed when the shoulders were in maximal external rotation ($p = 0.123$).

Kim et al. [20] investigated the vascularity in the rotator interval by comparing 39 patients diagnosed with adhesive capsulitis vs. a control group of 35 healthy individuals. They used superb microvascular imaging (Canon Medical Systems, Otawara, Japan) and power Doppler ultrasound to assess blood flow in the subcoracoid fat triangle. The results indicated that the area of vascular flow detected with superb microvascular imaging was significantly larger in the adhesive capsulitis group compared to the control group (2.95 mm^2 versus 0 mm^2, $p < 0.01$). Furthermore, superb microvascular imaging was more effective than power Doppler ultrasound in detecting vascular flow in the subcoracoid fat triangle ($p < 0.01$). In the adhesive capsulitis group, the area of vascular flow as measured by superb microvascular imaging was inversely correlated with external rotation and forward flexion ($p < 0.05$).

1.5 Ultrasound-guided Injection

For rotator cuff tears or related pathologies, subacromial-subdeltoid bursa injection is preferable. Corticosteroids can be used for bursitis [21], while platelet-rich plasma [22] may be considered for smaller rotator cuff tears. Ultrasound-guided injections for the subdeltoid bursa can be administered using various in-plane approaches, with the patient typically positioned in a neutral posture. After identifying the bursa above the supraspinatus tendon in the axial view, the needle can be inserted via the lateral-to-medial in-plane approach, allowing for broad coverage of the supraspinatus or even the infraspinatus tendons (Fig. 1.28a). For lesions of the rotator cuff, particularly supraspinatus tears located beneath the acromion, a lateral approach is preferable, especially for myotendinous tears. Positioning the transducer between the acromion and humerus facilitates a caudal-to-cephalic injection, targeting the subdeltoid bursa beneath the lateral acromion (Fig. 1.28b). If the posterior supraspinatus or infraspinatus tendon is involved, the transducer should be positioned on the middle facet to visualize both tendons. This placement facilitates a posterior-to-anterior injection using a long needle (Fig. 1.28c).

Regarding the injection treatment for adhesive capsulitis, Arrambide-Garza et al. [23] conducted a meta-analysis to compare the effectiveness of corticosteroid injections into the glenohumeral joint via the rotator interval vs. the posterior approach. The meta-analysis incorporated five clinical trials with a total of 323 primary adhesive capsulitis patients. The results indicated that corticosteroid injections into the

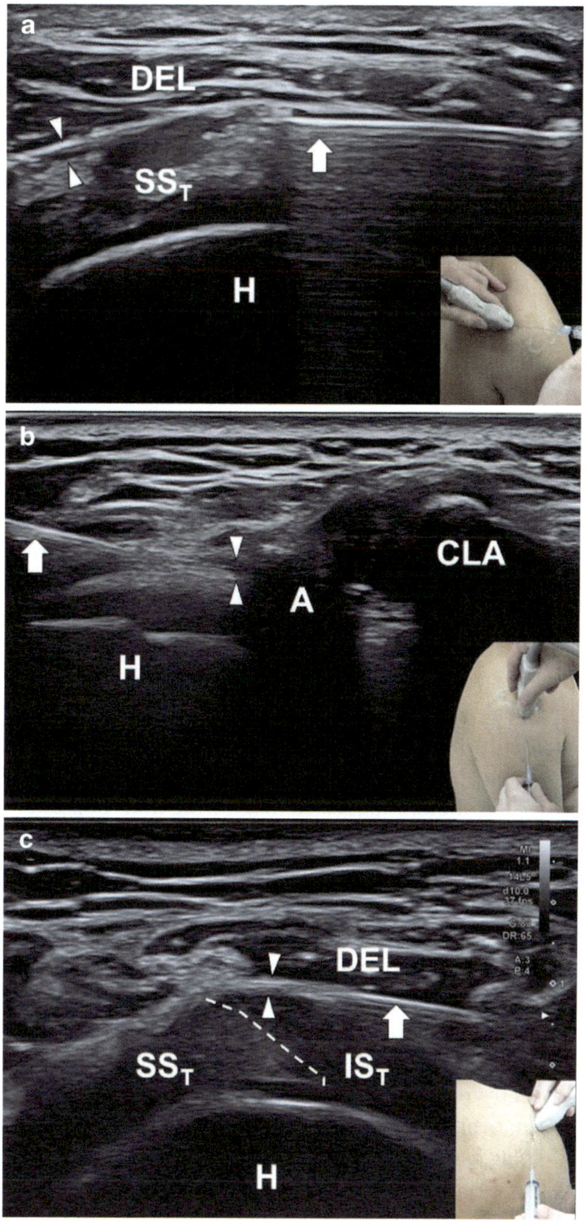

Fig. 1.28 Ultrasound-guided injection into the subdeltoid bursa using an in-plane approach via lateral-to-medial (**a**), caudal-to-cephalic (**b**), and posterior-to-anterior (**c**) directions. White arrows: needle; white arrowheads: subdeltoid bursa; SS_T supraspinatus tendon; IS_T infraspinatus tendon; dashed line: approximate border between the supraspinatus and infraspinatus tendons; DEL deltoid; A acromion; CLA clavicle; H humerus

glenohumeral joint via the rotator interval provided significantly better pain relief than injections using the posterior approach. Furthermore, injections through the rotator interval showed a notable improvement in shoulder function compared to the posterior approach, with these benefits observed after a 12-week follow-up period. These findings suggest that the rotator interval could be a better target for administering corticosteroid injections.

Similarly, in 64 adhesive capsulitis patients, Wang et al. [24] compared the effectiveness of hydrodilatation with triamcinolone acetonide through the posterior glenohumeral recess vs. the rotator cuff interval. The injection comprised a mixture of 4 ml of triamcinolone acetonide (40 mg), 4 ml of 2% lidocaine hydrochloride, and 12 ml of normal saline. Analyzed by the Shoulder Pain and Disability Index, visual analog scale for pain, and shoulder range of motion, both groups showed improvements during the 12-week follow-up. Hydrodilatation through the rotator cuff interval was more effective in reducing pain during shoulder movements.

In a cadaveric study, Kozlowski et al. [25] explored how various injection techniques in the rotator interval affected the distribution of methylene blue dye within the glenohumeral joint, i.e., intra-articular, intracapsular/extrasynovial, and pericapsular regions. One group received dye injections from medial to lateral, while the other group received injections from lateral to medial. The latter technique resulted in consistent staining across all three regions. However, the medial-to-lateral approach often misses some structures. The lateral-to-medial injections produced darker staining in intracapsular/extrasynovial areas like the superior glenohumeral ligament and the long head tendon of the biceps brachii. On the other hand, the medial-to-lateral approach caused more intense staining in pericapsular areas like the supraspinatus tendon and the coracohumeral ligament. Given these observations, the authors suggested that, owing to its consistent and comprehensive staining of key shoulder structures, the lateral-to-medial injection technique might be more effective for pain management in adhesive capsulitis.

To perform a lateral-to-medial injection in the rotator interval, the patient is typically positioned in a modified Crass posture (Fig. 1.29a), with the ultrasound transducer aligned horizontally. As the needle is inserted laterally, it first passes through the anterior edge of the supraspinatus tendon and then reaches the space between the coracohumeral ligament and the long head tendon of the biceps brachii. The glenohumeral capsule covers the upper surface of this tendon. When the needle is correctly positioned within the capsule, slight distension and bilateral flow of the injectate along the long head tendon of the biceps brachii should be visible. In cases of adhesive capsulitis, adhesions within the intracapsular space may increase resistance during injection. If thickening of a specific bundle of the coracohumeral ligament is observed, the transducer can be pivoted along the long axis of the target bundle (e.g., lateral bundle of the coracohumeral ligament). This allows for infiltration of the entire bundle (Fig. 1.29b).

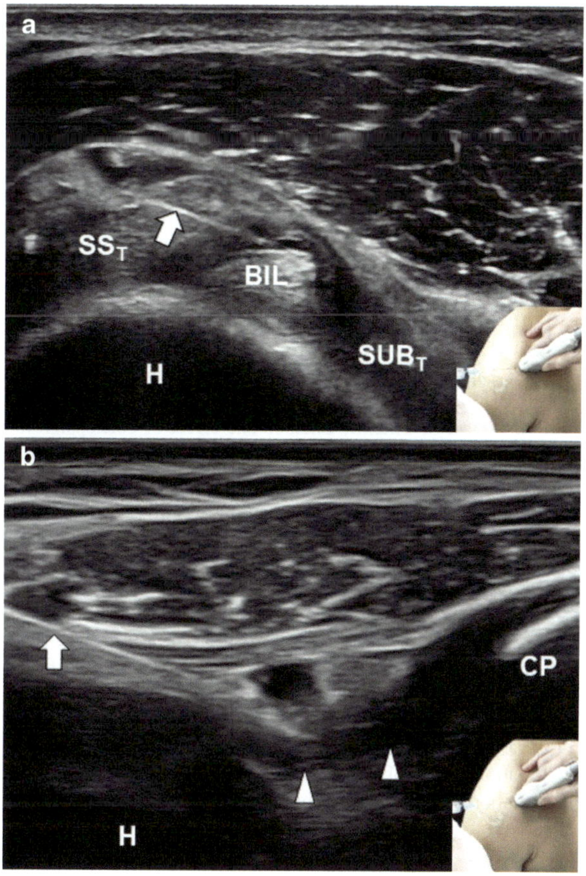

Fig. 1.29 Ultrasound-guided injection into the rotator interval (**a**) and the lateral bundle of the coracohumeral ligament (white arrowheads) (**b**) using an in-plane lateral-to-medial approach. White arrows: needle; BIL long head tendon of the biceps brachii; SS$_T$ supraspinatus tendon; SUB$_T$ subscapularis tendon; CP coracoid process; H humerus

1.6 Conclusion

In cases of anterior shoulder pain, particularly following trauma or sports injury, careful investigation of the rotator cuff tendons is essential to determine the severity and guide treatment decisions (including injections or surgery). The rotator interval can be effectively visualized with high-resolution ultrasound when the patient is properly positioned. In patients with adhesive capsulitis, the coracohumeral ligament within this interval often exhibits thickening, increased stiffness, and heightened vascularity. Research indicates that ultrasound-guided corticosteroid injections into the rotator interval may provide superior pain relief compared to traditional posterior glenohumeral injections.

Acknowledgments Images and illustrations adapted from cadaveric images provided by the Visible Human Project® of the National Library of Medicine. Excerpts featured in the VH Dissector are used with permission from Touch of Life Technologies Inc.

References

1. Farooqi AS, Lee A, Novikov D, et al. Diagnostic accuracy of ultrasonography for rotator cuff tears: a systematic review and meta-analysis. Orthop J Sports Med. 2021;9(10):23259671211035106.
2. Boyle-Walker KL, Gabard DL, Bietsch E, Masek-VanArsdale DM, Robinson BL. A profile of patients with adhesive capsulitis. J Hand Ther. 1997;10(3):222–8.
3. Jacob L, Gyasi RM, Koyanagi A, Haro JM, Smith L, Kostev K. Prevalence of and risk factors for adhesive capsulitis of the shoulder in older adults from Germany. J Clin Med. 2023;12(2)
4. Suh CH, Yun SJ, Jin W, et al. Systematic review and meta-analysis of magnetic resonance imaging features for diagnosis of adhesive capsulitis of the shoulder. Eur Radiol. 2019;29(2):566–77.
5. Wu H, Tian H, Dong F, et al. The role of grey-scale ultrasound in the diagnosis of adhesive capsulitis of the shoulder: a systematic review and meta-analysis. Med Ultrason. 2020;22(3):305–12.
6. Sun Y, Liu S, Chen S, Chen J. The effect of corticosteroid injection into rotator interval for early frozen shoulder: a randomized controlled trial. Am J Sports Med. 2018;46(3):663–70.
7. Gleason PD, Beall DP, Sanders TG, et al. The transverse humeral ligament: a separate anatomical structure or a continuation of the osseous attachment of the rotator cuff? Am J Sports Med. 2006;34(1):72–7.
8. Minagawa H, Itoi E, Konno N, et al. Humeral attachment of the supraspinatus and infraspinatus tendons: an anatomic study. Arthroscopy. 1998;14(3):302–6.
9. Hunt SA, Kwon YW, Zuckerman JD. The rotator interval: anatomy, pathology, and strategies for treatment. J Am Acad Orthop Surg. 2007;15(4):218–27.
10. Petchprapa CN, Beltran LS, Jazrawi LM, Kwon YW, Babb JS, Recht MP. The rotator interval: a review of anatomy, function, and normal and abnormal MRI appearance. AJR Am J Roentgenol. 2010;195(3):567–76.
11. Arai R, Nimura A, Yamaguchi K, et al. The anatomy of the coracohumeral ligament and its relation to the subscapularis muscle. J Shoulder Elb Surg. 2014;23(10):1575–81.
12. Tamborrini G, Möller I, Bong D, et al. The rotator interval - a link between anatomy and ultrasound. Ultrasound Int Open. 2017;3(3):E107–e16.
13. Kask K, Põldoja E, Lont T, et al. Anatomy of the superior glenohumeral ligament. J Shoulder Elb Surg. 2010;19(6):908–16.
14. Bianchi S, Martinoli C. Shoulder. In: Ultrasound of the musculoskeletal system. Berlin, Heidelberg: Springer Berlin Heidelberg; 2007. pp. 189–331.
15. Morag Y, Jamadar DA, Boon TA, Bedi A, Caoili EM, Jacobson JA. Ultrasound of the rotator cable: prevalence and morphology in asymptomatic shoulders. AJR Am J Roentgenol. 2012;198(1):W27–30.
16. Spargoli G. Partial articular supraspinatus tendon avulsion (PASTA) lesion. Current concepts in rehabilitation. Int J Sports Phys Ther. 2016;11(3):462–81.
17. Homsi C, Bordalo-Rodrigues M, da Silva JJ, Stump XM. Ultrasound in adhesive capsulitis of the shoulder: is assessment of the coracohumeral ligament a valuable diagnostic tool? Skeletal Radiol. 2006;35(9):673–8.
18. Lee BC, Yeo SM, Do JG, Hwang JH. Sequential ultrasound assessment of Peri-articular soft tissue in adhesive capsulitis of the shoulder: correlations with clinical impairments-sequential ultrasound in adhesive capsulitis. Diagnostics (Basel). 2022;12(9)
19. Wu CH, Chen WS, Wang TG. Elasticity of the Coracohumeral ligament in patients with adhesive capsulitis of the shoulder. Radiology. 2016;278(2):458–64.
20. Kim DH, Choi YH, Oh S, Kim HJ, Chai JW. Ultrasound microflow imaging technology for diagnosis of adhesive capsulitis of the shoulder. J Ultrasound Med. 2020;39(5):967–76.
21. Chang KV, Wu WT, Han DS, Özçakar L. Static and dynamic shoulder imaging to predict initial effectiveness and recurrence after ultrasound-guided subacromial corticosteroid injections. Arch Phys Med Rehabil. 2017;98(10):1984–94.

22. Tanpowpong T, Thepsoparn M, Numkarunarunrote N, Itthipanichpong T, Limskul D, Thanphraisan P. Effects of platelet-rich plasma in tear size reduction in partial-thickness tear of the supraspinatus tendon compared to corticosteroids injection. Sports Med. 2023;9(1):11.
23. Arrambide-Garza FJ, Guerrero-Zertuche JT, Alvarez-Villalobos NA, et al. Rotator interval vs posterior approach ultrasound-guided corticosteroid injections in primary frozen shoulder: a meta-analysis of randomized controlled trials. Arch Phys Med Rehabil. 2024;105(4):760–9.
24. Wang JC, Tsai PY, Hsu PC, et al. Ultrasound-guided Hydrodilatation with triamcinolone Acetonide for adhesive capsulitis: a randomized controlled trial comparing the posterior Glenohumeral recess and the rotator cuff interval approaches. Front Pharmacol. 2021;12:686139.
25. Kozlowski BJ, Tran J, Peng PWH, Agur AMR, Mittal N. Comparison of the spread pattern of medial-to-lateral and lateral-to-medial rotator interval injections: a cadaveric study. Intervent Pain Med. 2022;1(4):100164.

Chapter 2
Deciphering Subcoracoid Pain's Mystery

Ke-Vin Chang, Wei-Ting Wu, Shao-Yu Chi, and Levent Özçakar

2.1 Introduction

Pain associated with or in proximity to the coracoid process is an underrecognized condition, characterized by anterior shoulder pain and tenderness over the coracoid apex, distinct from well-known shoulder conditions such as rotator cuff abnormalities. In 2016, Gigante et al. [1] conducted a survey to investigate the prevalence, clinical characteristics, and response to corticosteroid injections for coracoid pain. They enrolled patients with primary anterior shoulder pain localized to the coracoid trigger point, excluding those with signs of other shoulder disorders. Triamcinolone acetonide injections were administered to 15 patients aged 26–66 years, with the majority being women (86.67%). After 15 days, 40% reported complete resolution, while 60% had residual symptoms and received additional injections. The author suggested that the response to landmark-guided corticosteroid injections was suboptimal, underscoring the complexity of pain generators near the coracoid region. Ultrasound imaging allows for a detailed examination of tendons and ligaments attached to the coracoid process, enabling precise targeting for treatment. This chapter will explore the sonoanatomy of structures in the coracoid region, their common pathologies, and considerations for pertinent ultrasound-guided interventions.

K.-V. Chang (✉) · W.-T. Wu · S.-Y. Chi
Bei-Hu Branch, National Taiwan University Hospital, Taipei, Taiwan

L. Özçakar
Department of Physical and Rehabilitation Medicine, Hacettepe University Medical School, Ankara, Turkey

K.-V. Chang (ed.), *Ultrasonography of Musculoskeletal Pain*,
https://doi.org/10.1007/978-981-96-6787-1_2

2.2 Anatomy

The coracoid process is a sturdy, curved structure that connects to the upper section of the scapula through a broad base. Initially ascending in an upward and medial direction, it subsequently diminishes in size, changing its course to project forward and lateralward. It comprises a base, an ascending portion, a descending portion, and an apex [2] (Fig. 2.1).

The superior and medial aspect of the ascending portion serves as the attachment site for the coracoclavicular (trapezoid and conoid) ligament (Fig. 2.2). The trapezoid ligament originates approximately 2 cm from the distal coracoid process, extending towards the undersurface of the clavicle [3]. Simultaneously, the conoid ligament originates at the medial posterior margin of the coracoid process and extends towards the conoid tubercle on the clavicle, positioned posterior and medial to the attachment of the trapezoid ligament.

The medial border of the ascending portion and the lateral aspect of the descending portion contribute to the insertion of the coracohumeral ligament. This ligament extends not only over the rotator interval but also over the cranial part of the subscapularis muscle. It covers a broad area on the anterior surface of the subscapularis muscle [4] (Fig. 2.3).

On the other hand, the lateral aspect of the descending segment facilitates the connection of the coracoacromial ligament, linking the coracoid process and acromion. According to Rothenberg et al.'s study [5], the ligament exhibits five subtypes based on its morphology: Type I, Y-shaped; Type II, broad-banded; Type III, quadrangular; Type IV, V-shaped; Type V, multi-banded. The apex of the coracoid process serves as the insertion site for the tendons of the pectoralis minor, and the coracobrachialis, and the short head of the biceps brachii, arranged in a medial to lateral orientation.

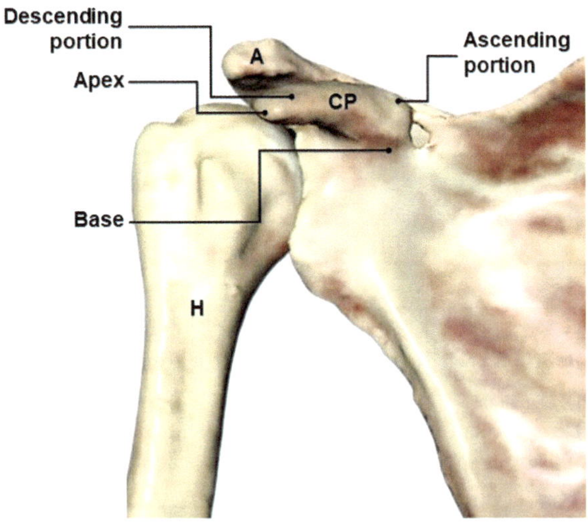

Fig. 2.1 The illustration shows the coracoid process and the surrounding bony structures. A acromion; CP coracoid process; H humerus

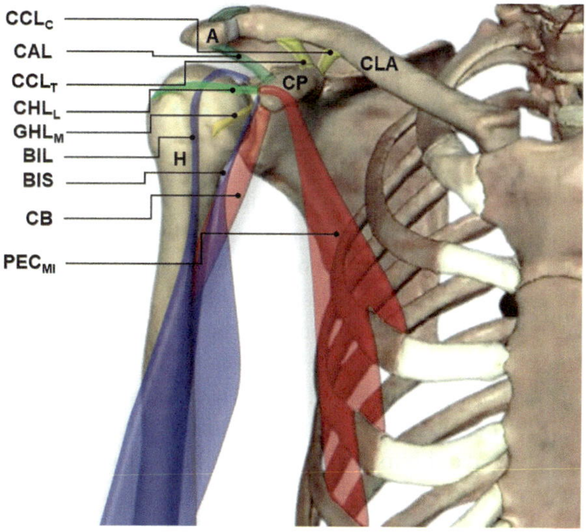

Fig. 2.2 The illustration shows the coracoid process and the inserting ligamentous and tendinous structures. CAL coracoacromial ligament; CCL_C conoid ligament of the coracoclavicular ligament; CCL_T trapezoid ligament of the coracoclavicular ligament; CHL_L lateral bundle of the coracohumeral ligament; GHL_M medial glenohumeral ligament; BIL long head tendon of the biceps brachii; BIS short head tendon of the biceps brachii; CB coracobrachialis; PEC_{MI} pectoralis minor; CLA clavicle; CP coracoid process; A acromion; H humerus

Fig. 2.3 The cadaveric image depicts the coracohumeral ligament in a coronal plane. Asterisk: long head tendon of the biceps brachii; white arrowhead: subscapularis tendon; black arrowhead: supraspinatus tendon; dashed lines: coracohumeral ligament; DEL deltoid; A acromion; CLA clavicle; CP coracoid process; H humerus

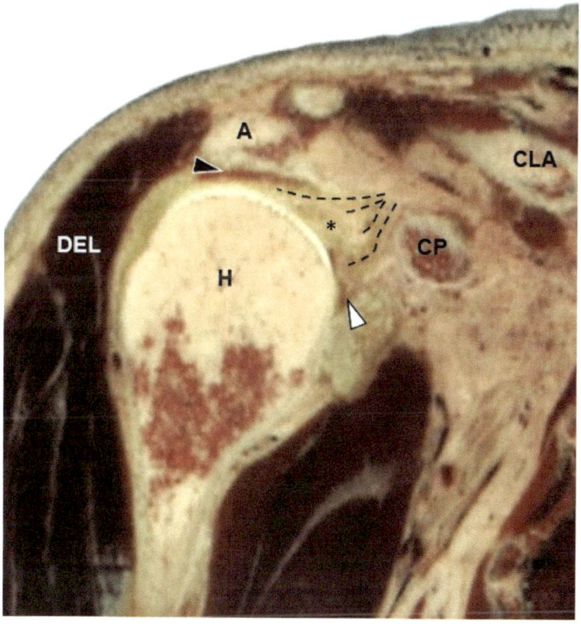

The pectoralis minor muscle, which is triangular in shape, is situated beneath the pectoralis major. It constitutes the anterior wall of the axilla and originates from the margins of the third to fifth ribs adjacent to the costochondral junction. The medial pectoral nerve provides motor innervation to the pectoralis minor [6]. The coracobrachialis muscle arises from the deep surface of the apex of the coracoid process, sharing its origin with the short head of the biceps brachii to form the conjoint tendon. The latter muscle converges with its long head and inserts on the radial tuberosity. Meanwhile, the coracobrachialis muscle inserts at the midpoint of the medial border of the humeral shaft, positioned between the attachments of the medial head of the triceps brachii and the brachialis. Both biceps brachii and coracobrachialis muscles receive innervation from the musculocutaneous nerve [7], originating from the lateral cord of the brachial plexus (Fig. 2.4).

Deep within the coracoid process lie two (i.e., subcoracoid and subscapular) synovial bursae [8]. The subscapular bursa acts as an extension of the glenohumeral joint, while the subcoracoid bursa is typically distinct from the subscapular bursa. Positioned between the anterior aspect of the glenohumeral joint and the deep surface of the subscapularis tendon, the subscapular bursa extends above the superior margin of the subscapularis tendon. In contrast, the subcoracoid bursa is situated between the deep surface of the coracoid process and the subscapularis muscle. The posterior wall of the subscapular bursa, attached to the joint capsule, remains stable, while its anterior wall moves along with the deep surface of the subscapularis muscle (coronal plane, Fig. 2.5a; sagittal plane, Fig. 2.5b).

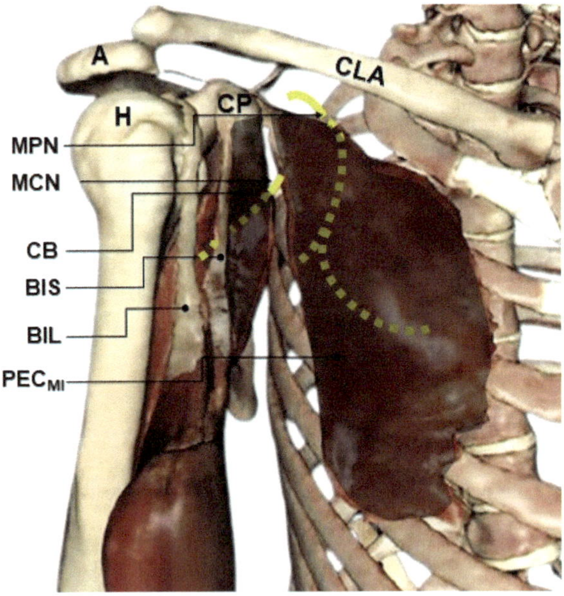

Fig. 2.4 The illustration displays the coracoid process, along with the muscles attached to it and the associated nerves. MPN medial pectoral nerve; MCN musculocutaneous nerve; BIL long head tendon of the biceps brachii; BIS short head of the biceps brachii; CB coracobrachialis; PEC$_{MI}$ pectoralis minor; CLA clavicle; CP coracoid process; A acromion; H humerus

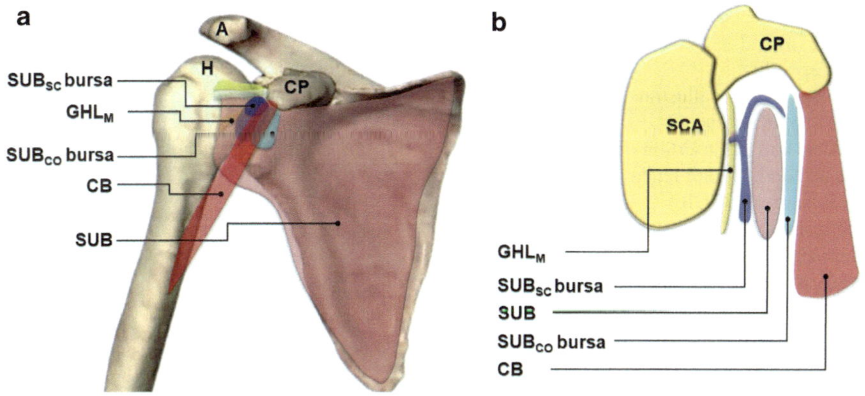

Fig. 2.5 The illustration shows the coracoid process and adjacent bursae in the coronal plane (**a**) and sagittal plane (**b**). SUB_{SC} bursa subscapular bursa; SUB_{CO} bursa subcoracoid bursa; GHL_M middle glenohumeral ligament; CB coracobrachialis; SUB subscapularis; A acromion; CP coracoid process; SCA scapula; H humerus

Branches originating from the subclavian and axillary arteries vascularize the coracoid process [9]. The suprascapular artery is responsible for supplying the ascending part of the coracoid process, while the descending part receives its supply from the thoracoacromial artery. The suprascapular artery, a branch of the thyrocervical trunk derived from the subclavian artery, gives off two branches. The major one runs into the suprascapular fossa, and the second one runs toward the vertical part of the coracoid process. The thoracoacromial artery is a branch of the axillary artery, originating from the medial edge of the pectoralis minor muscle. It currently gives off a medial thoracic branch and a lateral acromial one. The acromial branch runs upward and outward, coursing over the coracoid process.

2.3 Sonoanatomy

The transducer is initially positioned in the short-axis view, aligned with the proximal bicipital groove. Subsequently, it is maneuvered along the long axis of the subscapularis tendon towards the medial aspect to visualize the coracoid process tip. The hyperechoic structure above the coracoid process tip represents the conjoint tendon, i.e., the short head of the biceps brachii, proximal coracobrachialis, and proximal pectoralis minor tendons. Progressing distally with the transducer reveals the pectoralis minor muscle along with its tendinous portion, emerging obliquely from the medial aspect of the coracoid process tip (Fig. 2.6a, b). On the lateral side of the pectoralis minor, the coracobrachialis muscle/tendon can be observed

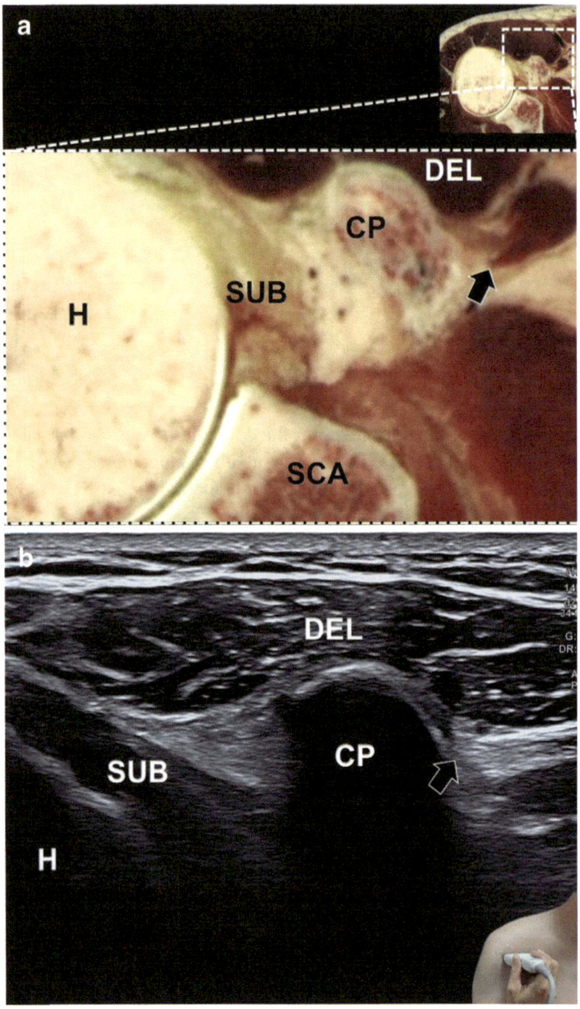

Fig. 2.6 The cadaveric image (**a**) and corresponding sonoanatomy (**b**) illustrate the tip of the coracoid process and the insertion of the pectoralis minor tendon (black arrows). SUB subscapularis; DEL deltoid; CP coracoid process; SCA scapula; H humerus

originating from the coracoid process tip (Fig. 2.7a, b). Moving the transducer slightly distally, the musculocutaneous nerve can be identified emerging from the lateral cord of the brachial plexus and piercing the coracobrachialis muscle (Fig. 2.8a, b). Farthest laterally, the axial view of the biceps short head tendon becomes visible, with its muscular portion not apparent—due to its myotendinous junction being more distal compared to the coracobrachialis and pectoralis minor muscles.

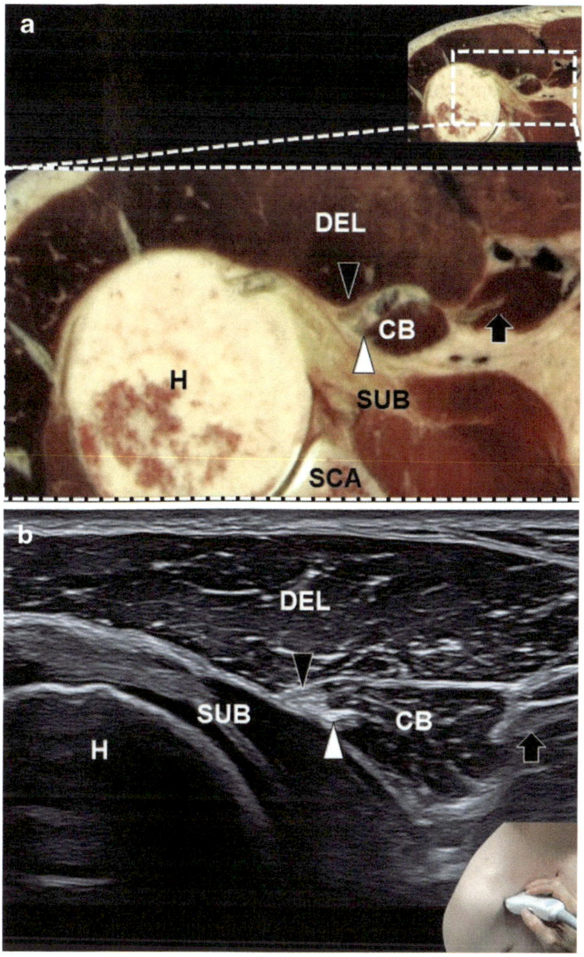

Fig. 2.7 The cadaveric image (**a**) and corresponding sonoanatomy (**b**) depict the conjoint tendon derived from the coracobrachialis (white arrowheads) and short head of the biceps brachii (black arrowheads). Black arrows: pectoralis minor tendon; CB coracobrachialis; DEL deltoid; SUB subscapularis; SCA scapula; H humerus

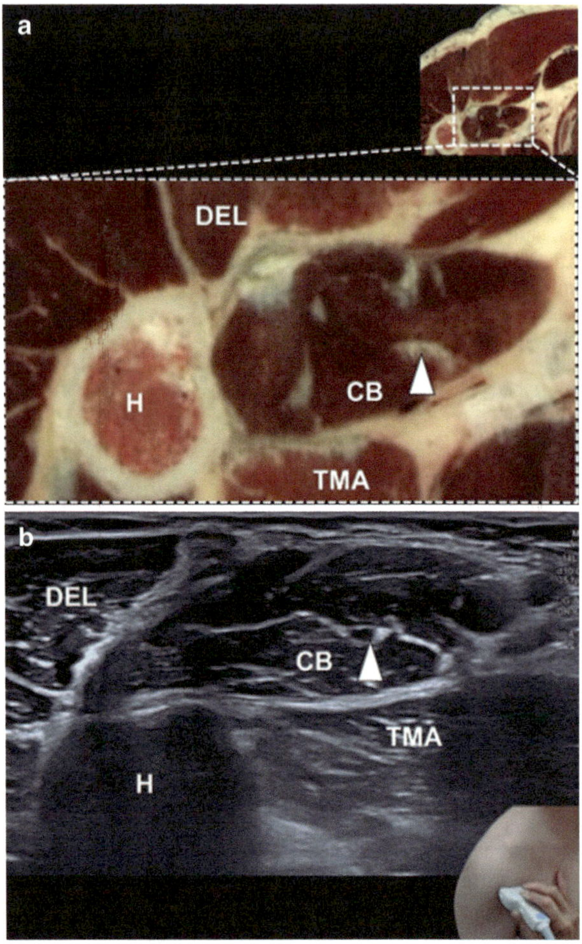

Fig. 2.8 The cadaveric image (**a**) and corresponding sonoanatomy (**b**) depict the coracobrachialis muscle and the musculocutaneous nerve (white arrowheads). CB coracobrachialis muscle; DEL deltoid; TMA teres major; H humerus

The described myotendinous complex can be observed in its long axis. For the pectoralis minor muscle, the transducer is initially positioned over the middle portion of the muscle in its short axis, enabling visualization of the three muscle bundles originating from the third to fifth ribs in a single view (Fig. 2.9a, c). Next, the middle bundle of the pectoralis minor is centered on the screen by adjusting the transducer. Then its lateral end is pivoted toward the coracoid process, allowing clear visualization of the middle bundle originating from the fourth rib in the long-axis view. The remaining bundles can be visualized in the same manner (Fig. 2.9b, d).

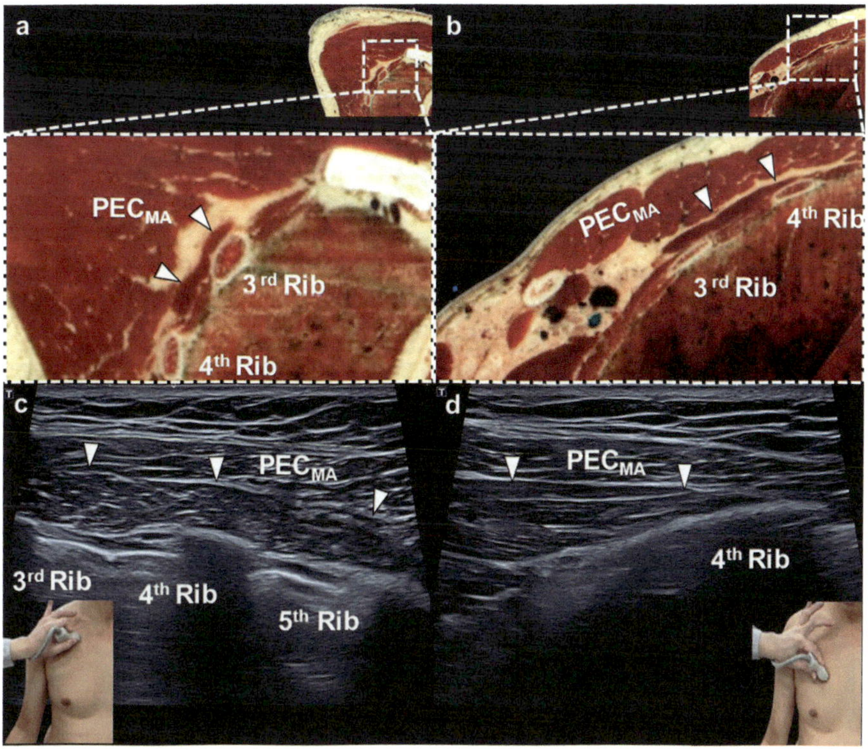

Fig. 2.9 The cadaveric images and corresponding sonoanatomy illustrate the middle portion of the pectoralis minor (white arrowheads) in the short-axis views (**a**, **c**) and the long-axis views (**b**, **d**), respectively. PEC$_{MA}$ pectoralis major

Beneath the long axis of the pectoralis minor muscle, the cord levels of the brachial plexus, surrounding the axillary artery, become distinctly visible (Fig. 2.10a, c). In certain instances, the proximal extent of the pectoralis minor tendon may be observed extending laterally towards the rotator interval (Fig. 2.10b, d). Similarly, after identifying the short axis of the coracobrachialis muscle, the transducer can be

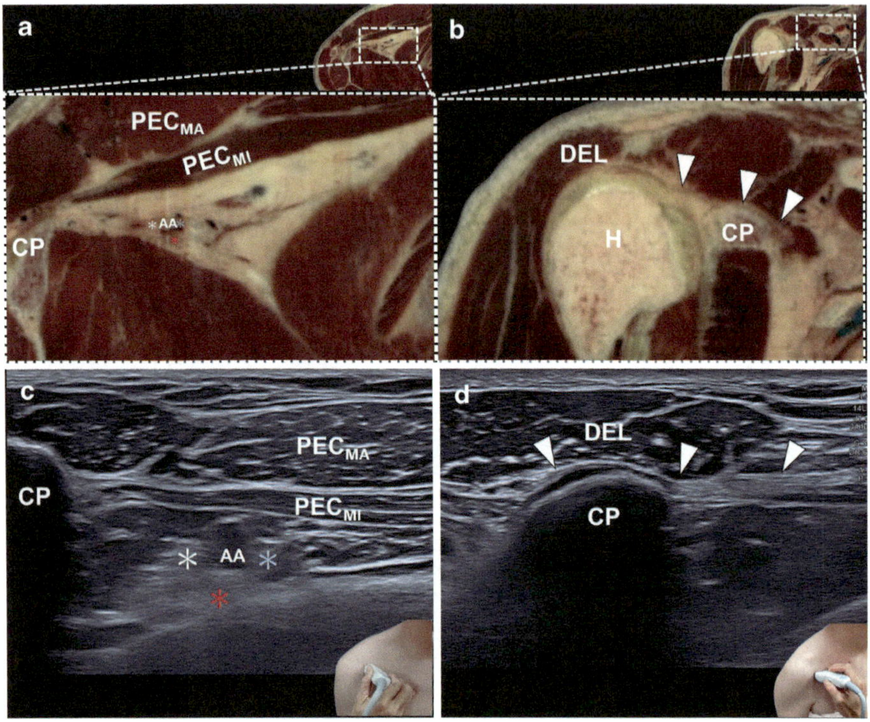

Fig. 2.10 The cadaveric image and corresponding sonoanatomy (**a**, **c**) illustrate the pectoralis minor muscle and the underlying brachial plexus, highlighting the lateral cord (white asterisks), posterior cord (red asterisks), and medial cord (blue asterisks). The cadaveric image and corresponding sonoanatomy (**b**, **d**) show the pectoralis minor tendon (white arrowheads) extending laterally to the rotator interval. PEC_{MI} pectoralis minor; PEC_{MA} pectoralis major; DEL deltoid; CP coracoid process; AA axillary artery; H humerus

rotated 90 degrees to visualize its long axis (Fig. 2.11a, c). By shifting the transducer laterally, the conjoint tendon—formed by the tendons of the short head of the biceps brachii and the coracobrachialis—can be visualized in the long axis (Fig. 2.11b, d). Additionally, locating the short axis of the biceps brachii tendon and repositioning the transducer toward the mid-arm enables visualization of the distal

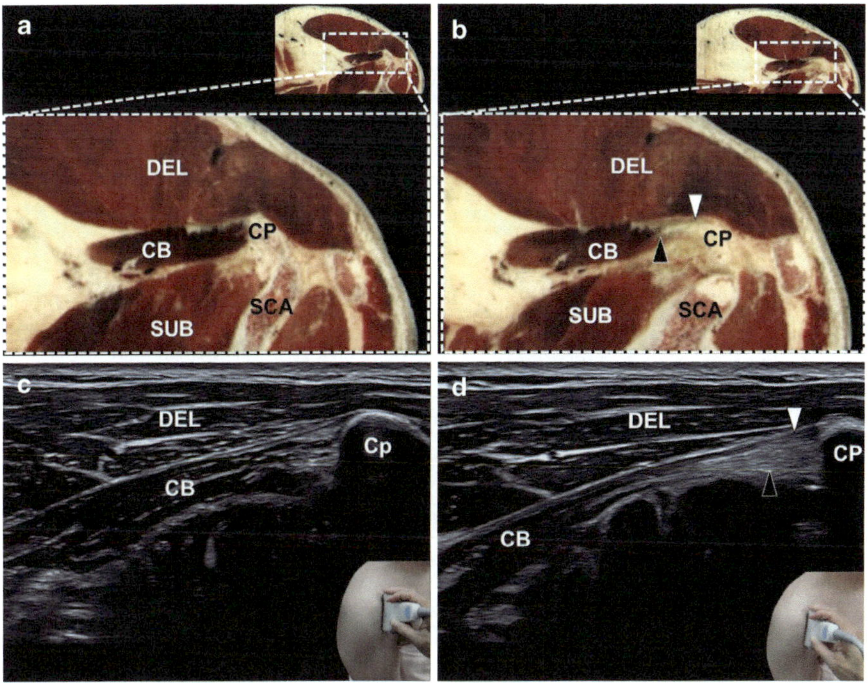

Fig. 2.11 The cadaveric image and corresponding sonoanatomy (**a**, **c**) depict the coracobrachialis muscle in its long axis. The cadaveric image and corresponding sonoanatomy (**b**, **d**) illustrate the conjoint tendon formed by the short head tendon of the biceps brachii (white arrowheads) and the coracobrachialis tendon (black arrowheads) when the transducer is moved more laterally. CB coracobrachialis; DEL deltoid; SUB subscapularis; CP coracoid process; SCA scapula

insertion of the coracobrachialis muscle (in its short-axis view) on the humerus (Fig. 2.12a, c). Pivoting the transducer along the long axis of the humerus provides a longitudinal view of the coracobrachialis muscle insertion (Fig. 2.12b, d).

Returning to the horizontal plane for the coracoid process, the transducer is moved to the middle of its descending portion. The lateral edge of the transducer is then pivoted cranially toward the acromion, revealing the coracoacromial ligament (Fig. 2.13a, c). Deeper than the coracoacromial ligament, the coracohumeral ligament can be found diving deeply to insert on the humeral head, and external rotation facilitates the visualization of the coracohumeral ligament (Fig. 2.13b, d). Further pivoting the cranial end of the transducer to pass the acromioclavicular joint first and then to reach the clavicle, the trapezoid ligament is seen (Fig. 2.14a, b). Moving the transducer and pivoting its cranial end more medially, the conoid ligament is

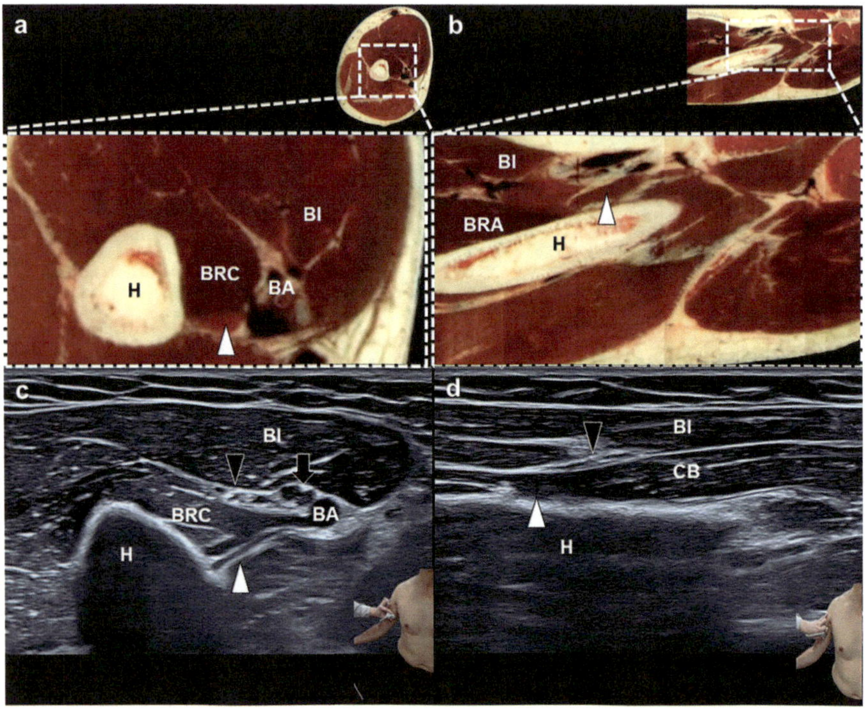

Fig. 2.12 The cadaveric image and the corresponding sonoanatomy depict the insertion of the coracobrachialis (white arrowheads) in the short-axis (**a**, **c**) and long-axis (**b**, **d**) views, respectively. Black arrow: median nerve; black arrowheads: musculocutaneous nerve; BRC brachialis; BI biceps brachii; BA brachial artery; H humerus

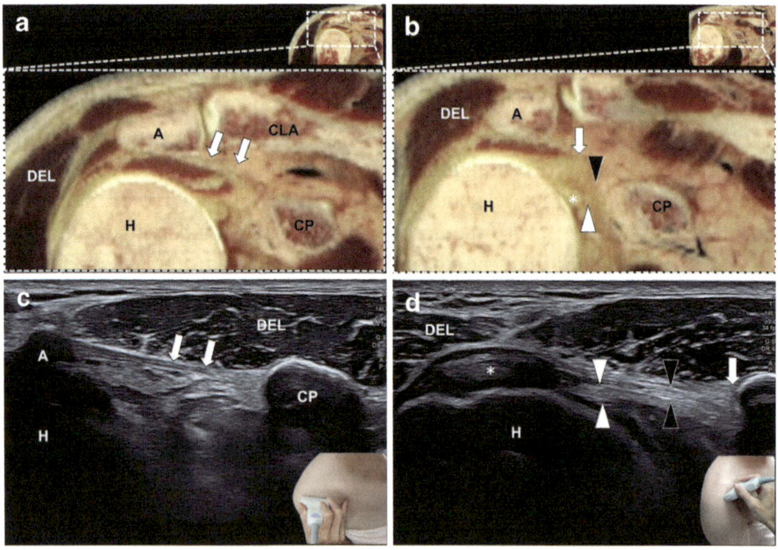

Fig. 2.13 The cadaveric images and corresponding sonoanatomy illustrate the coracoacromial ligament (**a**, **c**) and the coracohumeral ligament (**b**, **d**), respectively. White arrows: coracoacromial ligament; black arrowheads: lateral bundle of the coracohumeral ligament; white arrowheads: medial bundle of the coracohumeral ligament; asterisks: long head tendon of the biceps brachii; DEL deltoid; A acromion; CLA clavicle; CP coracoid process; H humerus

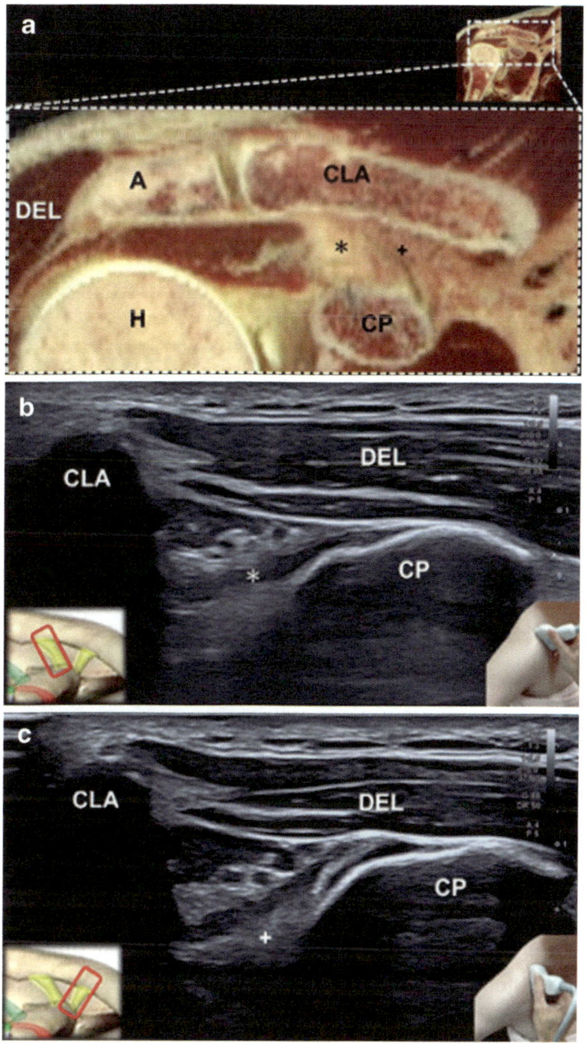

Fig. 2.14 The cadaveric image (**a**) and corresponding sonoanatomy illustrate the trapezoid (asterisk) (**b**) and conoid (cross) (**c**) components of the coracoclavicular ligament. DEL deltoid; CLA clavicle; CP coracoid process; A acromion; H humerus

identified, with its depth deeper than the trapezoid ligament (Fig. 2.14a, c). Extending the arm posteriorly and anteriorly tilting the scapula tightens the two components of the coracoclavicular ligament, facilitating their visualization. After identifying the ligament's long axis, the transducer can be rotated 90 degrees to investigate the insertion of both ligaments on the coracoid process in short axis (Fig. 2.15a, b).

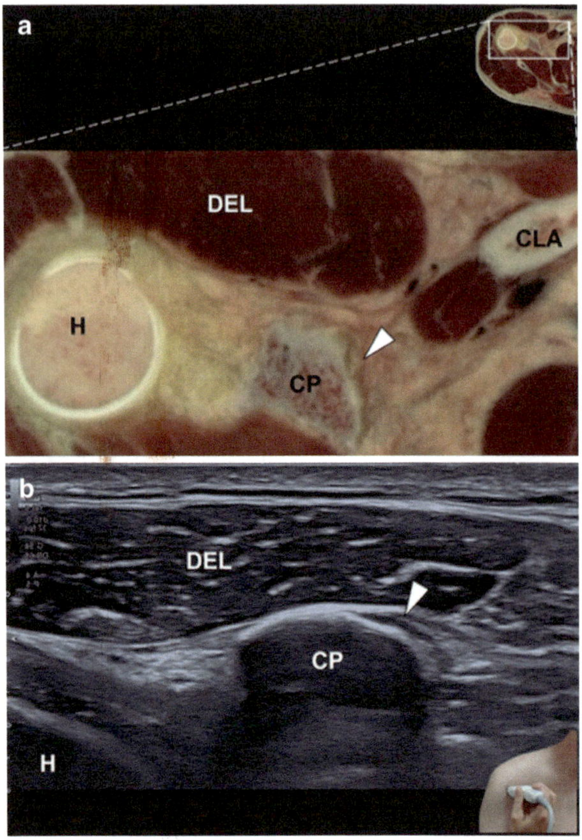

Fig. 2.15 The cadaveric image (**a**) and corresponding sonoanatomy (**b**) depict the short-axis view of the common insertion (white arrowheads) of the coracoclavicular ligament, including the trapezoid and conoid ligaments, on the coracoid process. DEL deltoid; CLA clavicle; CP coracoid process; H humerus

When examining the coracoclavicular ligament, one may observe the acromial branch of the thoracoacromial artery coursing over the descending portion of the coracoid process or atop the coracoclavicular ligament (Fig. 2.16a, c). By tracing the artery branch in a more medial direction, the examiner can identify its connection to the main trunk, which emerges from the medial border of the pectoralis minor muscle and passes beneath the pectoralis major or anterior deltoid muscle (Fig. 2.16b, d).

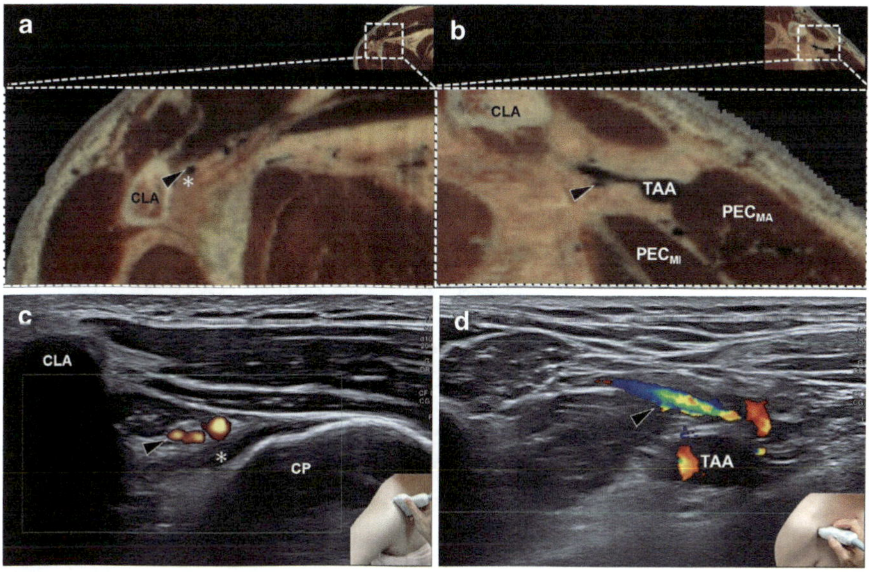

Fig. 2.16 The cadaveric images and the corresponding sonographic images illustrate the acromial branch (black arrowheads) of the thoracoacromial artery overlying the trapezoid ligament (asterisks) (**a**, **c**) and the origin of the acromial branch from its main trunk, the thoracoacromial artery (TAA) (**b**, **d**). CLA clavicle; CP coracoid process; PEC$_{MA}$ pectoralis major; PEC$_{MI}$ pectoralis minor

2.4 Pathology

The most prevalent pathologies affecting the coracoid region involve effusion within the subscapular or subcoracoid bursa. The subscapular bursa, which arises from the undersurface of the subscapularis tendon and curves around its superior edge, may partially overlap with the subcoracoid bursa (long axis, Fig. 2.17a; short axis, Fig. 2.17b). To distinguish between the two bursae, positioning the transducer in the sagittal plane is crucial. When fluid is observed both anterior and posterior to the subscapularis tendon, it is likely associated with the subscapular bursa. Conversely, if there is no effusion extending to the deeper surface of the subscapularis muscle, it is more probable that the fluid originates from the subcoracoid bursa (long axis,

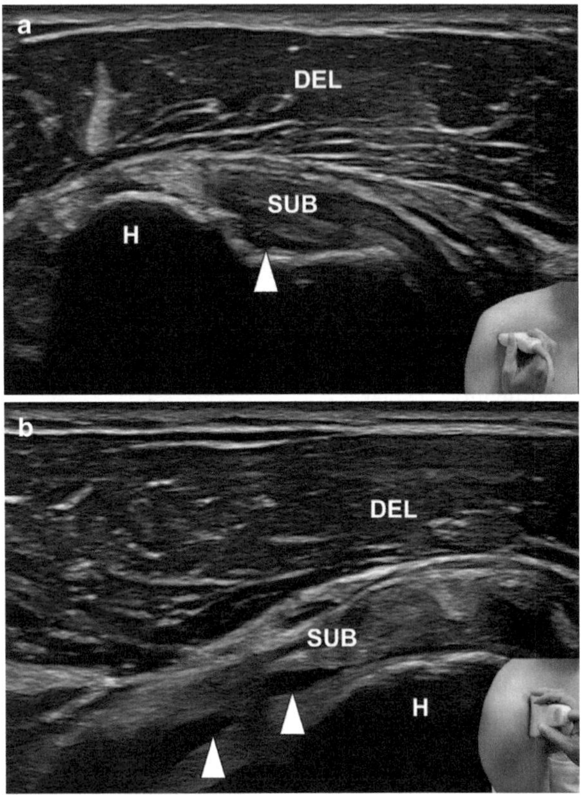

Fig. 2.17 The ultrasound images of the subscapular bursa (white arrowheads) in the long-axis (**a**) and short-axis (**b**) views of the subscapularis tendon. SUB subscapularis; DEL deltoid; H humerus

Fig. 2.18a; short axis, Fig. 2.18b). Considering the typical anastomosis between the subcoracoid bursa and the subdeltoid-subacromial bursa, the transducer can be oriented in the horizontal view to assess whether fluid extends into the fascial space between the anterior deltoid muscle and the subscapularis tendon [10]. In addition to bursal effusion, hypoechoic pannus (synovial hypertrophy) with or without intralesional hypervascularity and hyperechoic loose bodies exhibiting acoustic shadowing can also be present. Effusion in the subacromial region may indicate rupture of the subscapularis tendon for the assessment of which the transducer can be rotated to the horizontal plane (see Chap. 1).

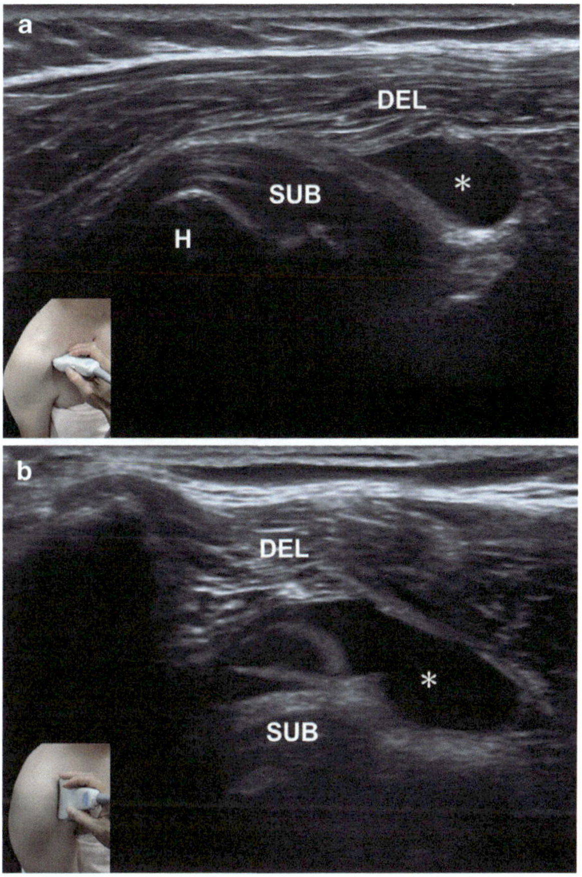

Fig. 2.18 The ultrasound images show effusion (asterisk) within the subcoracoid bursa in the long-axis (**a**) and short-axis (**b**) views of the subscapularis tendon. DEL deltoid; SUB subscapularis; H humerus

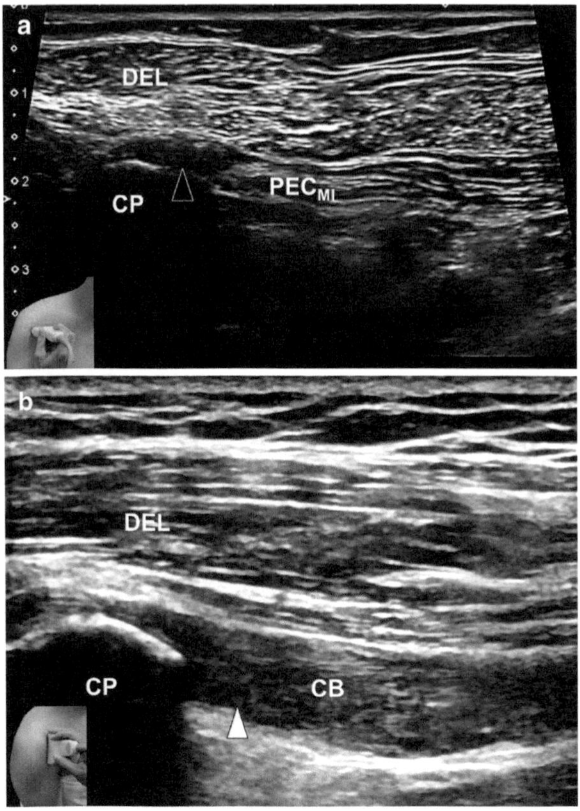

Fig. 2.19 The ultrasound images show tendinopathy of the pectoralis minor tendon (black arrowhead) (**a**) and a partial tear of the coracobrachialis muscle (white arrowhead) (**b**). CP coracoid process; PEC_{MI} pectoralis minor; CB coracobrachialis; DEL deltoid

In individuals experiencing anterior shoulder pain, ultrasound examination may reveal tendinopathy and various grades of tendon tears at the attachment sites of the pectoralis minor (Fig. 2.19a), coracobrachialis (Fig. 2.19b), and the short head of the biceps brachii tendon on the coracoid process (short axis, Fig. 2.20a; long axis, Fig. 2.20b). Hyperechoic calcifications within the tendon attachments, along with thickening and hypoechoic changes can be identified. Moreover, in patients with calcification of the distal subscapularis tendon, the calcific plaque may impinge the

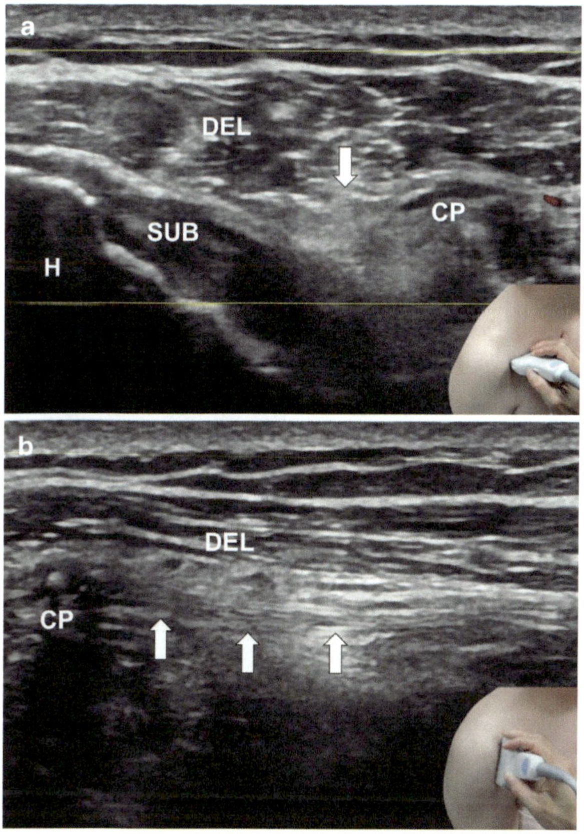

Fig. 2.20 The ultrasound images show tendinopathy (white arrows) of the short head of the biceps brachii in the short-axis (**a**) and long-axis (**b**) views. DEL deltoid; SUB subscapularis; CP coracoid process; H humerus

short head tendon of the biceps brachii during internal and external arm rotations (external rotation, Fig. 2.21a; internal rotation, Fig. 2.21b). This interaction may be accompanied by a thickened subcoracoid bursa and anterior displacement of the short head tendon of the biceps brachii during dynamic movement.

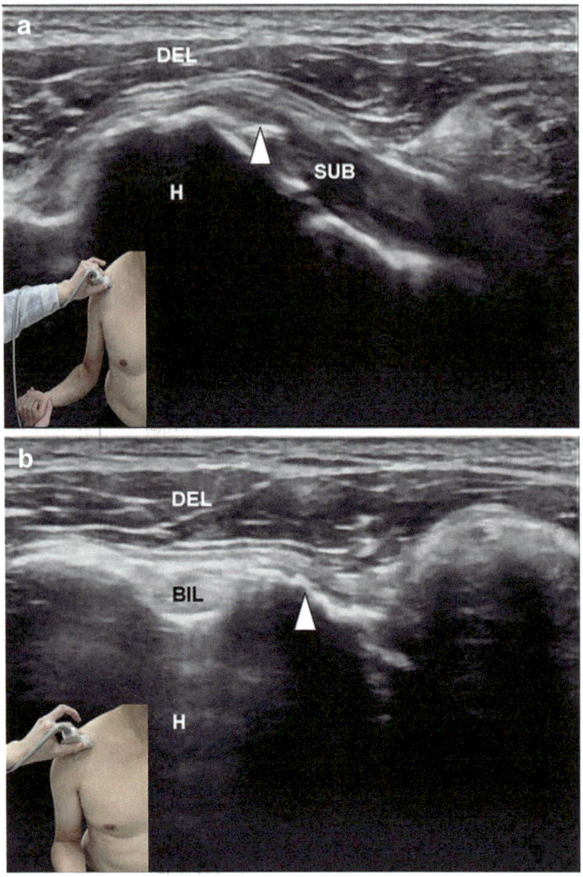

Fig. 2.21 Dynamic ultrasonography images demonstrate the transition from external rotation (**a**) to internal rotation (**b**), highlighting the calcific plaque (white arrowheads) in the subscapularis tendon and its associated impingement on the coracoid process. BIL long head tendon of the biceps brachii; DEL deltoid; SUB subscapularis; H humerus

In cases of trauma, ultrasound examination may reveal thickening and hypoechoic changes in the coracoclavicular ligament, including the trapezoid (Fig. 2.22a) and conoid (Fig. 2.22b) components, as well as the coracoacromial ligament (Fig. 2.23). Such findings suggest intra-ligamentous edema and fiber disorganization. Higher-grade injuries may exhibit complete ligamentous disruption, presenting a large hypoechoic area due to local posttraumatic hematoma. A noticeable widening of the

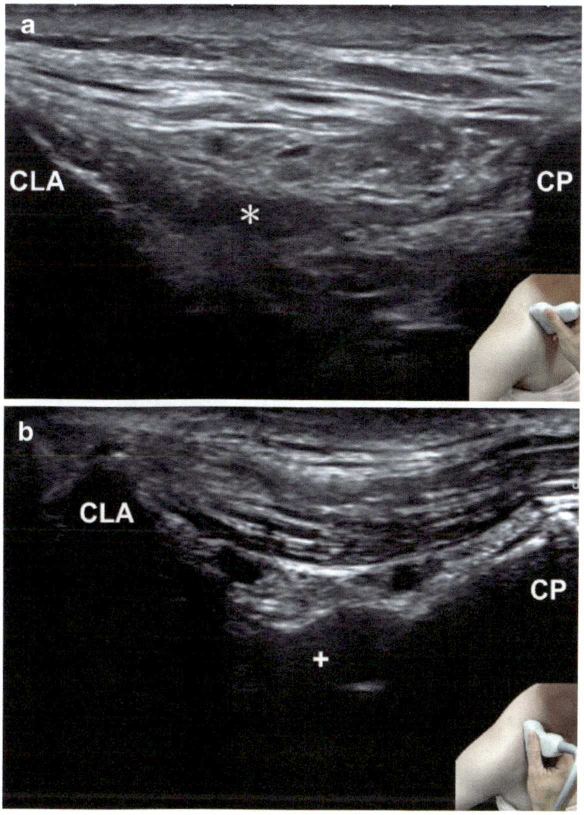

Fig. 2.22 The ultrasound images show partial tears of the trapezoid ligament (asterisk) (**a**) and the conoid ligament (cross) (**b**) in the ligamentous long-axis views. CLA clavicle; CP coracoid process

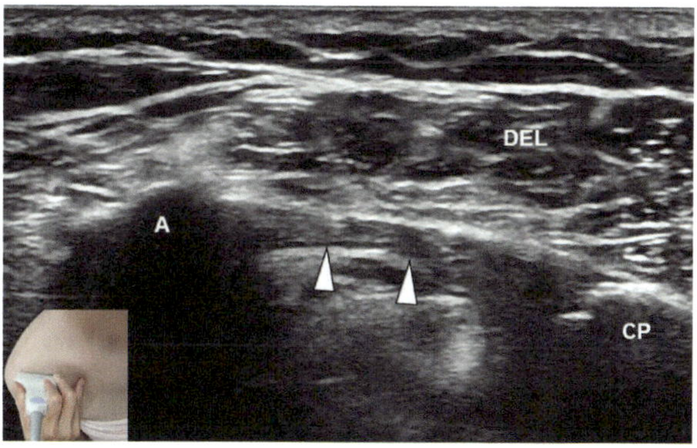

Fig. 2.23 The ultrasound image demonstrates hypoechoic changes and increased thickness (white arrows) of the coracoacromial ligament in the ligamentous long-axis view. DEL deltoid; A acromion; CP coracoid process

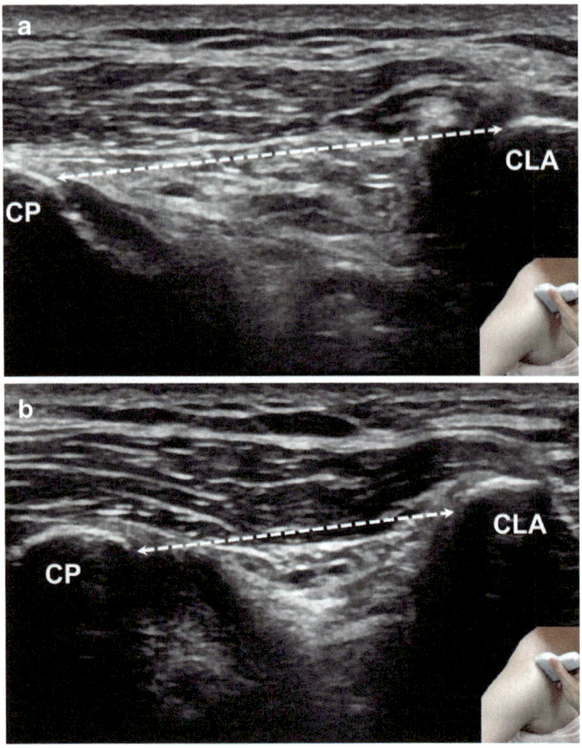

Fig. 2.24 The ultrasound images show a widened space (dashed lines) between the clavicle and coracoid process (**a**) compared to the asymptomatic side (**b**). CLA clavicle; CP coracoid process

space between the clavicle and coracoid process on the injured side (Fig. 2.24a), compared to the asymptomatic side (Fig. 2.24b), may be observed. Furthermore, the acromioclavicular joint may present with pathological findings such as acromioclavicular ligament sprain (Fig. 2.25a), joint dislocation with ligament inflammation (Fig. 2.25b), and ligament tear with articular disc rupture (Fig. 2.25c). In patients with frozen shoulder [11], ultrasound imaging may reveal involvement of the coracohumeral ligament which tends to be thickened, hypoechoic, and hypervascular (see Chap. 1).

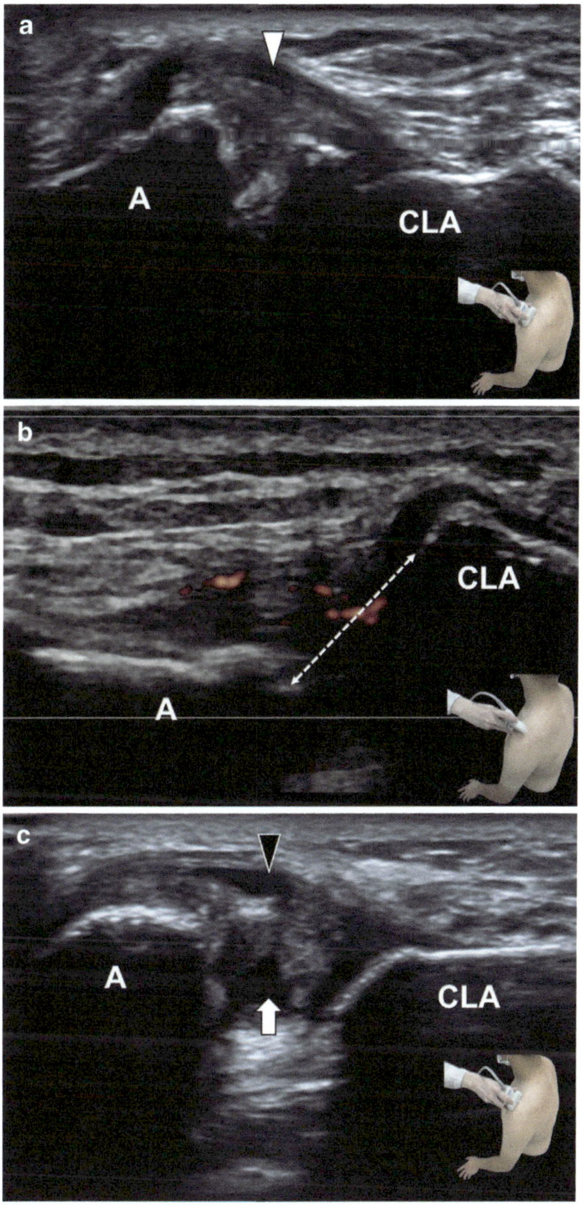

Fig. 2.25 The ultrasound images depict an acromioclavicular ligament sprain (white arrowhead) (**a**), joint dislocation with widening of the acromioclavicular distance (dashed line) and ligament hypervascularity (**b**), and a ligament tear (black arrowhead) with articular disc rupture (white arrow) (**c**). A acromion; CLA clavicle

2.5 Ultrasound-Guided Injection

In individuals presenting with effusion within the subcoracoid or subscapular bursa, ultrasound-guided aspiration followed by corticosteroid injection can be performed. The needle can be introduced using an in-plane approach from lateral to medial, with the transducer placed in the horizontal plane, targeting the subcoracoid bursa between the short head tendon of the biceps brachii and the subscapularis tendon (Fig. 2.26a). For patients with enthesopathy affecting the pectoralis minor, coracobrachialis, and short head tendon of the biceps brachii, ultrasound-guided administration of a 15–25% dextrose solution can be carried out using peppering injection maneuvers (Fig. 2.26b). In cases of sprain or tears in the coracohumeral ligament or the coracoclavicular ligament, ultrasound-guided platelet-rich plasma can be introduced into the ligament (Fig. 2.26c), with caution exercised to avoid injury to the acromial branch of the thoracoacromial artery. In instances of frozen shoulder (where the coracohumeral ligament is thickened), ultrasound-guided corticosteroid injections can be administered to the rotator cuff interval, which is formed by the coracohumeral ligament, long head tendon of the biceps brachii, and the superior glenohumeral ligament (see Chap. 1).

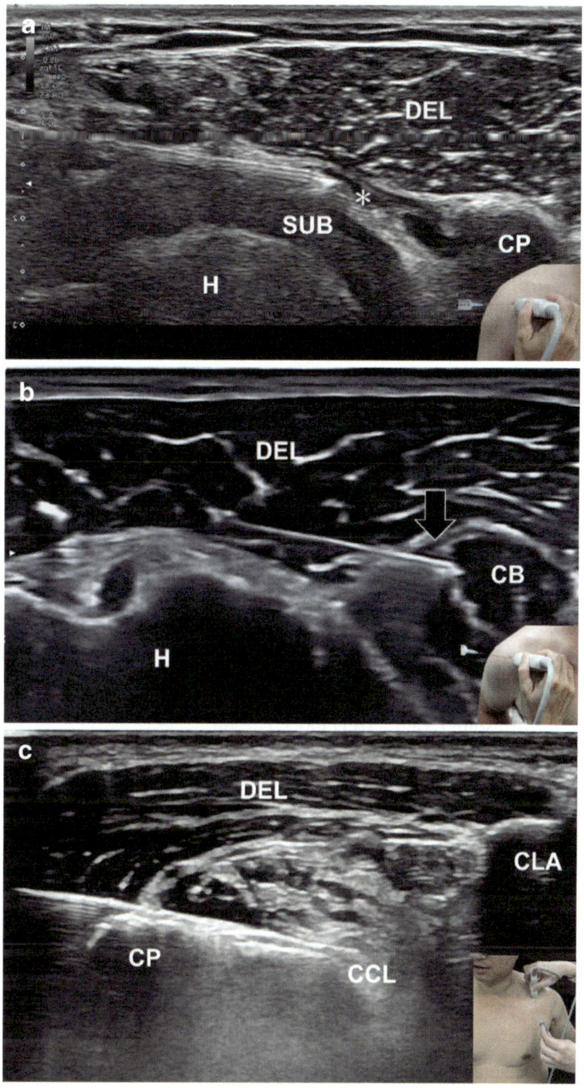

Fig. 2.26 The ultrasound images show injections into the subcoracoid bursa (asterisk) (**a**), coracobrachialis tendon (black arrow) (**b**), and coracoclavicular ligament (**c**) using an in-plane approach. CCL coracoclavicular ligament; SUB subscapularis; CLA clavicle; CP coracoid process; CB coracobrachialis; DEL deltoid; H humerus

2.6 Conclusion

There are four (trapezoid, conoid, coracoacromial, and coracohumeral) ligaments and three (pectoralis minor, coracobrachialis, and short head of the biceps brachii) tendons that attach to the coracoid process, all of which can be thoroughly examined using ultrasound. The most common pathology in the coracoid region is effusion within the subcoracoid or subscapular bursa. With ultrasound imaging, the condition is easily distinguishable by its association with the superior margin of the subscapularis tendon. Ultimately, ultrasound-guided injections can be safely administered in the coracoid region, with special attention to avoid injury to the acromial branch of the thoracoacromial artery.

Acknowledgments Images and illustrations adapted from cadaveric images provided by the Visible Human Project® of the National Library of Medicine. Excerpts featured in the VH Dissector are used with permission from Touch of Life Technologies Inc.

References

1. Gigante A, Bottegoni C, Barbadoro P. Coracoid syndrome: a neglected cause of anterior shoulder pain. Joints. 2016;4(1):31–8.
2. Bianchi S, Jacob D, Lambert A, Draghi F. Sonography of the coracoid process region. J Ultrasound Med. 2017;36(2):375–88.
3. Takase K. The coracoclavicular ligaments: an anatomic study. Surg Radiol Anat. 2010;32(7):683–8.
4. Arai R, Nimura A, Yamaguchi K, et al. The anatomy of the coracohumeral ligament and its relation to the subscapularis muscle. J Shoulder Elb Surg. 2014;23(10):1575–81.
5. Rothenberg A, Gasbarro G, Chlebeck J, Lin A. The Coracoacromial ligament: anatomy, function, and clinical significance. Orthop J Sports Med. 2017;5(4):2325967117703398.
6. Maldonado KA, Tadi P. Anatomy, thorax, medial pectoral nerves. In: StatPearls. Treasure Island (FL) ineligible companies. Disclosure: Prasanna Tadi declares no relevant financial relationships with ineligible companies.: StatPearls Publishing Copyright © 2024, StatPearls Publishing LLC.; 2024.
7. Desai SS, Arbor TC, Varacallo M. Anatomy, shoulder and upper limb, musculocutaneous nerve. In: StatPearls. Treasure Island (FL) ineligible companies. Disclosure: Tafline Arbor declares no relevant financial relationships with ineligible companies. Disclosure: Matthew Varacallo declares no relevant financial relationships with ineligible companies.: StatPearls Publishing Copyright © 2024, StatPearls Publishing LLC.; 2024.
8. Grainger AJ, Tirman PF, Elliott JM, Kingzett-Taylor A, Steinbach LS, Genant HK. MR anatomy of the subcoracoid bursa and the association of subcoracoid effusion with tears of the anterior rotator cuff and the rotator interval. AJR Am J Roentgenol. 2000;174(5):1377–80.
9. Hamel A, Hamel O, Ploteau S, Robert R, Rogez JM, Malinge M. The arterial supply of the coracoid process. Surg Radiol Anat. 2012;34(7):599–607.
10. Drakes S, Thomas S, Kim S, Guerrero L, Lee SW. Ultrasonography of subcoracoid bursal impingement syndrome. PM R. 2015;7(3):329–33.
11. Do JG, Hwang JT, Yoon KJ, Lee YT. Correlation of ultrasound findings with clinical stages and impairment in adhesive capsulitis of the shoulder. Orthop J Sports Med. 2021;9(5):23259671211003675.

Chapter 3
Pectoralis Major Muscles: Revealing the Layers of Pain

Ke-Vin Chang, Wei-Ting Wu, Shao-Yu Chi, and Levent Özçakar

3.1 Introduction

Over the past two decades, injuries to the pectoralis major muscle have become more common. This rise in prevalence is associated with the growing participation in weightlifting activities, both for recreation and in sports contexts. Oftentimes, such injuries ensue at the tendinous insertions (65%) and the musculotendinous junction (27%) [1]. The typical patient is a muscular male aged 20 to 40 years who often reports a tearing sensation, accompanied by an audible pop during weightlifting [2]. Symptoms manifest as localized pain, swelling, weakness, and ecchymosis in the axillary region and the upper arm. This injury is commonly associated with the eccentrically loaded pectoralis major during the descending phase of a bench press exercise. Clinical strength testing reveals weakness in adduction and internal rotation of the affected arm. Magnetic resonance imaging of the chest—in addition to radiographs initially used to detect acute fractures, dislocations, or bony avulsions—is generally used for the diagnosis. Herewith, ultrasound, being a readily available and cost-effective imaging modality, serves as a valuable tool for screening muscle tears [3]. In this chapter, we aim to investigate the sonoanatomy of the pectoralis major muscle with its associated nerves and present the use of ultrasound-guided injections for managing relevant painful conditions.

K.-V. Chang (✉) · W.-T. Wu · S.-Y. Chi
Bei-Hu Branch, National Taiwan University Hospital, Taipei, Taiwan

L. Özçakar
Department of Physical and Rehabilitation Medicine, Hacettepe University Medical School, Ankara, Turkey

K.-V. Chang (ed.), *Ultrasonography of Musculoskeletal Pain*,
https://doi.org/10.1007/978-981-96-6787-1_3

3.2 Anatomy

The pectoralis major tendon is composed of two layers, which convolutes to attach over the proximal humerus. The first layer originates from the clavicular head, while the second layer is formed by the common tendon emerging from the sternocostal and abdominal portions. Notably, the clavicular head attaches more distally on the humerus, while the conjoint tendon attaches more proximally. At the attachment site, these different layers intertwine, presenting an anterior-to-posterior laminated structure. The pectoralis major tendon forms a characteristic U shape and has anterior and posterior tendon layers that are continuous at their distal ends [4]. The arrangement places the clavicular head superficially, followed by the sternocostal and then the abdominal heads (Fig. 3.1).

Collectively, these three muscular portions form a broad, flat, and sturdy tendon that inserts on the greater tubercle of the humerus near the bicipital groove. Each layer exhibits distinct orientations, mirroring the diverse alignment of muscle fibers in the three heads. For instance, the clavicular head follows a cranial-medial to caudal-lateral direction, the sternocostal head adopts a horizontal orientation, and the abdominal head shows a caudal-medial to cranial-lateral direction.

The pectoralis major is enveloped by a thin layer known as the pectoral fascia, which originates from the clavicle and sternum [5]. This fascia seamlessly integrates with the fascial layers extending over the muscles of the shoulder, thorax, abdomen, and back. At the caudal border of the pectoralis major, the fascia splits

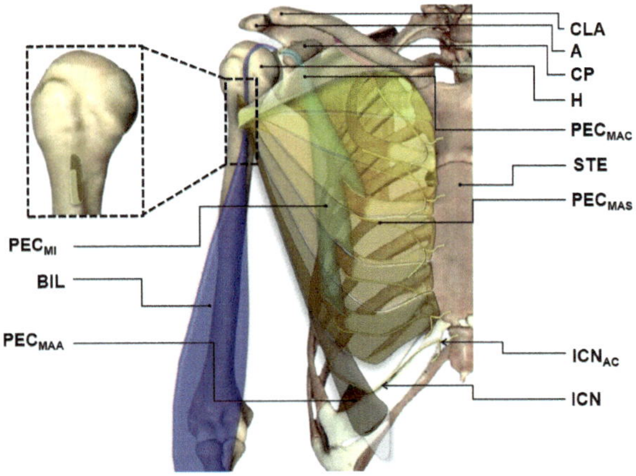

Fig. 3.1 The illustration highlights the pectoralis major muscle and its tendinous insertion on the humerus, forming a characteristic U shape, as depicted in the upper left subgraph. BIL long head of the biceps brachii; PEC$_{MI}$ pectoralis minor; PEC$_{MAA}$ abdominal head of the pectoralis major; PEC$_{MAC}$ clavicular head of the pectoralis major; PEC$_{MAS}$ sternocostal head of the pectoralis major; ICN intercostal nerve; ICN$_{AC}$ anterior cutaneous branches of the intercostal nerve; CP coracoid process; STE sternum; A acromion; CLA clavicle; H humerus

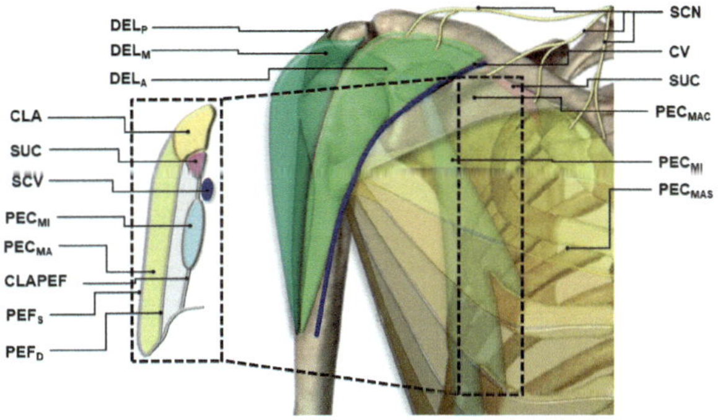

Fig. 3.2 The illustration depicts the superficial and deep layers of the pectoral fascia, the supraclavicular nerves, and the associated muscles. DEL$_A$ anterior head of the deltoid; DEL$_M$ middle head of the deltoid; DEL$_P$ posterior head of the deltoid; SUC subclavius; SCV subclavian vein; SCN supraclavicular nerve; PMC$_{MI}$ pectoralis minor; PEC$_{MA}$ pectoralis major; PEC$_{MAC}$ clavicular head of the pectoralis major; PEC$_{MAS}$ sternocostal head of the pectoralis major; CLA clavicle; PEF$_S$ superficial layer of the pectoral fascia; PEF$_D$ deep layer of the pectoral fascia; CLAPEF clavipectoral fascia; CV cephalic vein

into two layers; the superficial layer, which folds back to cover the posterior surface of the pectoralis major, and the deep layer that connects with the fascia of the pectoralis minor and the coracoclavicular fascia (also known as the clavipectoral fascia) (Fig. 3.2). The fibers of the pectoral fascia run perpendicular to those of the pectoralis major muscle.

The standard anatomical innervation of the pectoralis major is provided by the medial and lateral pectoral nerves [6] (Fig. 3.3). The latter typically arises from the lateral cord of the brachial plexus—to a lesser extent, from the medial cord. Its primary function is to innervate the clavicular head of the pectoralis major [7]. In contrast, the medial pectoral nerve predominantly originates from the medial cord of the brachial plexus [7]. Initially, it gives the main branch to the pectoralis minor muscle before branching further into the abdominal and sternocostal heads of the pectoralis major. This nerve is mainly associated with the caudal segments of the pectoralis major muscle, specifically the sternocostal and abdominal heads. The blood supply to the pectoralis major is facilitated by four arteries: the pectoral branch of the thoracoacromial artery, the lateral and superior thoracic artery, and the intercostal arteries (Fig. 3.4).

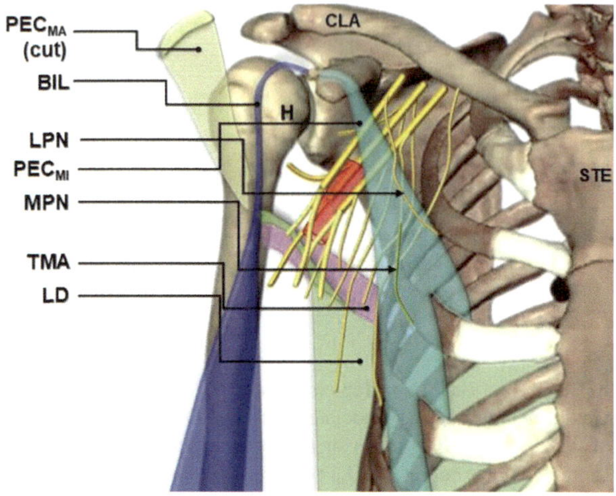

Fig. 3.3 The illustration depicts the lateral and medial pectoral nerves along with the surrounding anatomical structures. LPN lateral pectoral nerve; MPN medial pectoral nerve; BIL long head of the biceps brachii; LD latissimus dorsi; PEC$_{MI}$ pectoralis minor; TMA teres major; PEC$_{MA}$ pectoralis major; CLA clavicle; STE sternum; H humerus

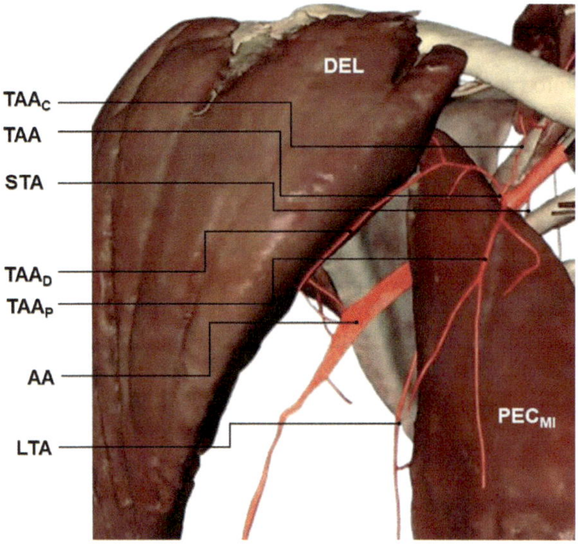

Fig. 3.4 The illustration depicts the arterial supply surrounding the pectoralis muscle group. DEL deltoid; PEC$_{MI}$ pectoralis minor; AA axillary artery; TAA thoracoacromial artery; TAA$_{C}$ the clavicular branch of the thoracoacromial artery; TAA$_{D}$ the deltoid branch of the thoracoacromial artery; TAA$_{P}$ the pectoral branch of the thoracoacromial artery; STA superior thoracic artery; LTA lateral thoracic artery

3.3 Sonoanatomy

The transducer is positioned in the horizontal plane, slightly caudal to the outermost point of the clavicle. Upon gentle compression, the cephalic vein—a branch of the subclavian vein—can be seen (Fig. 3.5a). The anterior deltoid muscle lies on the lateral side of the cephalic vein, while the clavicular head of the pectoralis major muscle is positioned medially (Fig. 3.5b). Pivoting the transducer to the sagittal plane reveals the proximal origin of the clavicular head emerging from the clavicle (Fig. 3.5c).

In the subcutaneous layer, hypoechoic monofascicular structures representing the distal branches of the supraclavicular nerve, derived from the superficial cervical plexus, may be identified. These structures can be visualized at the supraclavicular (Fig. 3.6a), clavicular (Fig. 3.6b), and infraclavicular levels (Fig. 3.6c).

The long axis of the clavicular head of the pectoralis major muscle can be visualized by angling the lateral end of the transducer toward the proximal humerus, positioning its lateral end distal to the medial end, and slightly deviating from the horizontal plane. The transducer is then advanced laterally until it aligns with the crest adjacent to the bicipital groove. In this view, the axial plane of the long head (lateral side) and short head (medial side) of the biceps brachii muscle can be seen beneath the long axis of the pectoralis major tendon, particularly under the clavicular head (Fig. 3.7a). The distal attachment of the clavicular head appears as a small arc, defined by the myotendinous junction of the long head of the biceps brachii (Fig. 3.7b). Visualization of the conjoint tendon of the teres major and latissimus dorsi, emerging from the posterior aspect of the axillary fossa, is enhanced by maximal external rotation of the humerus. The connection between the fibers from the distal pectoralis major tendon and the conjoint tendon of the teres major and latissimus dorsi might be observed (Fig. 3.8a), encircling the lateral aspect of the short axis of the biceps brachii (Fig. 3.8b).

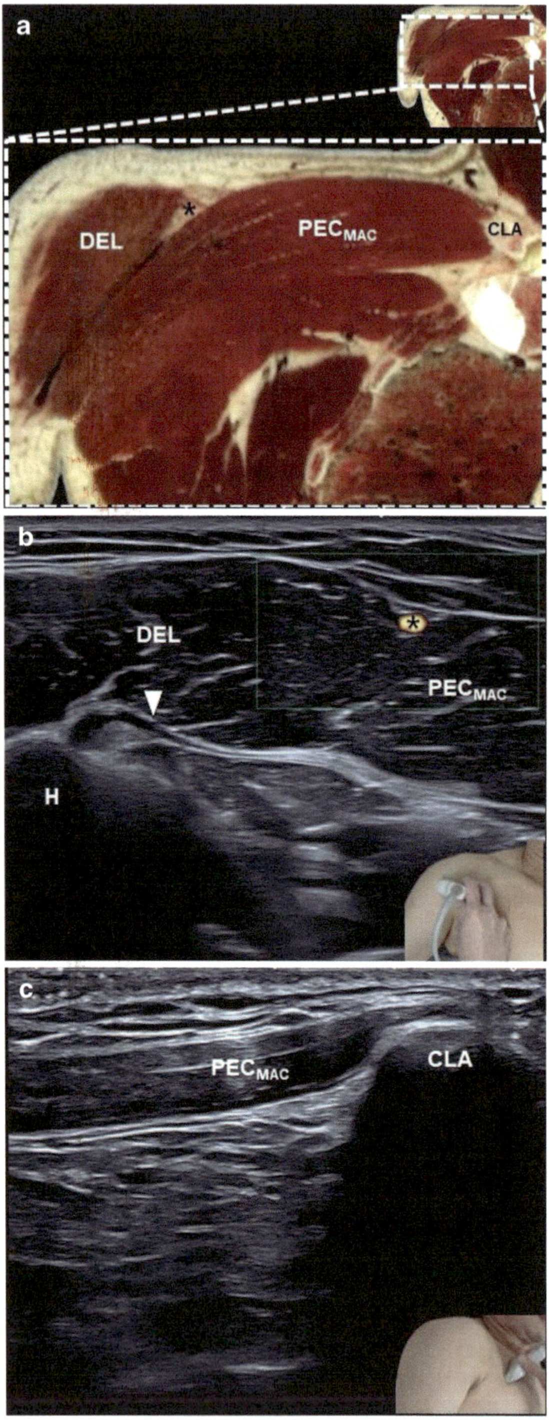

Fig. 3.5 The cadaveric image (**a**) and the corresponding sonoanatomy illustrate the clavicular head of the pectoralis major in an oblique-axis view (**b**) and a long-axis view (**c**). White arrowhead: pectoralis major tendon, primarily from its clavicular head; asterisk: cephalic vein; DEL deltoid; PEC$_{MAC}$ clavicular head of the pectoralis major muscle; CLA clavicle; H humerus

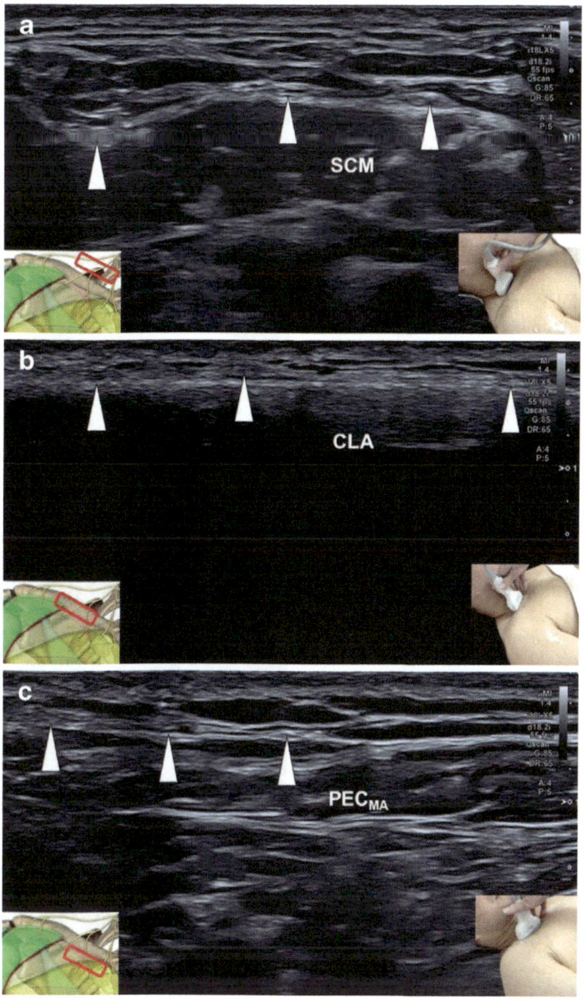

Fig. 3.6 Ultrasound images show the branches of the supraclavicular nerve (white arrowheads) at three levels: supraclavicular (**a**), clavicular (**b**), and infraclavicular (**c**). PEC_{MA} pectoralis major; SCM sternocleidomastoid muscle; CLA clavicle

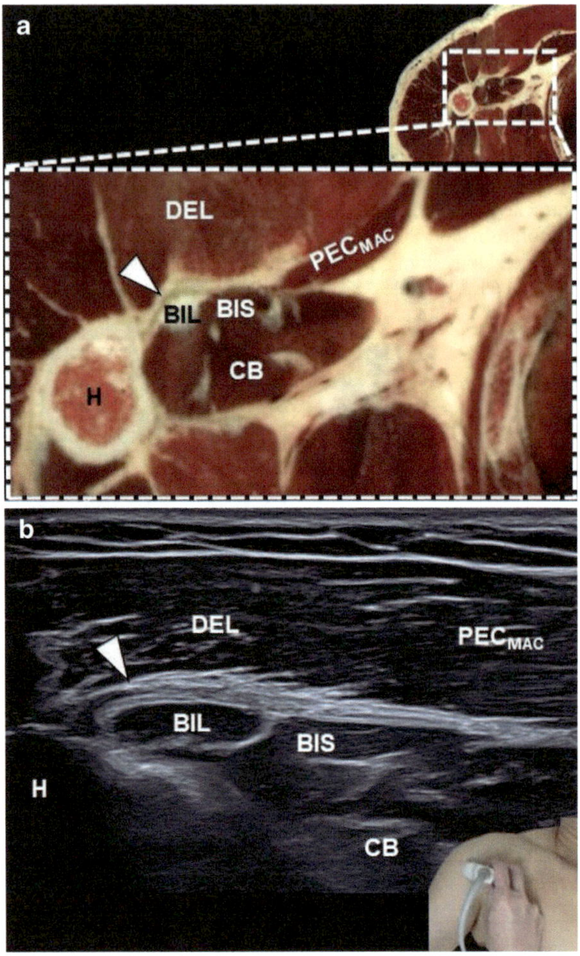

Fig. 3.7 The cadaveric image (**a**) and corresponding sonoanatomy (**b**) demonstrate the tendon of the clavicular head of the pectoralis major (white arrowheads) in the long axis. BIL long head of the biceps brachii; BIS short head of the biceps brachii; DEL deltoid; PEC_{MAC} clavicular head of the pectoralis major; CB coracobrachialis muscle; H humerus

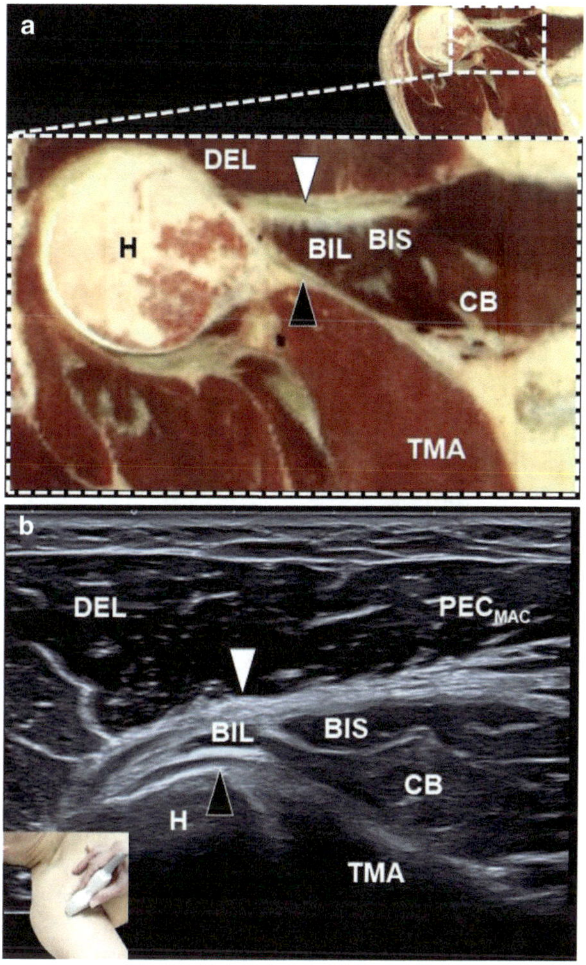

Fig. 3.8 The cadaveric image (**a**) and corresponding sonoanatomy (**b**) demonstrate the pectoralis major tendon, primarily originating from its clavicular head (white arrowheads), connecting with the conjoint tendon (black arrowheads) of the teres major and latissimus dorsi in the long axis. DEL deltoid; TMA teres major; CB coracobrachialis; PEC$_{MAC}$ clavicular head of the pectoralis major; BIL long head of the biceps brachii; BIS short head of the biceps brachii; H humerus

To examine the sternocostal head of the pectoralis major muscle, positioning the transducer beside the sternum in the sagittal plane provides a view of its short axis (Fig. 3.9a, c). Pivoting the transducer to the horizontal plane reveals the proximal origin of the sternocostal head emerging from the periosteum of the sternum (Fig. 3.9b, d). Beneath the short axis of this muscle, the intercostal muscle between

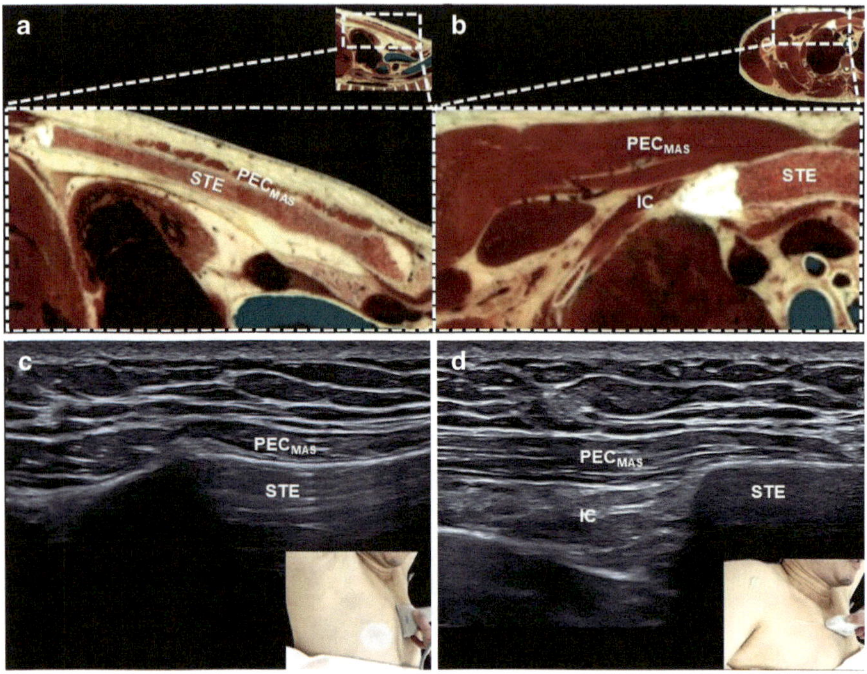

Fig. 3.9 The cadaveric images and corresponding sonoanatomy illustrate the origin of the sternocostal head of the pectoralis major muscle (PEC_{MAS}) in short-axis (**a**, **c**) and long-axis (**b**, **d**) views. IC intercostal muscles; STE sternum

the ribs is visible (Fig. 3.10a), with the internal thoracic artery (also known as the internal mammary artery) located deeper, running along the sternum (Fig. 3.10b).

Returning to the long axis of the sternocostal head and sliding the transducer laterally toward the proximal humerus reveals its humeral attachment. The tendon fibers appear straighter compared to those of the clavicular head (Fig. 3.11a, c). For optimal visualization, the lateral end of the transducer should be positioned more cranially than the medial end, rather than in a horizontal orientation. Once the long axis of the sternocostal head is identified, the transducer can be aligned with the long axis of the proximal humerus. The short axis of the clavicular head appears distal and superficial to the sternocostal head, with a portion of the long axis of the long head of the biceps brachii visible beneath both heads of the pectoralis major muscle (Fig. 3.11b, d). Within the subcutaneous layer of the sternocostal head of the

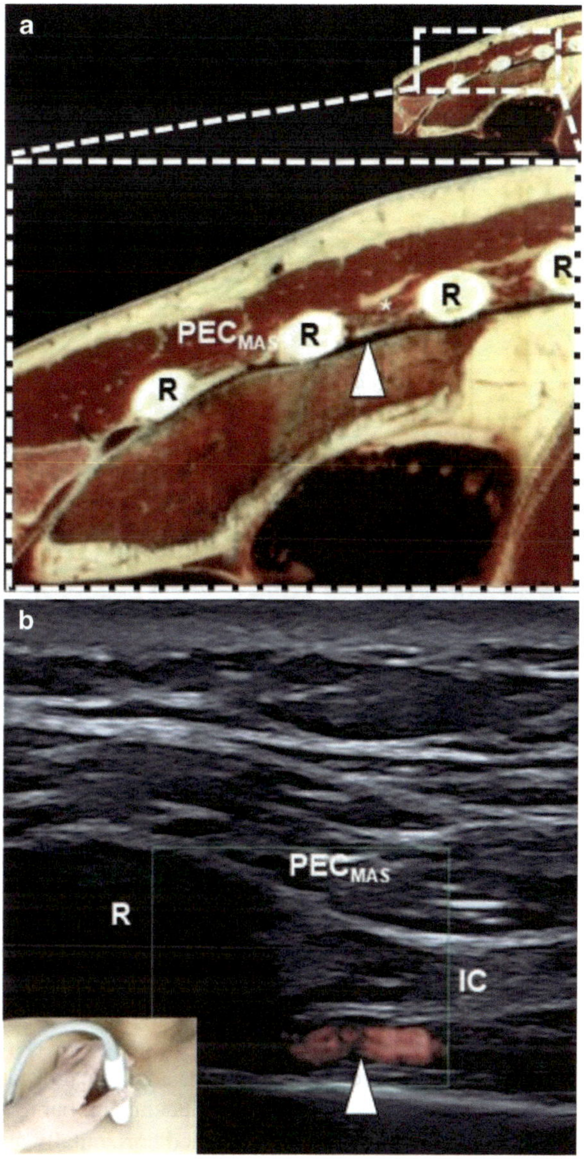

Fig. 3.10 The cadaveric image (**a**) and corresponding sonoanatomy (**b**) demonstrate the internal thoracic artery (white arrowheads) in its long-axis views. IC and asterisk: intercostal muscles; PEC_{MAS} sternocostal head of the pectoralis major; R rib

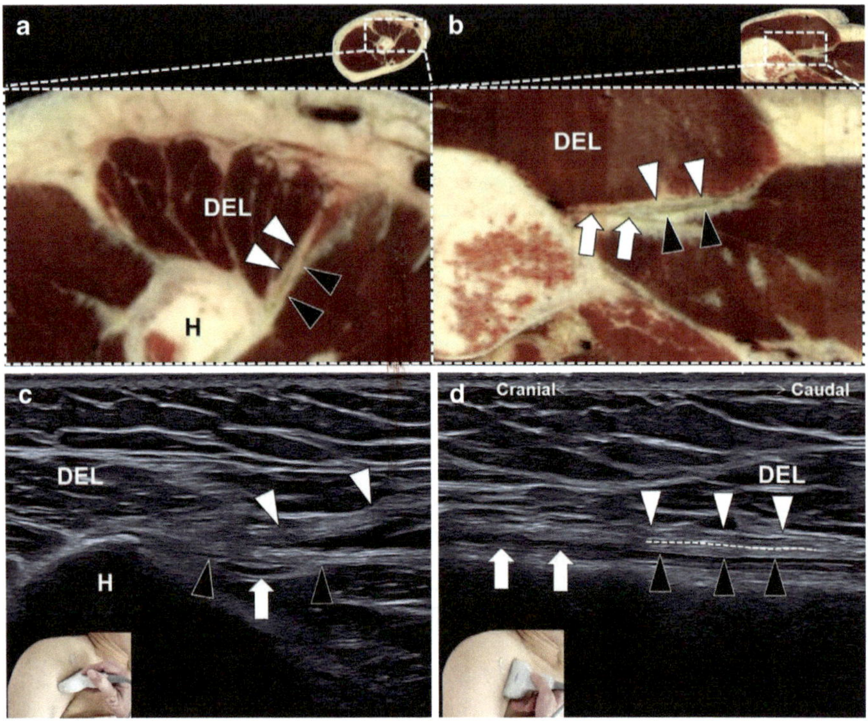

Fig. 3.11 The cadaveric images and corresponding sonoanatomy illustrate the insertion of the sternocostal head (black arrowheads) of the pectoralis major at the greater tuberosity in the long-axis (**a**, **c**) and short-axis (**b**, **d**) views of the pectoralis major tendon. White arrowheads: tendon of the clavicular head of the pectoralis major; dashed line: separation plane between the clavicular and sternocostal heads; white arrows: long head tendon of the biceps brachii; DEL deltoid; H humerus

pectoralis major muscle, hypoechoic monofascicular structures may be observed (Fig. 3.12a). These structures correspond to the anterior cutaneous branches of the intercostal nerves, visualized in short-axis (Fig. 3.12b) and long-axis views (Fig. 3.12c).

It is challenging to differentiate the abdominal head of the pectoralis major from the sternocostal head at its humeral attachment, but its proximal origin can be identified. The transducer is first positioned horizontally at the level of the xiphoid process and gradually moved laterally, with its lateral end slightly angled cranially. This maneuver provides an oblique view, revealing the external oblique abdominal muscle overlying the lower ribs. Above the aponeurosis of the external oblique muscle, the proximal fibers of the abdominal head of the pectoralis major become

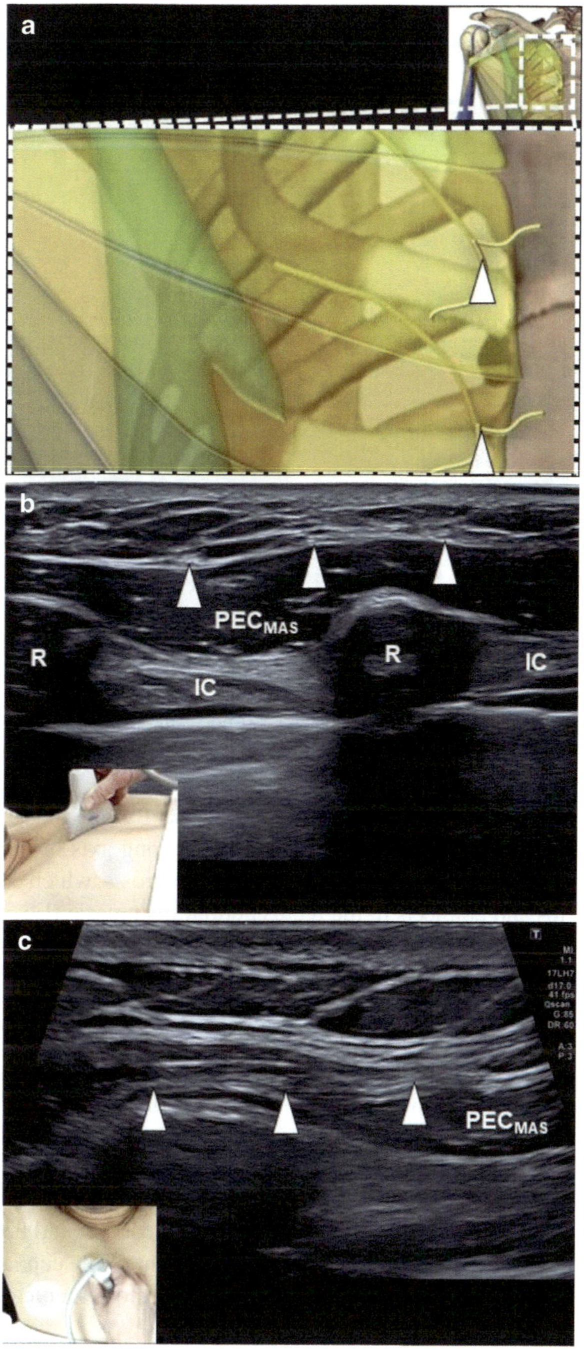

Fig. 3.12 The illustration (**a**) and corresponding sonoanatomy showing the anterior cutaneous branches of the intercostal nerves (white arrowheads) in the short-axis (**b**) and long-axis (**c**) views. IC intercostal muscles; PEC$_{MAS}$ sternocostal head of the pectoralis major; R rib

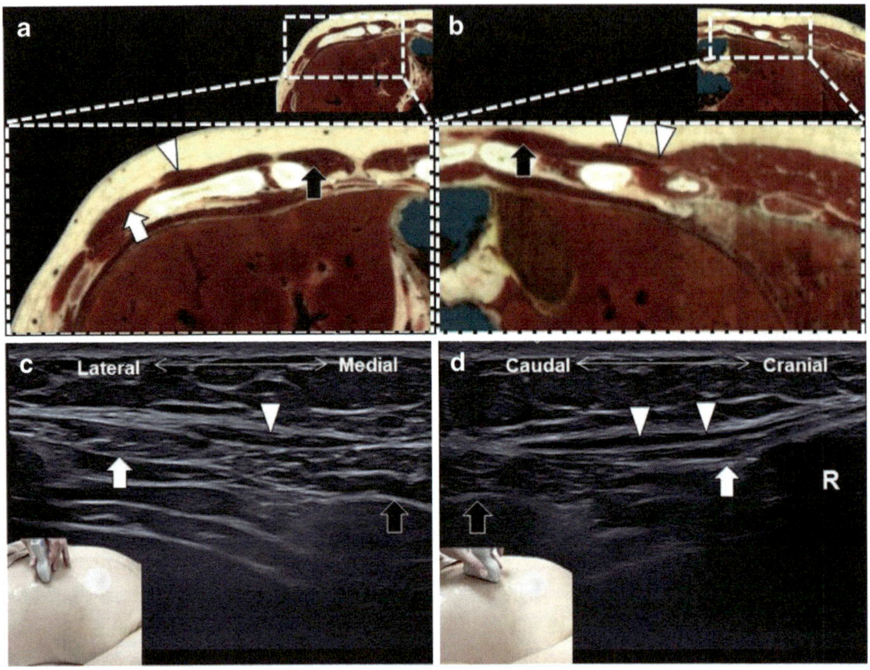

Fig. 3.13 The cadaveric images and corresponding sonoanatomy demonstrate the origin of the abdominal head (white arrowheads) of the pectoralis major in short-axis (**a**, **c**) and long-axis (**b**, **d**) views. White arrows: external oblique abdominal muscle; black arrows: rectus abdominis; R rib

visible in its axial plane (Fig. 3.13a, c). By pivoting the transducer from a lateral-cranial to medial-caudal direction, the long axis of the abdominal head's origin is visualized as it transitions into an aponeurosis, which crosses the seventh and eighth ribs and connects to the rectus abdominis muscle (Fig. 3.13b, d).

Ultrasound imaging proves to be a valuable modality for visualizing the nerves innervating the pectoralis major muscle [7]. The transducer is strategically placed medial to the coracoid process in the horizontal plane to identify the thoracoacromial artery, emanating as a bifurcation from the infraclavicular segment of the axillary artery. The subsequent divisions of the thoracoacromial artery give rise to pectoral, acromial, deltoid, and clavicular branches. The pectoral branch courses between the pectoralis major and minor muscles—often accompanied by the lateral pectoral nerve, presenting as a hypoechoic ovoid structure. (Fig. 3.14b). Originating from the medial cord, the medial pectoral nerve traverses beneath the pectoralis minor muscle (Fig. 3.14c). Another approach would be to locate the intersection of the axillary artery and the branching point of the cephalic vein from the subclavian vein, potentially revealing the medial pectoral nerve positioned amidst these anatomical structures.

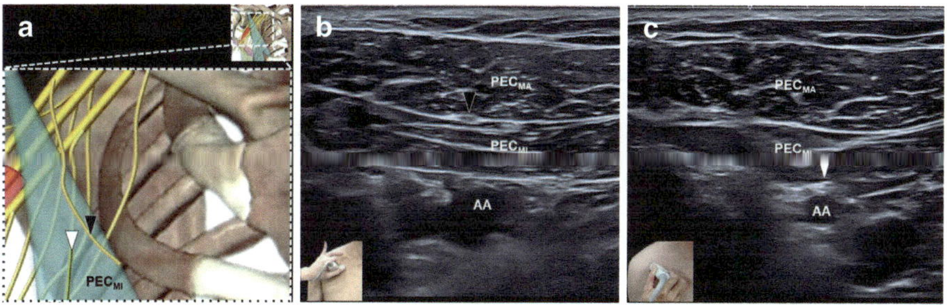

Fig. 3.14 The illustration (**a**) and corresponding sonoanatomy show the lateral pectoral nerve (black arrowhead) (**b**) and the medial pectoral nerve (white arrowhead) (**c**) in the short-axis views. PEC_{MA} pectoralis major; PEC_{MI} pectoralis minor; AA axillary artery

3.4 Pathology

The primary mechanism of pectoralis major muscle injury is often that of forced external rotation, extension, and abduction of the humerus during bench-press exercises. Complete tears have been reported as more prevalent than partial tears, particularly occurring at the distal humeral insertion (enthesis) rather than the myotendinous junction [4, 8]. In cases of a complete tear, ultrasound imaging may reveal a substantial intramuscular gap with or without retraction (short axis, Fig. 3.15a; long axis, Fig. 3.15b), increased echogenicity due to fat infiltration in the muscle belly, and a subacute hematoma adjacent to the torn site.

For patients with partial tears of the pectoralis major, the rupture typically involves muscle fibers without extending to full thickness (clavicular head, Fig. 3.16a; sternocostal head, Fig. 3.16b), possibly accompanied by an intramuscular hematoma. In instances of a muscle strain, ultrasound imaging indicates focal hyperechoic changes (edema) with blurred distinction between perimysium and background muscle bundles. Moreover, ultrasound examination may show involvement of the tendinous portion of the pectoralis major, displaying loss of fibrillar pattern and increased thickness of the pectoralis major tendon near its insertion on the humerus (affected side, Fig. 3.17a; non-affected side, Fig. 3.17b). In patients with pain near the attachment of the pectoralis major tendon, not all have pathologies affecting the pectoralis major tendon itself. Occasionally, a rupture of the long head of the biceps brachii tendon accompanied by hematoma formation (Fig. 3.18a) may be observed, along with involvement of the conjoint tendon of the latissimus dorsi and teres major (Fig. 3.18b).

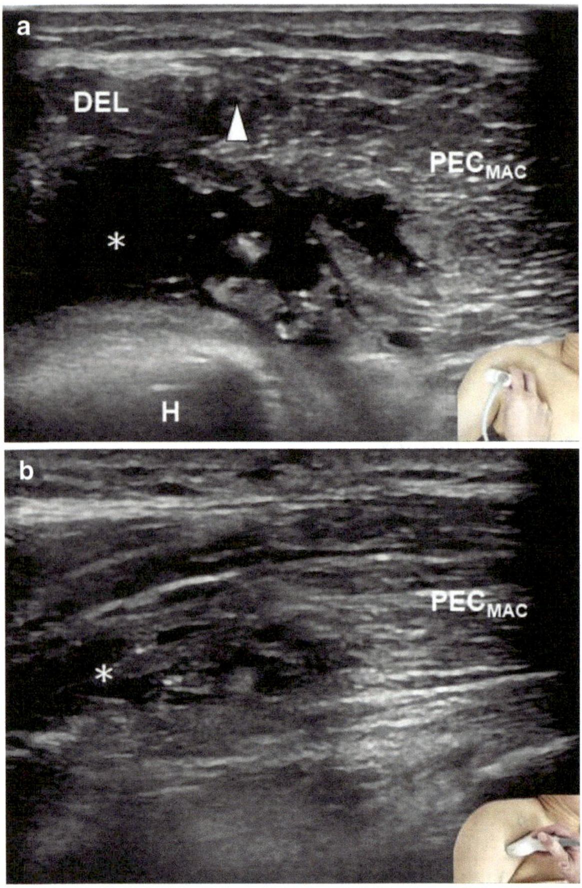

Fig. 3.15 The ultrasound images demonstrate a complete tear of the pectoralis major muscle, with deficient muscle fibers and effusion (asterisks) in short- (**a**) and long-axis (**b**) views. White arrowhead: cephalic vein; DEL deltoid; PEC$_{MAC}$ clavicular head of the pectoralis major; H humerus

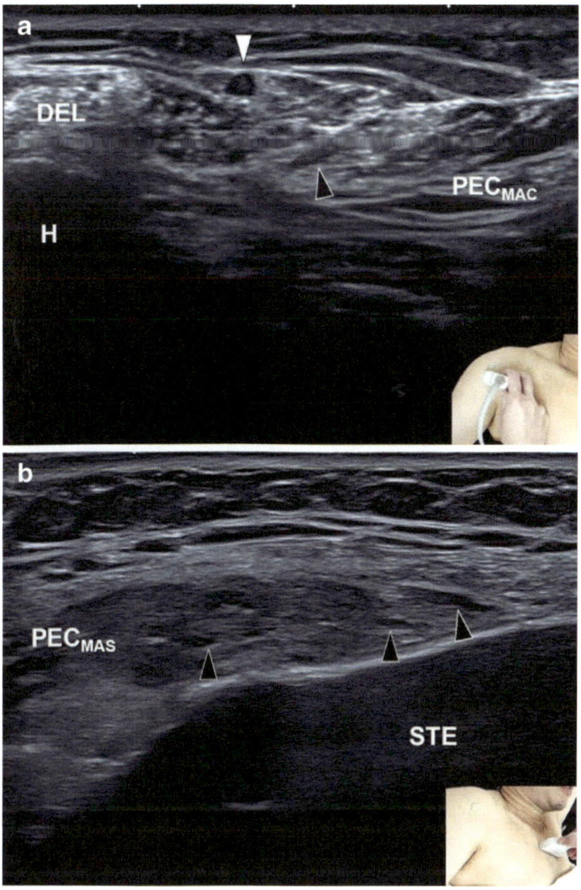

Fig. 3.16 The ultrasound images show a partial tear (black arrowheads) at the myotendinous junction of the clavicular head of the pectoralis major (**a**) and at the origin of the sternocostal head of the pectoralis major in the long-axis view (**b**). White arrowhead: cephalic vein; DEL deltoid; PEC$_{MAC}$ clavicular head of the pectoralis major; PEC$_{MAS}$ sternocostal head of the pectoralis major; STE sternum; H humerus

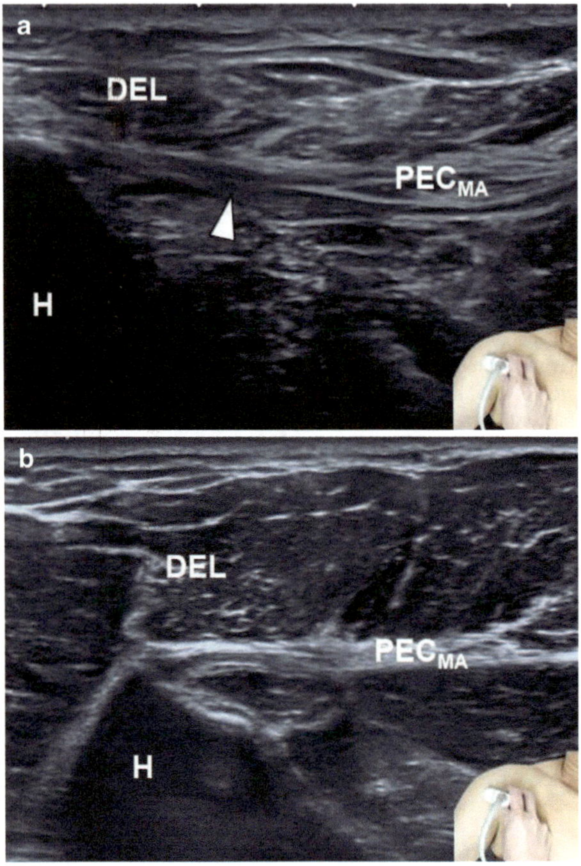

Fig. 3.17 The ultrasound image in the tendon's long axis demonstrates thickening and loss of the fibrillar pattern (arrowhead) in the pectoralis major tendon, primarily the sternocostal head (**a**), compared to the healthy side (**b**). DEL deltoid; PEC_{MA} pectoralis major; H humerus

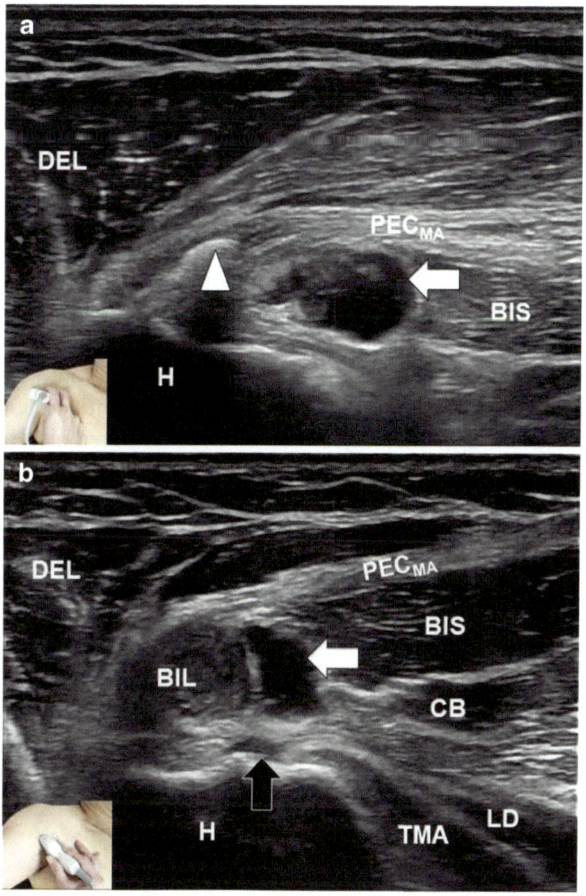

Fig. 3.18 The ultrasound images show calcific tendinosis of the pectoralis major (white arrowhead) and a concomitant tear of the long head of the biceps brachii tendon with hematoma formation (white arrows) (**a**). In the same case, a tear of the conjoint tendon (black arrow) of the latissimus dorsi and teres major is also observed while externally rotating the patient's arm (**b**). BIL long head of the biceps brachii; BIS short head of the biceps brachii; CB coracobrachialis; PEC_{MA} pectoralis major; DEL deltoid; LD latissimus dorsi; TMA teres major; H humerus

3.5 Ultrasound-Guided Intervention

Shin et al. [9] conducted an uncontrolled, prospective clinical trial that focused on addressing myofascial pain in individuals who had undergone mastectomy and had discomfort in the pectoralis major muscle. The study included nineteen participants diagnosed with at least one active myofascial trigger point in either the subscapularis or pectoralis muscles. For those requiring injections into the pectoralis muscle, patients were positioned supine with the arm at their side and the hand supinated. Visualization of the pectoralis major muscle was achieved through ultrasound guidance in a horizontal plane. A 25-gauge, 3.8-cm needle, connected to a 5-mL syringe containing 0.5% lidocaine, was then carefully inserted into the myofascial trigger point region of the pectoralis muscle using the out-of-plane approach. Repeat needling targeted various loci in the region to identify latent trigger points. Ultrasound-guided trigger point injections were administered in all affected muscles at one-week intervals. Additional injections were considered only if patients expressed dissatisfaction with the reduction in discomfort. They reported significant improvement in pain and shoulder motions (including external rotation and abduction) immediately after the initial injection and three months following the last injection. In addition to administering injectate into the muscular portion of the pectoralis major (Fig. 3.19a),

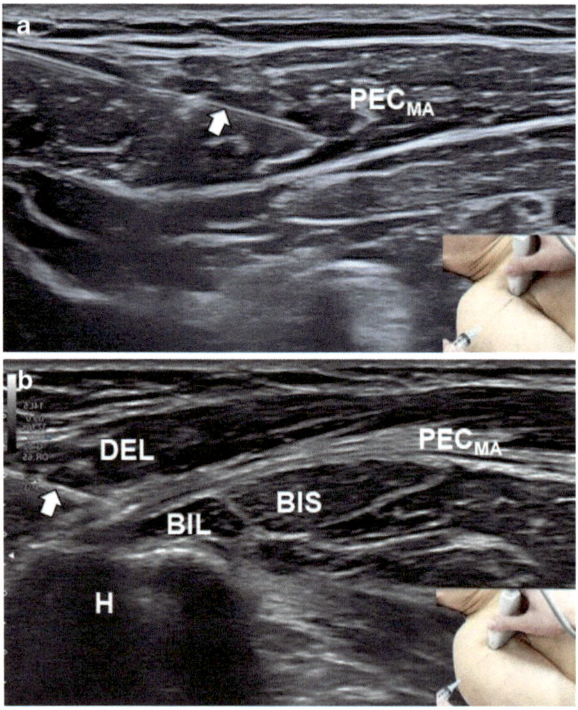

Fig. 3.19 Ultrasound images show injections into the pectoralis major muscle (**a**) and tendon (**b**) using the in-plane approach. White arrows: needle; DEL deltoid; PEC$_{MA}$ pectoralis major; BIL long head of the biceps brachii; BIS short head of the biceps brachii; H humerus

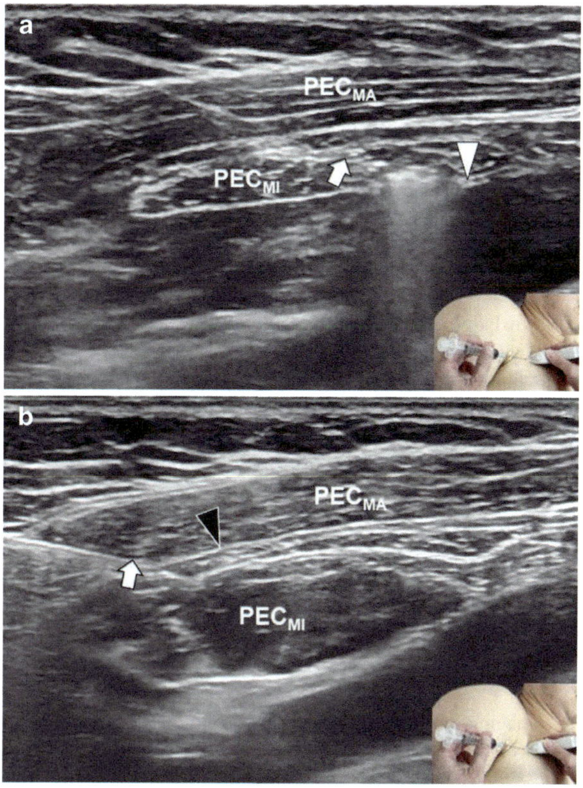

Fig. 3.20 Ultrasound images illustrate injections targeting the medial pectoral nerve (white arrowhead) beneath the pectoralis minor muscle (**a**) and the lateral pectoral nerve (black arrowhead) between the pectoralis major and minor muscles (**b**) using an in-plane approach. White arrows: needle; PEC_{MA} pectoralis major; PEC_{MI} pectoralis minor

if pain is localized to the tendinous portion of the pectoralis major and the area appears thickened or hypoechoic, suggesting tendinopathy, an ultrasound-guided intratendinous injection can be performed using a dextrose solution or platelet-rich plasma (Fig. 3.19b).

While addressing pain in the pectoral region, pectoral nerve blocks can also be administered [10]. Initially, the transducer is positioned in the sagittal plane, slightly distal to the coracoid process. Subsequently, the transducer's distal end is pivoted towards the axillary line. The nerve block is conducted with the patient in the supine position, either with the arm resting next to the chest or abducted 90 degrees. The needle is introduced from a caudal to cranial direction to target the fascial plane underneath the pectoralis minor or between the pectoralis minor and serratus anterior muscles for blocking the medial pectoral nerve (Fig. 3.20a). Once the injectate, e.g., 10 mL of 1% lidocaine, is delivered to the specified fascial plane, the needle is withdrawn to the fascial plane situated between the pectoralis major and minor muscles. An additional 10 mL of 1% lidocaine can be administered to block the lateral pectoral nerve as well (Fig. 3.20b).

3.6 Conclusion

In summary, ultrasound imaging has proven effective in evaluating pectoralis muscle injuries. It provides an accurate assessment for individual muscle components as well as for the myotendinous junction or the enthesis. Additionally, ultrasound-guided interventions—including intramuscular trigger point injections, intratendinous injections, and pectoral nerve blocks—have shown efficacy for the management of associated painful conditions.

Acknowledgment Images and illustrations adapted from cadaveric images provided by the Visible Human Project® of the National Library of Medicine. Excerpts featured in the VH Dissector are used with permission from Touch of Life Technologies Inc.

References

1. Giordano JR, Klein B, Hershfeld B, Gruber J, Trasolini R, Cohn RM. A review of chronic pectoralis major tears: what options are available? Clin Shoulder Elb. 2023;26(3):330–9.
2. Stefanou N, Karamanis N, Bompou E, Vasdeki D, Mellos T, Dailiana ZH. Pectoralis major rupture in body builders: a case series including anabolic steroid use. BMC Musculoskelet Disord. 2023;24(1):264.
3. Lin TY, Chang KV, Wu WT, Özçakar L. Right arm pain after strength training: ultrasound imaging for pectoralis major tendon strain. J Yeungnam Med Sci. 2023;40(1):109–11.
4. Lee YK, Skalski MR, White EA, et al. US and MR imaging of pectoralis major injuries. Radiographics. 2017;37(1):176–89.
5. Stecco A, Masiero S, Macchi V, Stecco C, Porzionato A, De Caro R. The pectoral fascia: anatomical and histological study. J Bodyw Mov Ther. 2009;13(3):255–61.
6. Solari F, Burns B. Anatomy, Thorax, pectoralis major major. In: StatPearls. Treasure Island (FL) ineligible companies. Disclosure: Bracken Burns declares no relevant financial relationships with ineligible companies.: StatPearls Publishing Copyright © 2024, StatPearls Publishing LLC.; 2024.
7. Chang KV, Lin CP, Lin CS, Wu WT, Karmakar MK, Özçakar L. Sonographic tracking of trunk nerves: essential for ultrasound-guided pain management and research. J Pain Res. 2017;10:79–88.
8. Rehman A, Robinson P. Sonographic evaluation of injuries to the pectoralis muscles. AJR Am J Roentgenol. 2005;184(4):1205–11.
9. Shin HJ, Shin JC, Kim WS, Chang WH, Lee SC. Application of ultrasound-guided trigger point injection for myofascial trigger points in the subscapularis and pectoralis muscles to post-mastectomy patients: a pilot study. Yonsei Med J. 2014;55(3):792–9.
10. Wu WT, Chang KV, Özçakar L. Dynamic ultrasound imaging and guidance for pectoral nerve block in the management of arterial thoracic outlet syndrome. Med Ultrason. 2022;24(3):378–9.

Chapter 4
Navigating Complexities of the Axillary Region

Ke-Vin Chang, Wei-Ting Wu, and Yuan-Yuan Tsai

4.1 Introduction

Pain in the axillary region is a commonly encountered issue with diverse etiologies. One prevalent cause of discomfort in this area is muscle sprain, often arising from sports-related injuries and manifesting as armpit pain. For example, the teres major [1], a substantial muscle in the axillary region, may be injured due to traumatic incidents like forceful traction on an outstretched arm or during a throwing motion.

In addition, lymphadenopathy is frequently observed in the axillary area. Understanding the intricate interplay between enlarged lymph nodes and neighboring neuromuscular structures aids in identifying the source of pain. Conversely, persistent axillary pain can result from axillary nerve compression caused by both exogenous factors (such as humeral head spur) and endogenous factors (such as intraneural neoplasm). A case reported by Hung et al. [2] highlighted axillary pain radiating to the posterior shoulder, ultimately diagnosed as an axillary nerve schwannoma.

Axillary web syndrome is a common complication post-breast cancer surgery, particularly following ipsilateral lymphadenectomy [3]. This condition presents as a single or multiple thin cords in the subcutaneous tissues of the ipsilateral axilla, often leading to painful shoulder abduction and restricted shoulder range of motion.

Considering the various causes of axillary pain, utilizing imaging tools becomes paramount to accurately identify the underlying issue. This chapter will delve into the sonoanatomy of the axillary region, provide concise descriptions of relevant pathologies, and discuss the application of ultrasound-guided injections for pain relief.

K.-V. Chang (✉) · W.-T. Wu · Y.-Y. Tsai
Bei-Hu Branch, National Taiwan University Hospital, Taipei, Taiwan

K.-V. Chang (ed.), *Ultrasonography of Musculoskeletal Pain*,
https://doi.org/10.1007/978-981-96-6787-1_4

4.2 Anatomy

The axilla is a concave region situated beneath the skin, bounded posteriorly by the latissimus dorsi and teres major muscles, and anteriorly by the pectoralis major muscle. Its floor is formed by the humeral head and the glenoid of the scapula. As it extends toward the arm, the coracobrachialis muscle serves as the anterior boundary, while the long head of the triceps brachii forms the posterior boundary, projecting away from the trunk [4]. The floor of the axilla is further supported by the inferior glenohumeral joint, which is reinforced by the inferior glenohumeral ligament originating from the inferior portion of the glenoid labrum and the adjacent scapular neck (sagittal plane, Fig. 4.1a; coronal plane, Fig. 4.1b) [5]. This inferior glenohumeral ligament attaches distally to the medial side of the surgical neck of the humerus, with its most distal fibers reaching up to 2 cm distal to the cartilage of the humeral head. The laxity of the inferior glenohumeral ligament is noticeable when the shoulder is adducted, tightening during abduction. Together with the synovial membrane, it forms the inferior capsulosynovial recess. The labrum, a triangular and hyperechoic fibrocartilaginous structure, directly contacts the glenoid margin of the scapula.

The latissimus dorsi originates from the spinous processes of vertebrae T7-L5, thoracolumbar fascia, iliac crest, inferior 3 or 4 ribs, and the inferior angle of the scapula, extending superiorly and laterally [6]. The latissimus dorsi wraps around the distal part of the teres major muscle [7] (Fig. 4.2a), passing along the lateral edge of the scapula. The conjoint tendon [8], formed by the latissimus dorsi and teres major muscles, inserts on the medial side of the intertubercular groove. The

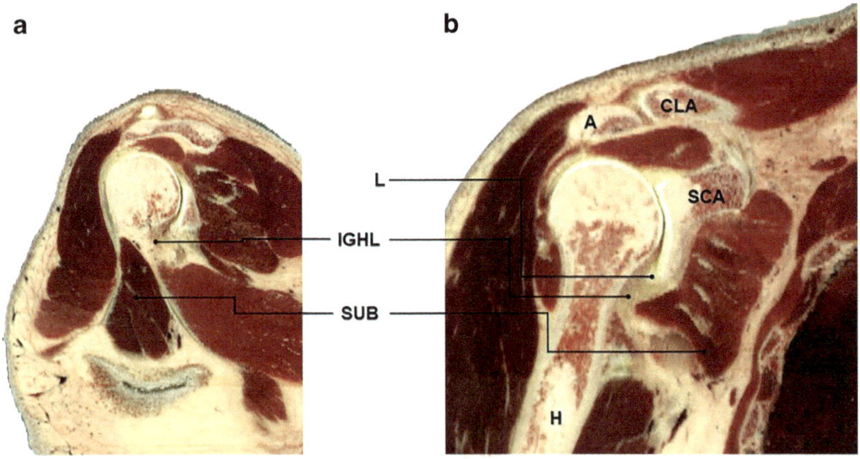

Fig. 4.1 The cadaveric cross-sections of the inferior glenohumeral ligament (GHL_I) demonstrate its origin from the inferior part of the glenoid labrum and the adjacent scapula, shown in the (**a**) sagittal plane and (**b**) coronal plane. SUB subscapularis; CLA clavicle; A acromion; SCA scapula; H humerus

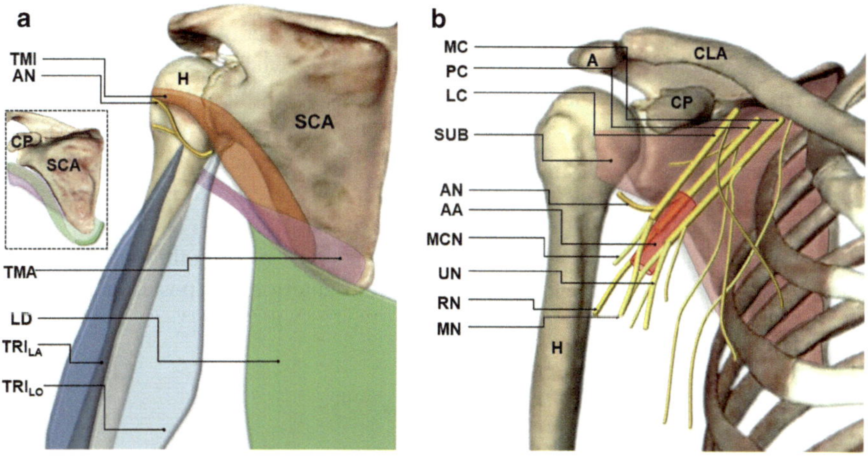

Fig. 4.2 The illustrations depict some relevant muscles in the axillary region (**a**) and branches of the brachial plexus nearby (**b**). The dashed subgraph specifically demonstrates the latissimus dorsi and teres major from the anterior view. AA axillary artery; LD latissimus dorsi; TMA teres major; TMI teres minor; TRI_{LA} lateral head of the triceps brachii muscle; TRI_{LO} long head of the triceps brachii muscle; AN axillary nerve; MCN musculocutaneous nerve; MN median nerve; UN ulnar nerve; RN radial nerve; PC posterior cord; LC lateral cord; MC medial cord; SUB subscapularis; CLA clavicle; CP coracoid process; A acromion; SCA scapula; H humerus

subscapularis muscle belly, situated cranial to the latissimus dorsi and teres major muscles, displays a multipennate architecture. Its superior muscular fibers converge to form tendinous bands that merge laterally into the terminal tendon. Notably, the inferior portion consists of parallel fibers that neither form fibrous bands nor contribute to the terminal tendon [9]. The teres major, latissimus dorsi, and subscapularis muscle belly collectively serve as the floor for the neurovascular bundle of the axillary region.

Beyond the pectoralis minor, the axillary artery and the cord segment of the brachial plexus accompany the upper limb course together along the anterior surface of the subscapularis muscle. The myotendinous junction of the subscapularis muscle lies beneath the axillary neurovascular bundle (comprising the axillary nerve and posterior humeral circumflex vessels) and above the anterior-inferior aspect of the humeral head (Fig. 4.2b). Distally, the axillary neurovascular bundle traverses the space between the subscapularis and the conjoint tendon of the latissimus dorsi and teres major muscles.

The posterior cord of the brachial plexus issues branches such as the radial and axillary nerves posterior to the axillary artery [10]. The lateral cord, giving rise to the musculocutaneous nerve and part of the median nerve, courses laterally and superficially to the axillary artery. In contrast, the medial cord, supplying the ulnar nerve and part of the median nerve, takes a medial and deep trajectory beneath the axillary artery.

The axillary nerve diverges early from the plexus, traversing inferiorly across the glenohumeral joint from the anterior to the posterior aspect of the shoulder [11]. It innervates the deltoid and teres minor muscles, along with the skin on the lateral shoulder, extending from the inferior capsule of the joint through the quadrilateral space (Fig. 4.3). This space is demarcated by the teres minor muscle superiorly, teres major muscle inferiorly, long head of the triceps medially, and humeral shaft laterally. Running parallel to the axillary nerve, the posterior humeral circumflex artery, a branch of the axillary artery, follows a similar course.

The axillary nerve divides into several branches after passing through the quadrilateral space, where it typically bifurcates into anterior and posterior branches

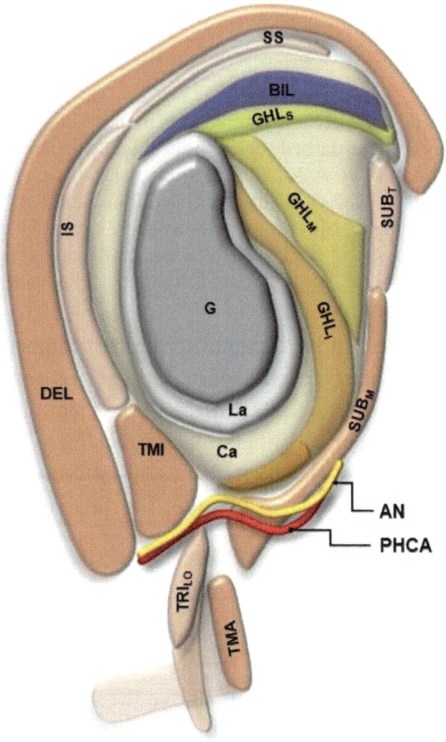

Fig. 4.3 The illustration shows the main trunk of the axillary nerve as it traverses the inferior glenohumeral capsule, along with the surrounding muscle structures. BIL long head tendon of the biceps brachii; SUB_T tendon of the subscapularis; SUB_M muscle of the subscapularis; SS supraspinatus; IS infraspinatus; TMI teres minor; TMA teres major; TRI_{LO} long head of triceps brachii; DEL deltoid; GHL_S superior glenohumeral ligament; GHL_M middle glenohumeral ligament; GHL_I inferior glenohumeral ligament; AN axillary nerve; PHCA posterior humeral circumflex artery; G glenoid; La labrum; Ca capsule

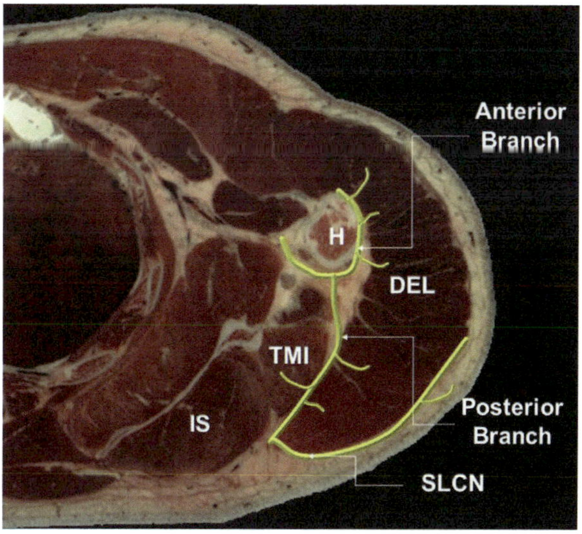

Fig. 4.4 The illustration highlights the main branches of the axillary nerve. SLCN superior lateral cutaneous nerve of the arm, TMI teres minor, IS infraspinatus; DEL deltoid; H humerus

(Fig. 4.4) [12]. The anterior branch provides motor innervation to the anterior part of the deltoid muscle and gives off cutaneous branches to the overlying skin. The posterior branch innervates the teres minor and the posterior part of the deltoid and extends as the superior lateral cutaneous nerve of the arm, which supplies sensory innervation to the skin over the lower two-thirds of the deltoid and adjacent upper arm. Additionally, the axillary nerve gives rise to an articular branch that provides sensory fibers to the shoulder joint.

4.3 Sonoanatomy

4.3.1 Infra-axilla Approach

In the examination of the axillary region, it is recommended that the examiner elevate the shoulder by placing their hand over the forehead, with the palm facing upward. This specific positioning facilitates the alignment of the teres major and latissimus dorsi muscles over the humeral head. Following the exposure of the entire axilla, the linear transducer is positioned horizontally over the axillary fold.

At this point, the latissimus dorsi muscle courses over the lateral border of the teres major, running atop it and becoming visible superficially. Meanwhile, the teres major muscle is identified beneath it (Fig. 4.5a, c). Shifting the transducer toward the lesser tubercle of the humerus reveals the long head of the triceps brachii muscle emerging posterolaterally to the teres major (Fig. 4.5b, d). Subsequently, the

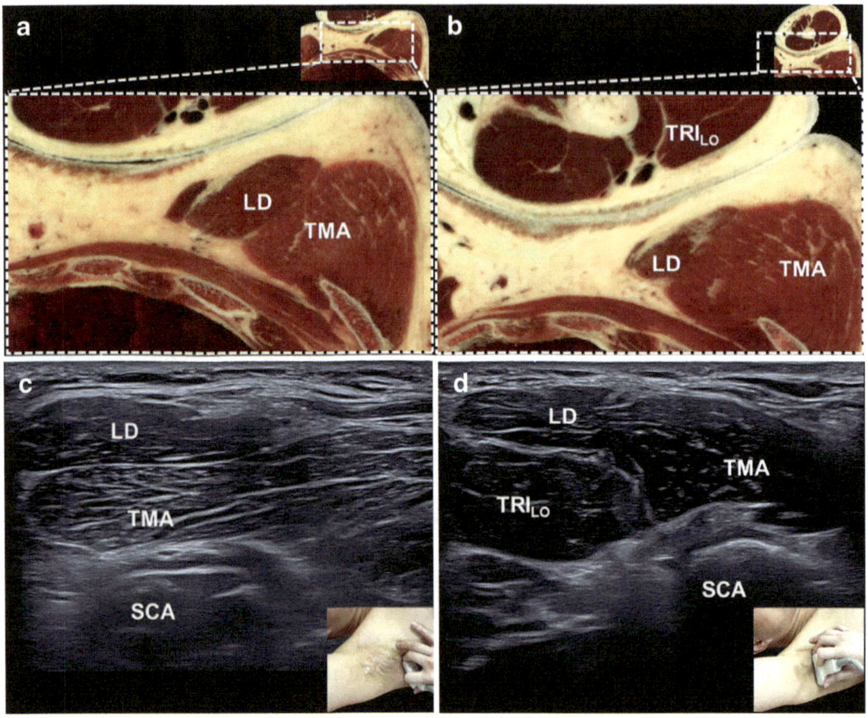

Fig. 4.5 The cadaveric images and corresponding sonographic anatomy illustrate the relationship between the teres major and latissimus dorsi muscles in the infra-axillary region, viewed from inferomedial (**a**, **c**) to superolateral (**b**, **d**). Note that the arm in the cadaver is not abducted, whereas it is abducted in the human volunteer and scanned from the armpit, which explains the discrepancy in the positioning of the long head of the triceps brachii between the ultrasound and cadaveric images. TMA teres major; LD latissimus dorsi; TRI$_{LO}$ long head of the triceps brachii; SCA scapula

latissimus dorsi muscle converges with the teres major to form a tendon (Fig. 4.6a, c). Although the teres major and latissimus dorsi muscles merge into the conjoint tendon, the footprints of both muscles can still be distinguished in most cases using a long-axis view (Fig. 4.6b, d).

Returning to a horizontal plane view and moving the transducer medially toward the trunk reveals the humeral head, characterized by hypoechoic cartilage overlaying the rounded bony cortex. The pulsating, tubular posterior humeral circumflex

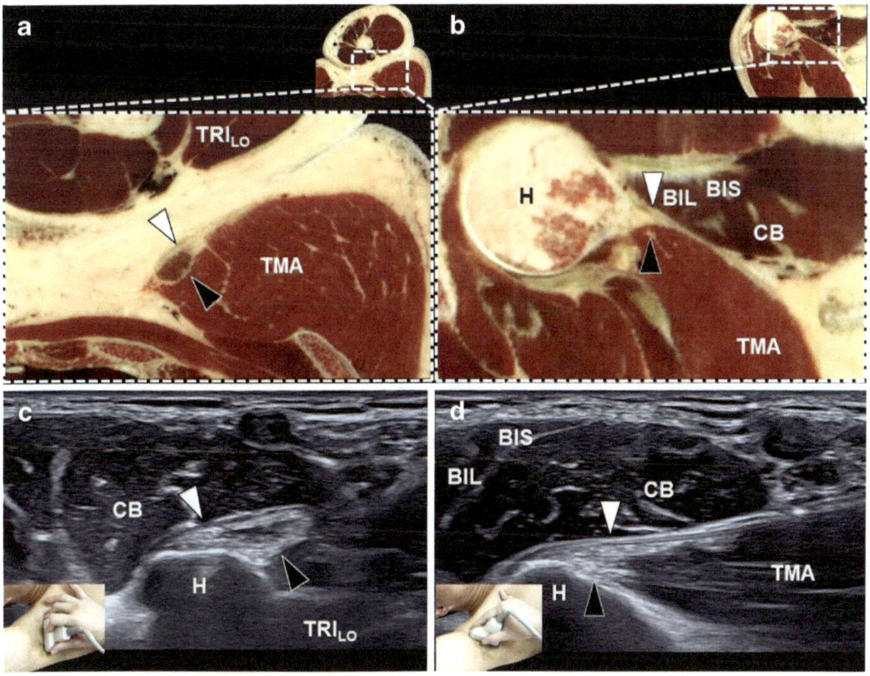

Fig. 4.6 The cadaveric image and corresponding sonoanatomy show the conjoint tendon of the teres major and latissimus dorsi in the short-axis (**a**, **c**) and long-axis (**b**, **d**) views. White arrowheads: tendon of the latissimus dorsi; black arrowheads: tendon of the teres major. TMA teres major; CB coracobrachialis; BIS short head of the biceps brachii; BIL long head of the biceps brachii; TRI_{LO} long head of the triceps brachii; H humerus

artery encircles the humeral head (Fig. 4.7a, b) and can be traced proximally to the axillary artery (Fig. 4.7c). By aligning the transducer parallel to the posterior humeral circumflex artery and gently swaying it, the axillary nerve becomes visible. Medial repositioning of the transducer, with slight adjustment of its anterior end, enables visualization of the axillary nerve in its long axis as it courses between the undersurface of the teres major muscle and the distal myotendinous junction of the subscapularis muscle (Fig. 4.8a, b), connecting with the posterior cord of the brachial plexus as it courses alongside the artery over the inferior glenohumeral joint capsule.

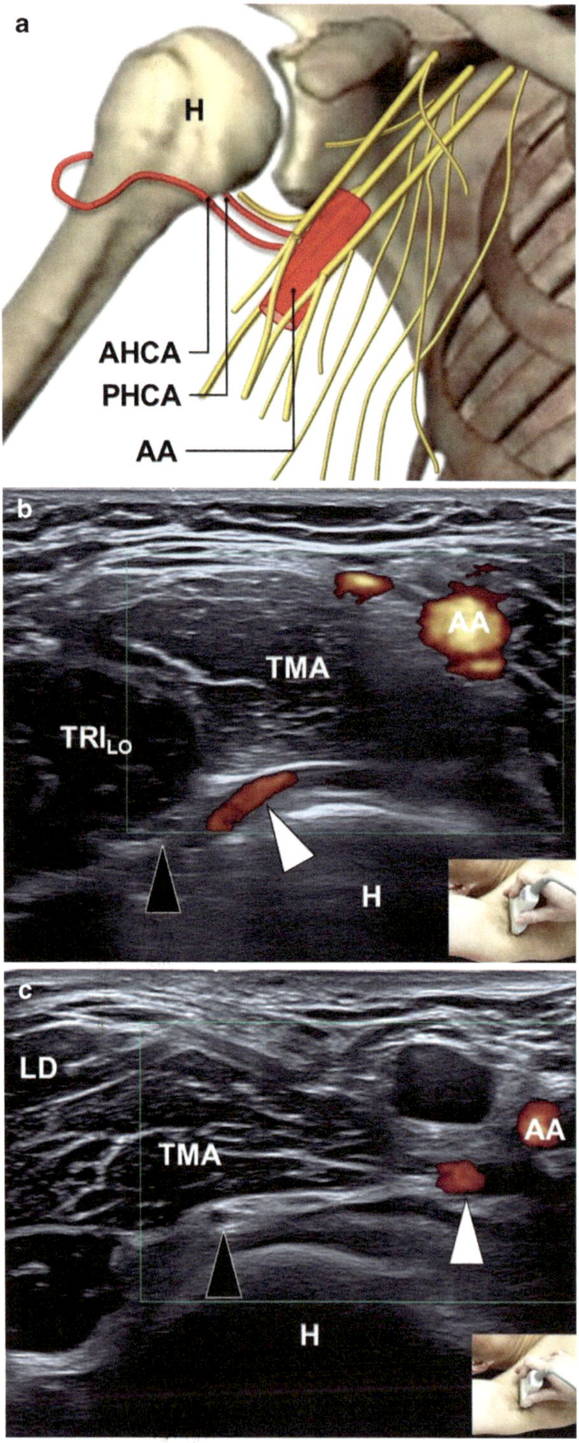

Fig. 4.7 The illustration (**a**) and corresponding sonographic anatomy show the tracing of the posterior humeral circumflex artery (PHCA, white arrowheads) from the distal region (**b**) to the proximal region (**c**), connecting back to the axillary artery (AA). Black arrowheads: axillary nerve; AHCA anterior humeral circumflex artery; H humerus

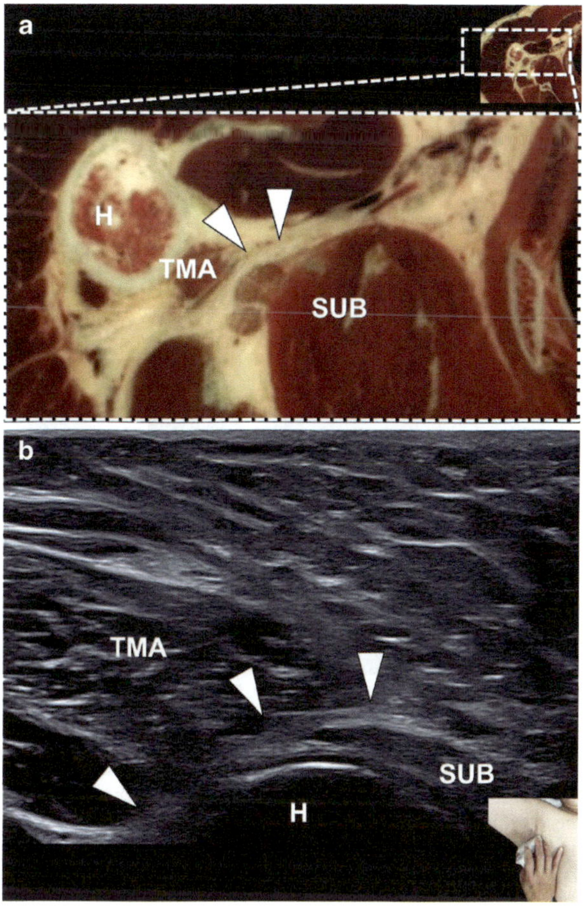

Fig. 4.8 The cadaveric image (**a**) and corresponding sonographic anatomy (**b**) show the axillary nerve (white arrowheads) located between the teres major (TMA) and the distal myotendinous junction of the subscapularis (SUB). H humerus

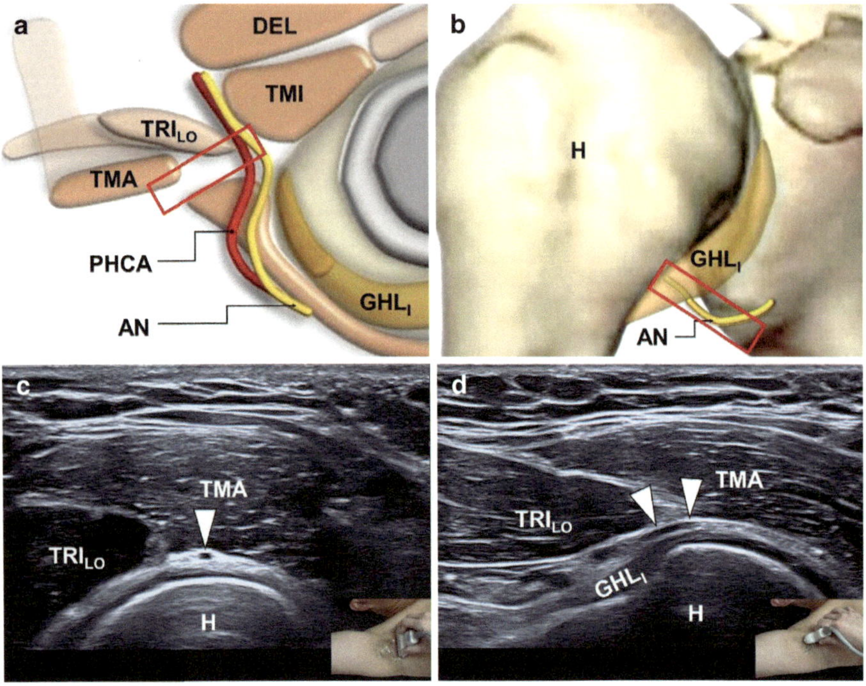

Fig. 4.9 The illustration and corresponding sonoanatomy show the typical infra-axillary view of the axillary nerve (AN and white arrowheads) located between the teres major and the head of the humerus, visualized in its short-axis (**a**, **c**) and long-axis (**b**, **d**) views. Red squares indicating the transducer's position have been added to the schematic drawing to enhance clarity. TRI$_{LO}$ long head of the triceps brachii muscle; TMA teres major; TMI teres minor; DEL deltoid; PHCA posterior humeral circumflex artery; GHL$_I$ inferior glenohumeral ligament; H humerus

Moving the transducer laterally, the axillary nerve could be noted leaving the overlying teres major muscle (Fig. 4.9a, c) and coursing between the long head of the triceps and the proximal humerus (Fig. 4.9b, d). The superior lateral cutaneous nerve of the arm (Fig. 4.10a), a branch from the main trunk, courses between the long head of the triceps brachii and deltoid muscles (Fig. 4.10b) before penetrating the deltoid fascia to supply the subcutaneous region (Fig. 4.10c).

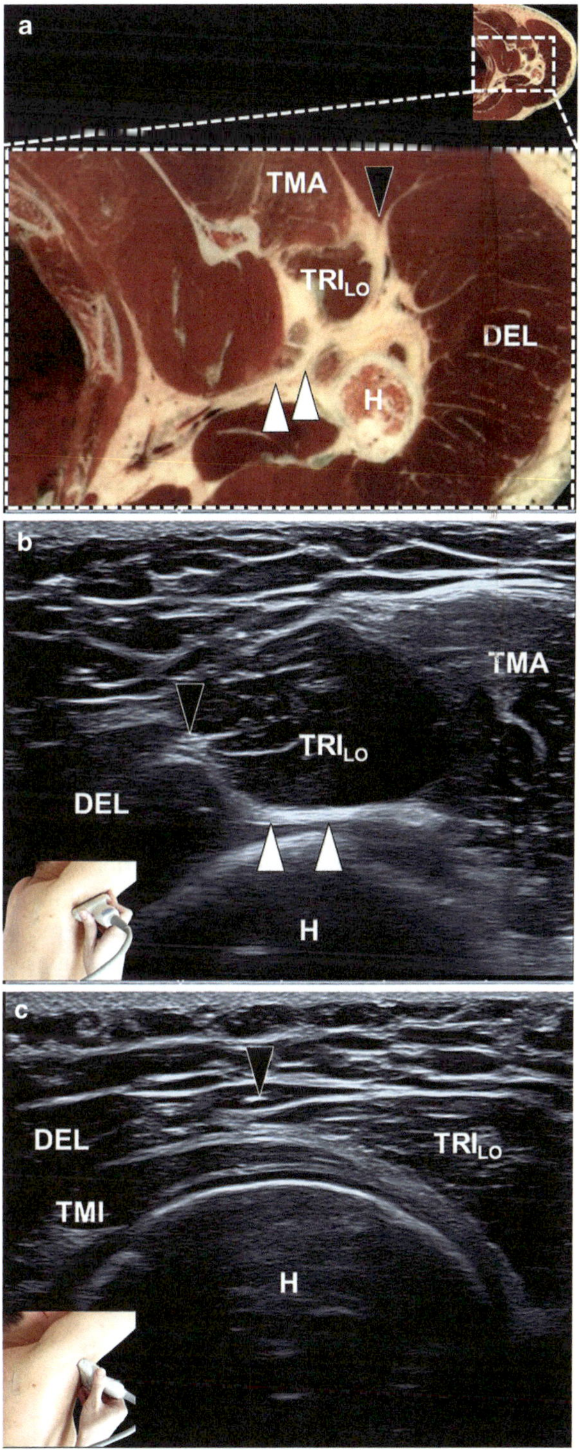

Fig. 4.10 The cadaveric image (**a**) and corresponding ultrasound anatomy show the superior lateral cutaneous nerve of the arm (black arrowheads) passing between the long head of the triceps brachii and the deltoid muscles (**b**) before piercing the deltoid fascia to reach the subcutaneous layer (**c**). White arrowheads: main trunk of the axillary nerve; TMA teres major; TMI teres minor; DEL deltoid; TRI_{LO} long head of the triceps brachii muscle; H humerus

4.3.2 Subscapularis Approach

Using the subscapularis approach, the axillary region can be assessed without exposing the armpit. The transducer is positioned at the anterior aspect of the shoulder, while the examinee's shoulder is abducted to 90 degrees with the arm externally rotated. Aligning the transducer in a horizontal plane over the proximal humerus, distal to the level of the coracoid process, allows visualization of the subscapularis tendon attaching to the lesser tubercle, medial to the bicipital groove.

Upon shifting the transducer more medially to the subscapularis myotendinous junction, identification of the axillary artery becomes possible, situated on top of it, where the cord level of the brachial plexus is observed. The posterior cord, housing the radial nerve and axillary nerve, is located at the posterior-lateral corner of the axillary artery (Fig. 4.11a, c). Maintaining the transducer at the horizontal plane and moving it more distally, as the subscapularis tendon disappears, the teres major muscle emerges. The axillary nerve courses alongside the posterior humeral circumflex artery, traversing the gap between the subscapularis and teres major muscles, ultimately reaching the plane between the teres major and the cartilage of the humeral head (Fig. 4.11b, d).

4.3.3 Triceps Approach

The triceps approach is designed to visualize the axillary nerve as it exits the quadrilateral space. The transducer is initially placed in the sagittal plane to identify the long head of the triceps brachii (Fig. 4.12a). As the transducer is moved laterally, the short axis of the axillary nerve and posterior humeral circumflex vessels become visible distal to the teres minor (Fig. 4.12b). Continuing lateral movement enhances the visibility of the axillary nerve over the lateral head of the triceps brachii by aligning the nerve's cross-section with the scanning plane, minimizing anisotropy (Fig. 4.12c). Once the nerve's short axis is identified, the transducer can be rotated to a horizontal plane to visualize the anterior terminal division of the axillary nerve, located primarily between the deltoid and the humerus (Fig. 4.12d).

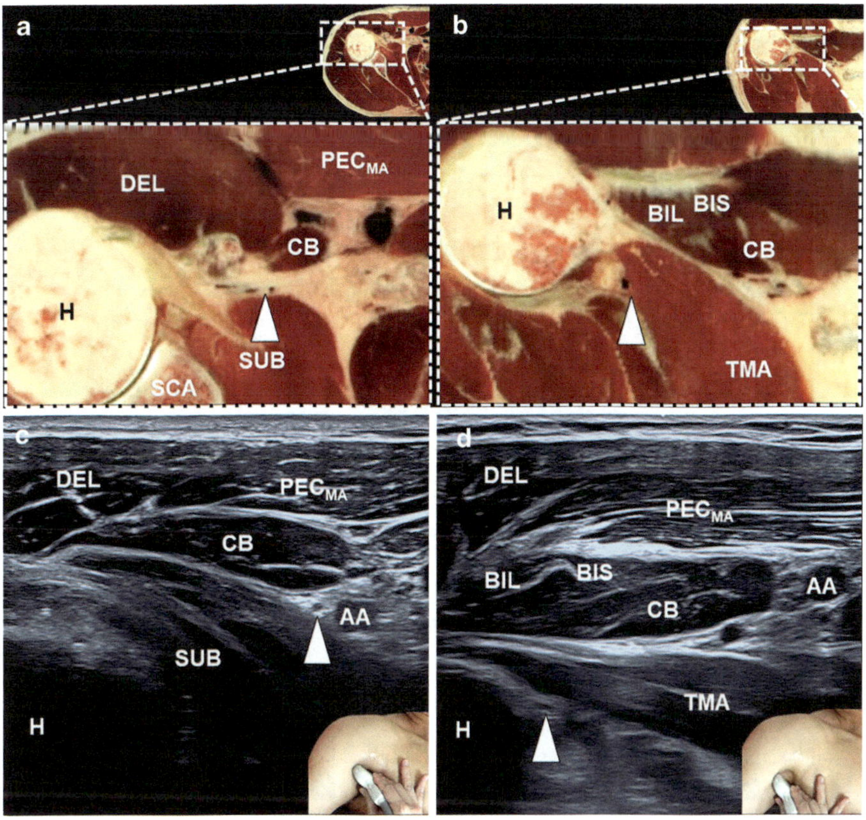

Fig. 4.11 The cadaveric images and corresponding sonographic anatomy demonstrate the division of the axillary nerve (white arrowheads) over the myotendinous junction of the subscapularis (SUB) (**a**, **c**) and between the teres major (TMA) and the head of the humerus (**b**, **d**). PEC$_{MA}$ pectoralis major; CB coracobrachialis; BIS short head of the biceps brachii; BIL long head of the biceps brachii; DEL deltoid; AA, axillary artery; SCA scapula; H humerus

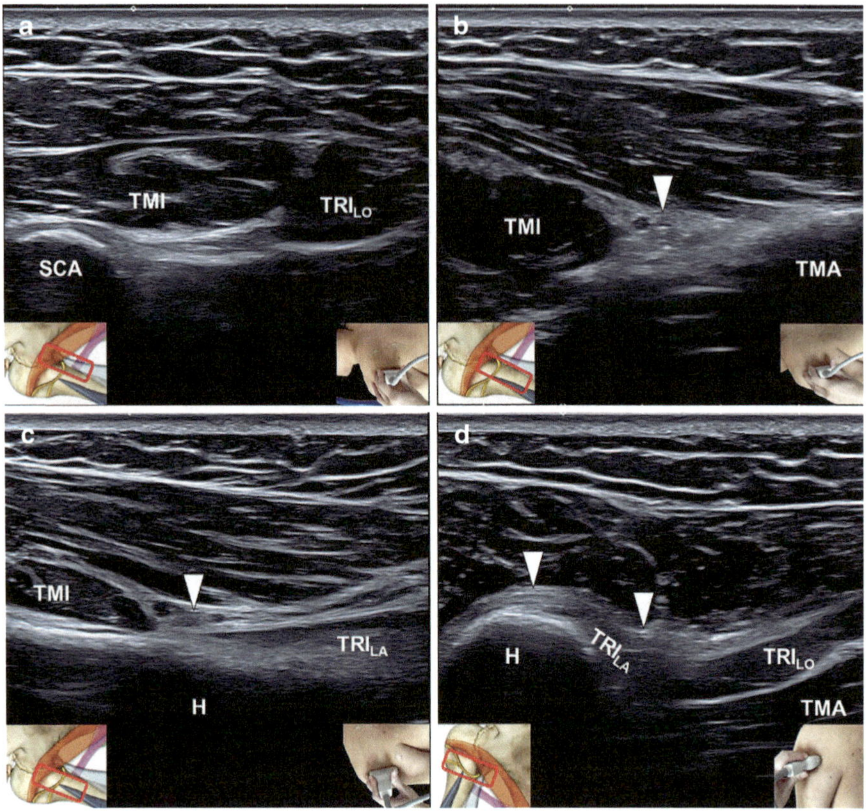

Fig. 4.12 The ultrasound images demonstrate the triceps approach. The transducer is aligned along the long axis of the long head of the triceps brachii (TRI_{LO}) (**a**). Lateral movement of the transducer reveals the short axis of the axillary nerve (white arrowheads) (**b**), positioned above the origin of the lateral head of the triceps brachii (TRI_{LA}) (**c**). After identifying the short axis of the axillary nerve, the transducer is rotated to the horizontal plane to visualize the nerve in its long axis (**d**). Red squares indicating the transducer's position have been added to the schematic drawing to enhance clarity. TMI teres minor; TMA teres major; SCA scapula; H humerus

4.4 Pathologies

Thickening of the inferior glenohumeral ligament represents a common pathology in the axillary region. The inferior glenohumeral joint capsule can be distended by the accumulation of fluid, typically gathering in the most dependent part of the shoulder joint—the inferior glenohumeral joint. Hypertrophic synovium, appearing as hypoechoic structures, becomes evident within the distended inferior glenohumeral joint due to fluid, presenting as anechoic.

Visualizing the vascularity of hypertrophic synovium may prove challenging for two reasons: (1) the deep location of the joint and (2) motion artifacts from the pulsation of the axillary artery. In individuals with adhesive capsulitis, the capsule of the glenohumeral joint is thickened (Fig. 4.13a, b) compared to the contralateral, non-involved side (Fig. 4.13c, d). A study involving 20 patients with magnetic resonance imaging-confirmed adhesive capsulitis found an average thickness of 4.0 mm

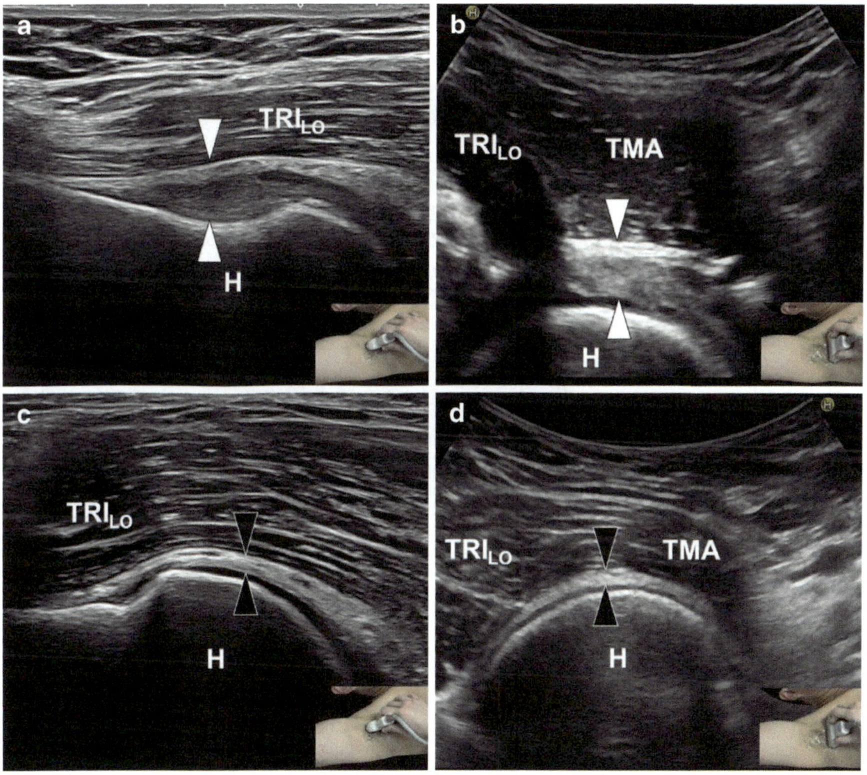

Fig. 4.13 Ultrasound images of adhesive capsulitis show thickening of the inferior glenohumeral capsule (white arrowheads) in the long axis (**a**) and short axis (**b**) of the humerus, compared to the normal side (black arrowheads) in the long axis (**c**) and short axis (**d**) of the humerus. TMA teres major; TRI_{LO} long head of triceps brachii muscle; H humerus

in shoulders with capsular contracture compared to 1.3 mm in asymptomatic contralateral shoulders [13].

Following an anteromedial dislocation of the shoulder, a traumatic sprain of the inferior glenohumeral ligament may occur. An injured inferior glenohumeral ligament appears thickened and hypoechoic, often accompanied by fluid accumulation (Fig. 4.14). Shoulder dislocation can result in axillary nerve injury, as indicated by an increased cross-sectional area of the nerve (Fig. 4.15a) compared to a distal entrapped segment (Fig. 4.15b). This is further characterized by focal enlargement prominently observed on the long-axis view of the axillary nerve (Fig. 4.15c).

In cases of trauma, an inferior glenoid fracture indicative of a Bankart lesion [14]—characterized by a fracture of the adjacent anteroinferior glenoid, often associated with anterior glenohumeral dislocation—can be identified on reconstructed computed tomography (Fig. 4.16a) and detected using ultrasound with a curved transducer due to its deep location (Fig. 4.16b). Additionally, a concomitant inferior labrum tear may appear as a slit within the hyperechoic triangular fibrocartilage (Fig. 4.16c) when compared to the intact contralateral side (Fig. 4.16d).

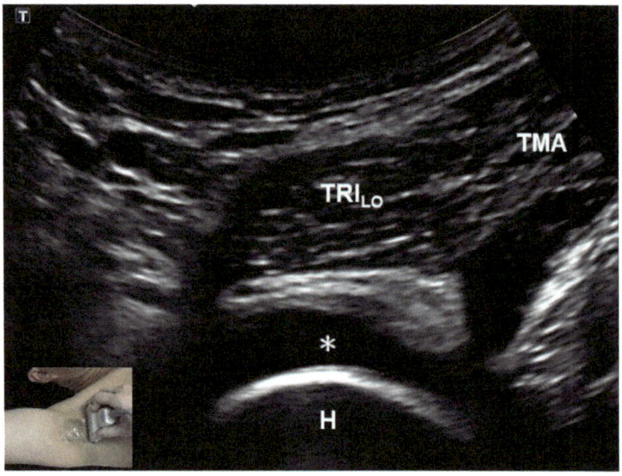

Fig. 4.14 The ultrasound image shows joint effusion (asterisk) within the glenohumeral joint, causing distension of the inferior glenohumeral recess. TRI_{LO} long head of the triceps brachii; TMA teres major; H humerus

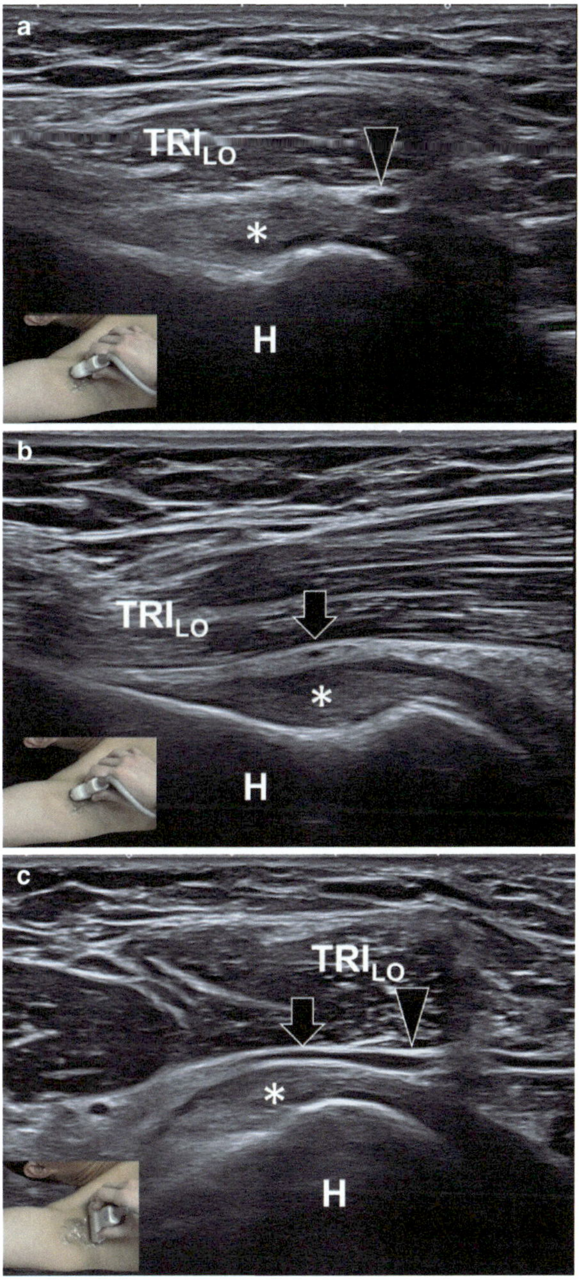

Fig. 4.15 The ultrasound images show a thickened segment (black arrowheads) of the axillary nerve proximal to the entrapment site (black arrow), caused by a swollen inferior glenohumeral capsule (asterisks). (**a**) The short-axis view of the thickened proximal segment of the axillary nerve. (**b**) The short-axis view of the entrapment site. (**c**) The long-axis view illustrates both the thickened and entrapped segments of the axillary nerve. TRI$_{LO}$ long head of the triceps brachii muscle; H humerus

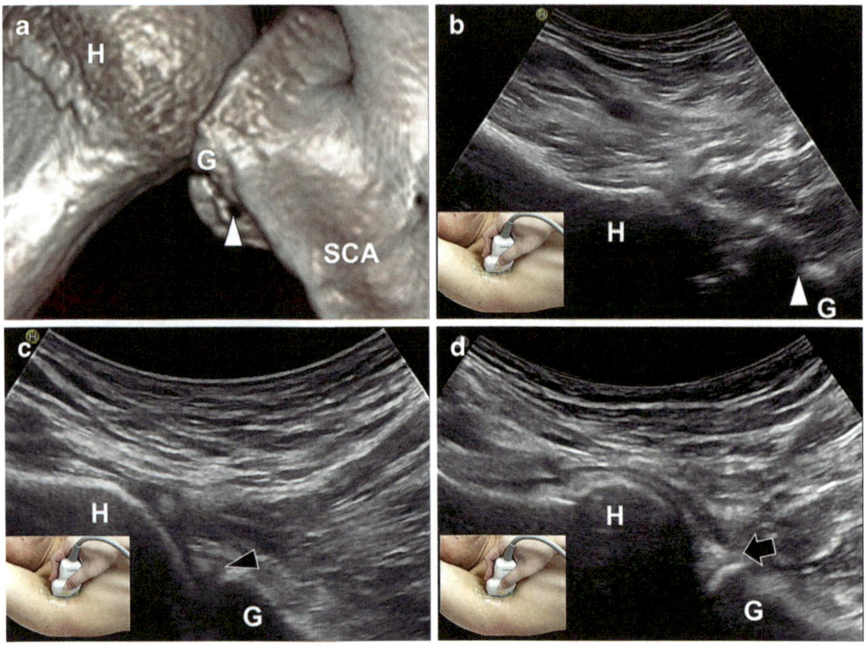

Fig. 4.16 (**a**) A 3D computed tomography scan and (**b**) a corresponding ultrasound image show a glenoid fracture (white arrowheads). (**c**) An ultrasound image illustrates a tear of the inferior labrum (black arrowhead), compared to (**d**) the intact labrum on the healthy side (black arrow). SCA scapula; G glenoid; H humerus

Damage to the brachial plexus during a traction injury can lead to enlargement of the posterior cord and the axillary nerve, which can be identified through ultrasound imaging. This can be demonstrated in the subscapularis approach (Fig. 4.17), the affected side in the horizontal plane using the triceps approach (Fig. 4.18a), and the non-affected side in the horizontal plane using the same view (Fig. 4.18b). In cases

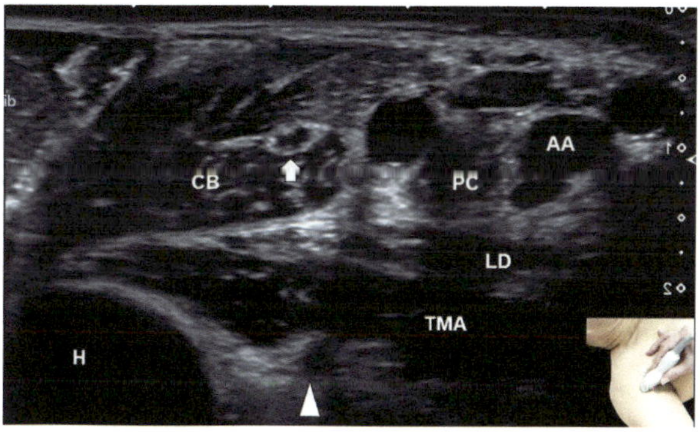

Fig. 4.17 The ultrasound image via the subscapularis approach depicts enlargement of the posterior cord (PC) of the brachial plexus and the axillary nerve (white arrowhead). White arrow: musculocutaneous nerve; TMA teres major; LD latissimus dorsi; CB coracobrachialis; AA axillary artery; H humerus

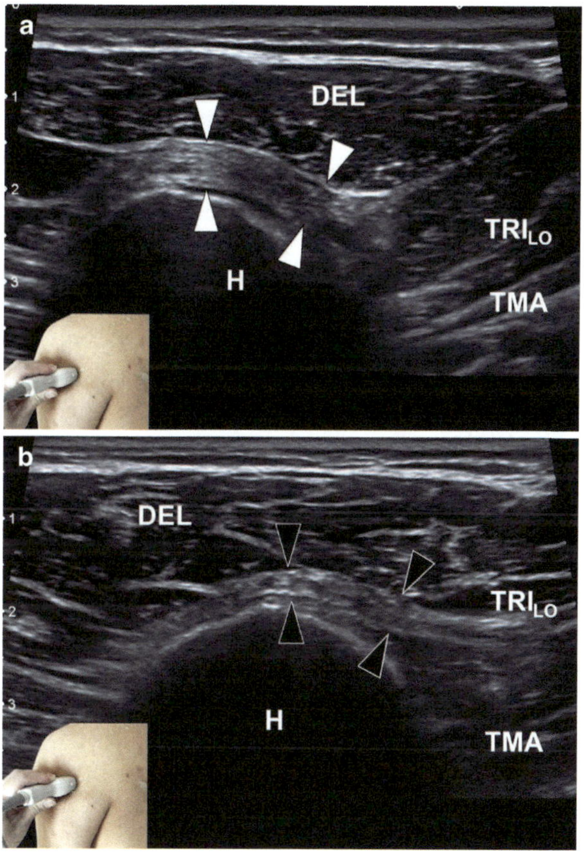

Fig. 4.18 (**a**) The ultrasound image via the triceps approach shows thickening of the axillary nerve (white arrowheads) on the affected side, compared to (**b**) the healthy side (black arrowheads). DEL deltoid; TMA teres major; H humerus

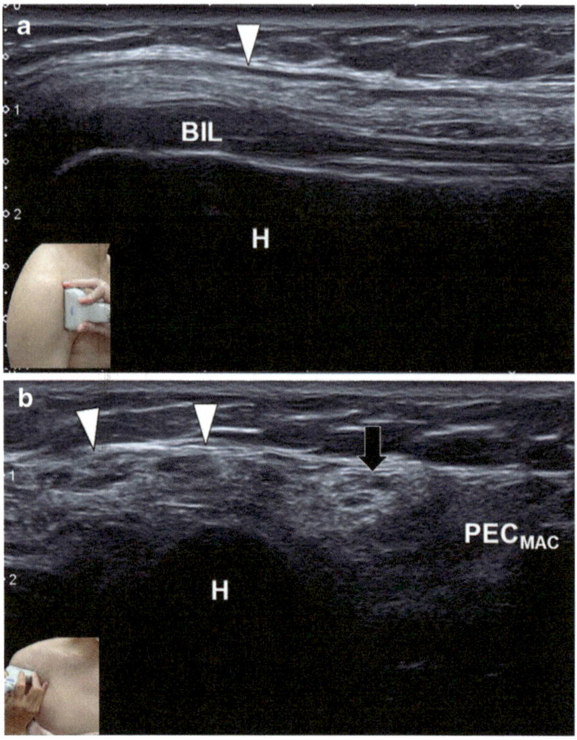

Fig. 4.19 The ultrasound images depict deltoid muscle atrophy (white arrowheads) in the long-axis (**a**) and short-axis (**b**) views. Black arrow: cephalic vein; BIL long head of the biceps brachii; PEC_{MAC} clavicular head of the pectoralis major; H humerus

of axillary nerve injury, muscles innervated by the axillary nerve, such as the teres minor and deltoid, may exhibit atrophy and increased echogenicity due to fatty infiltration, as seen in the long-axis view (Fig. 4.19a) and the short-axis view (Fig. 4.19b).

Besides, the investigator can compare the echotexture of the infraspinatus muscle [15], which is innervated by the suprascapular nerve rather than the axillary nerve, for patients with possible axillary nerve injury. In such a case, the infraspinatus muscle would exhibit normal thickness and echotexture, whereas the teres minor would appear thinner and hyperechoic in the short axis (Fig. 4.20a) and long axis (Fig. 4.20b).

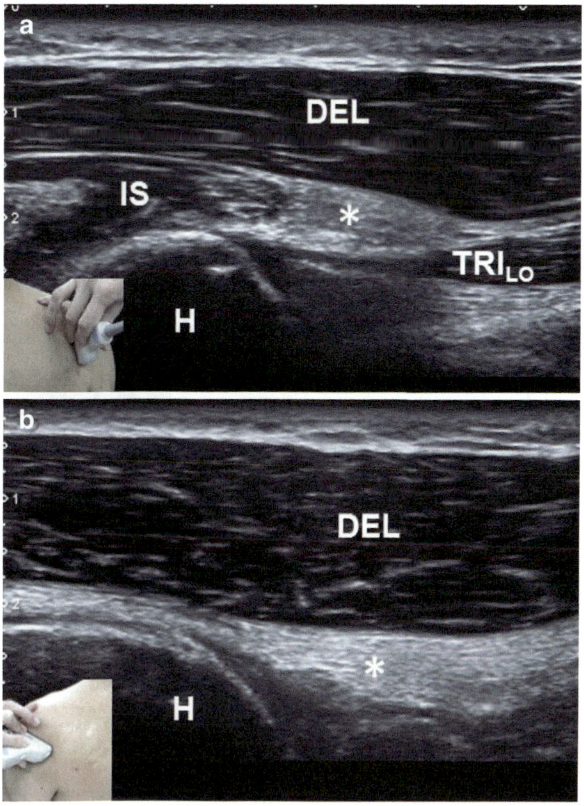

Fig. 4.20 The ultrasound images show muscle atrophy of the teres minor (asterisk) in the short-axis (**a**) and long axis (**b**) views. Given the normal echotexture of the deltoid muscle, the injury is more likely located at the posterior branch of the axillary nerve. TRI_{LO} long head of the triceps brachii muscle; IS infraspinatus; DEL deltoid; H humerus

Furthermore, persistent pain in the anterior axillary region, along with weakness in humeral extension and internal rotation, may suggest involvement of the teres major (supplied by the lower subscapular nerve) and latissimus dorsi (innervated by the thoracodorsal nerve) muscles. In chronic cases, the affected latissimus dorsi (Fig. 4.21a) and teres major (Fig. 4.21b) may appear thinner and hyperechoic.

Axillary web syndrome [16], also known as cording, commonly occurs after lymph node removal during breast cancer surgery. This condition is characterized

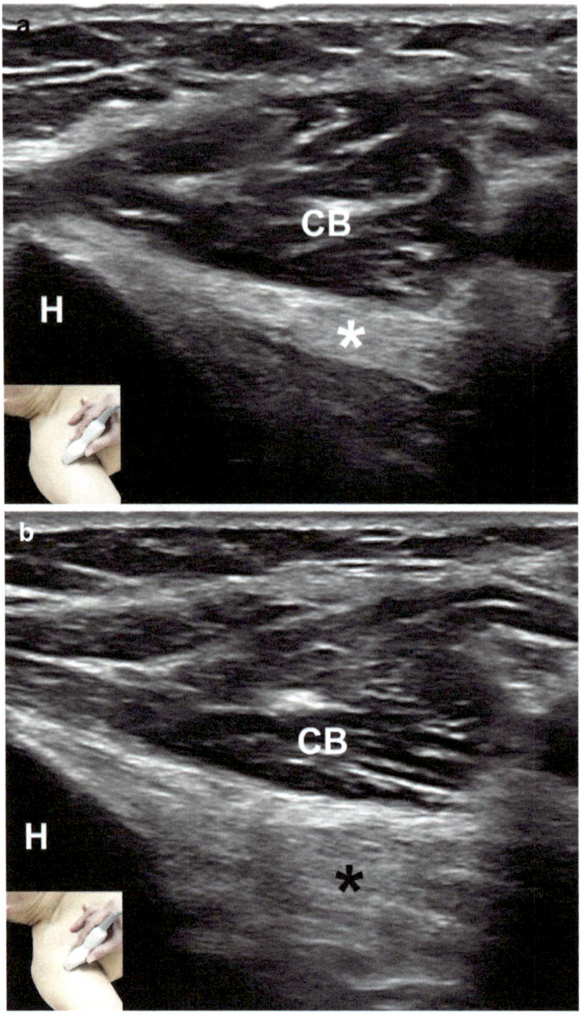

Fig. 4.21 The ultrasound images show atrophy and fatty infiltration of the latissimus dorsi (white asterisk) (**a**) and the teres major (black asterisk) in the long-axis view (**b**). CB coracobrachialis; H humerus

by tight, cord-like structures in the subcutaneous tissue of the axilla, often extending down the arm. These cords can cause pain and restrict shoulder and arm movement, particularly during abduction or stretching. On ultrasound imaging, one or more thin, hypoechoic cords are typically observed within the subcutaneous tissues in the short axis (Fig. 4.22a) and long axis (Fig. 4.22b).

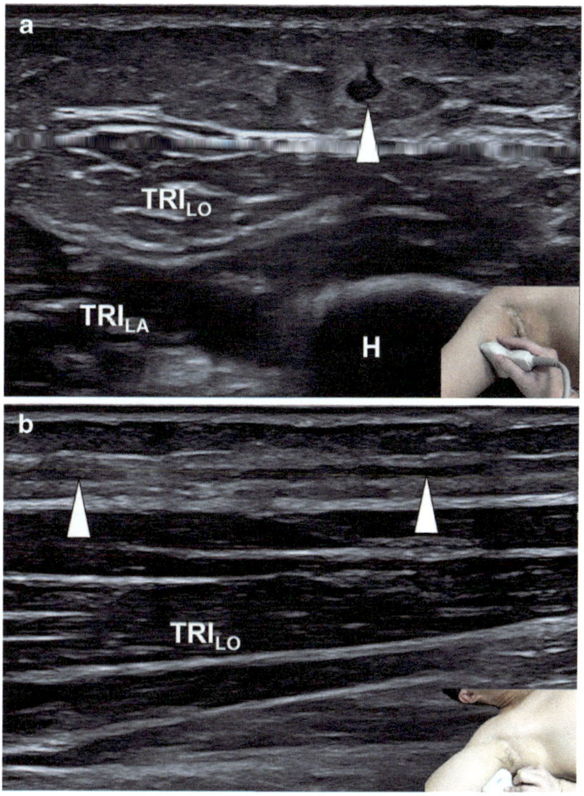

Fig. 4.22 The ultrasound images show a subcutaneous thin cord in the short-axis (**a**) and long-axis (**b**) views. TRI_{LO} long head of the triceps brachii muscle; TRI_{LA} lateral head of the triceps brachii muscle; H humerus

4.5 Ultrasound-Guided Injection

When injections are administered in the axillary region, a side-lying posture is assumed by the patient with the arm abducted to at least 90 degrees [17]. For targeting the axillary nerve, the transducer is positioned in the horizontal plane to visualize the nerve above the inferior glenohumeral capsule (Fig. 4.23a). The in-plane approach is then used, with the needle introduced from the posterior to the anterior aspect. In cases of frozen shoulder requiring hydrodilatation, once the needle penetrates the inferior glenohumeral capsule, the injectate (e.g., a mixture of 10 mL normal saline, 4 mL of 1% lidocaine and 40 mg of triamcinolone acetonide) is administered to hydrodilate the capsule (Fig. 4.23b).

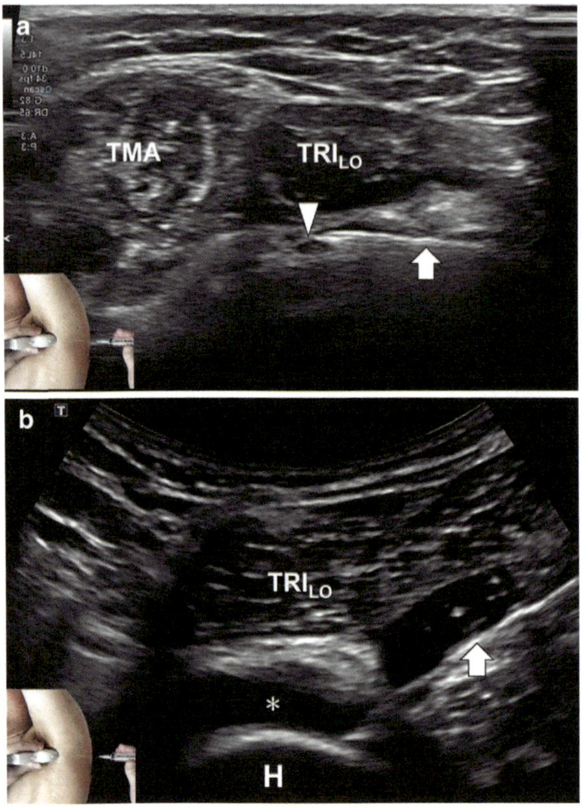

Fig. 4.23 The ultrasound images demonstrate the injection into the axillary nerve (white arrowhead) (**a**) and hydrodilation of the capsule with injectate (asterisk) (**b**), using an in-plane approach. White arrows: needle; TRI_{LO} long head of the triceps brachii muscle; TMA teres major; H humerus

If the focal point, such as a spur irritating the inferior glenohumeral capsule, is located at the inferior glenohumeral recess, it is advisable to redirect the transducer along the long axis of the humerus to visualize the inferior glenohumeral joint at the junction between the proximal humeral shaft and humeral head (Fig. 4.24a). The needle is then introduced using the in-plane approach until the tip penetrates the inferior glenohumeral ligament, after which the injectate is administered (Fig. 4.24b).

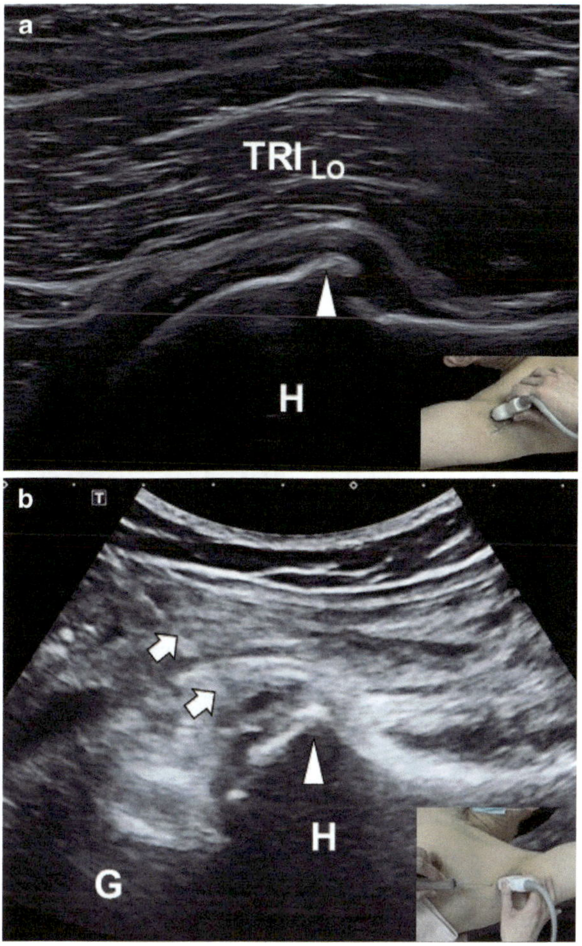

Fig. 4.24 The ultrasound image shows irritation of the inferior glenohumeral capsule due to the spur (white arrowhead) (**a**). The ultrasound-guided injection is performed along the long axis of the humerus to visualize the inferior glenohumeral joint using an in-plane approach (**b**). White arrows: needle; TRI_{LO} long head of the triceps brachii muscle; G glenoid; H humerus

If axillary nerve entrapment is identified after the nerve exits the quadrilateral space, an ultrasound-guided perineural injection can be administered in a cephalo-caudal direction. The traditional method (Fig. 4.25a), which uses the lateral head of the triceps brachii muscle over the proximal humerus as a landmark, is widely utilized. However, the approach just cephalically and laterally to the long head of the triceps brachii muscle is also acceptable (Fig. 4.25b).

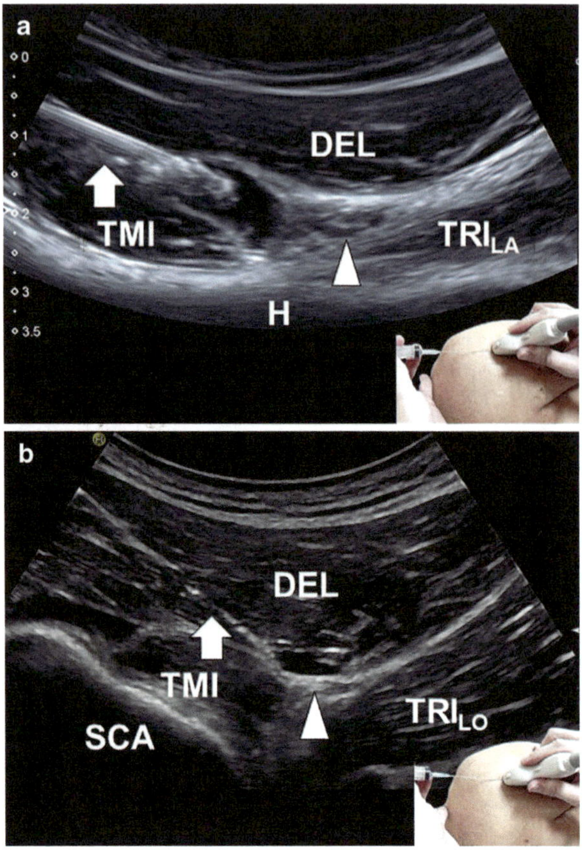

Fig. 4.25 The ultrasound-guided injection of the axillary nerve (white arrowheads) can be performed using an in-plane approach, positioned cephalically to the lateral head of the triceps brachii muscle (**a**) or just cephalically and laterally to the long head of the triceps brachii muscle (**b**). White arrows: needle; TMI teres minor; TRI_{LA} lateral head of the triceps brachii muscle; TRI_{LO} long head of the triceps brachii muscle; SCA scapula; DEL deltoid; H humerus

4.6 Conclusion

The axillary region serves as the convergence point for the teres major, latissimus dorsi, triceps long head, and subscapularis muscles, rendering it a frequent location for inferior shoulder pain. The axillary nerve, intricately linked with the inferior glenohumeral capsule, is not only the most critical nerve in this region but also a prime target for pain management. When performing ultrasound-guided interventions in the axillary region, it is imperative to exercise caution to prevent injury to the posterior humeral circumflex artery.

Acknowledgment Images and illustrations adapted from cadaveric images provided by the Visible Human Project® of the National Library of Medicine. Excerpts featured in the VH Dissector are used with permission from Touch of Life Technologies Inc.

References

1. Syros A, Rizzo MG. Anatomy, shoulder and upper limb, teres major muscle. In: StatPearls. Treasure Island (FL) ineligible companies. Disclosure: Michael Rizzo declares no relevant financial relationships with ineligible companies.: StatPearls Publishing Copyright © 2024, StatPearls Publishing LLC.; 2024.
2. Hung CY, Chang KV, Chen PT, et al. Sonoelastography for the evaluation of an axillary schwannoma in a case of quadrilateral space syndrome. Clin Imaging. 2014;38(3):360–3.
3. Mullen LA, Harvey SC. Review of axillary web syndrome: what the radiologist should know. Eur J Radiol. 2019;113:66–73.
4. Gordon A, Alsayouri K. Anatomy, shoulder and upper limb, axilla. In: StatPearls. Treasure Island (FL) ineligible companies. Disclosure: Khalid Alsayouri declares no relevant financial relationships with ineligible companies.: StatPearls Publishing Copyright © 2024, StatPearls Publishing LLC.; 2024.
5. Passanante GJ, Skalski MR, Patel DB, et al. Inferior glenohumeral ligament (IGHL) complex: anatomy, injuries, imaging features, and treatment options. Emerg Radiol. 2017;24(1):65–71.
6. Jeno SH, Varacallo M. Anatomy, back, Latissimus Dorsi. In: StatPearls. Treasure Island (FL) ineligible companies. Disclosure: Matthew Varacallo declares no relevant financial relationships with ineligible companies.: StatPearls Publishing Copyright © 2024, StatPearls Publishing LLC.; 2024.
7. Wang AA, Strauch RJ, Flatow EL, Bigliani LU, Rosenwasser MP. The teres major muscle: an anatomic study of its use as a tendon transfer. J Shoulder Elb Surg. 1999;8(4):334–8.
8. Beck PA, Hoffer MM. Latissimus dorsi and teres major tendons: separate or conjoint tendons? J Pediatr Orthop. 1989;9(3):308–9.
9. Aguirre K, Mudreac A, Kiel J. Anatomy, shoulder and upper limb, subscapularis muscle. In: StatPearls. Treasure Island (FL) ineligible companies. Disclosure: Andrew Mudreac declares no relevant financial relationships with ineligible companies. Disclosure: John Kiel declares no relevant financial relationships with ineligible companies.: StatPearls Publishing Copyright © 2024, StatPearls Publishing LLC.; 2024.
10. Chang KV, Lin CP, Lin CS, Wu WT, Karmakar MK, Ozcakar L. Sonographic tracking of trunk nerves: essential for ultrasound-guided pain management and research. J Pain Res. 2017;10:79–88.
11. Okwumabua E, Thompson JH. Anatomy, shoulder and upper limb, axillary nerve. In: StatPearls. Treasure Island (FL) ineligible companies. Disclosure: Johnathan Thompson declares no relevant financial relationships with ineligible companies.: StatPearls Publishing Copyright © 2024, StatPearls Publishing LLC.; 2024.
12. Galley IJ. Axillary nerve. In: Bain GI, Itoi E, Di Giacomo G, Sugaya H, editors. Normal and pathological anatomy of the shoulder. Berlin, Heidelberg: Springer Berlin Heidelberg; 2015. p. 315–30.
13. Michelin P, Delarue Y, Duparc F, Dacher JN. Thickening of the inferior glenohumeral capsule: an ultrasound sign for shoulder capsular contracture. Eur Radiol. 2013;23(10):2802–6.
14. Weisberg Z, Cole W, Rumps MV, Vopat B, Mulcahey MK. Bony Bankart lesion: diagnosis, management, and outcomes. JBJS Rev. 2024;12(5)
15. Williams JM, Sinkler MA, Obremskey W. Anatomy, shoulder and upper limb, infraspinatus muscle. In: StatPearls. Treasure Island (FL) ineligible companies. Disclosure: Margaret Sinkler declares no relevant financial relationships with ineligible companies. Disclosure: William Obremskey declares no relevant financial relationships with ineligible companies.: StatPearls Publishing Copyright © 2024, StatPearls Publishing LLC.; 2024.
16. Koehler LA, Haddad TC, Hunter DW, Tuttle TM. Axillary web syndrome following breast cancer surgery: symptoms, complications, and management strategies. Breast Cancer (Dove Med Press). 2019;11:13–9.
17. Chang KV, Lin CP, Lin CS, Wu WT, Ozcakar L. A novel approach for ultrasound guided axillary nerve block: the inferior axilla technique. Med Ultrason. 2017;19(4):457–61.

Part II
Elbow

Chapter 5
Demystifying Lateral Elbow Pain Beyond Tennis Elbow

Ke-Vin Chang, Wei-Ting Wu, Shao-Yu Chi, and Yuan-Yuan Tsai

5.1 Introduction

Lateral epicondylitis, commonly known as tennis elbow, is a prevalent condition that affects the tendons on the outer side of the elbow. The annual incidence ranges from 2.4 to 4.5 per 1000 people [1]. Despite its association with tennis, this condition can impact individuals of various backgrounds, particularly those engaged in repetitive arm motions or activities that strain the forearm muscles. Other risk factors include female sex, dominant-side involvement, and manual labor [2].

Most commonly observed in individuals between the ages of 30 and 50 [3], lateral epicondylitis is characterized by inflammation/degeneration of the tendons attached to the lateral epicondyle, the bony bump on the outer side of the elbow. While the term "tennis elbow" suggests a sports-related origin, it can affect anyone involved in activities that repetitively strain the forearm muscles.

The hallmark symptoms of lateral epicondylitis include pain, weakness in grip strength, and tenderness on the lateral part of the elbow. The pain may radiate down the forearm and is often exacerbated by activities requiring wrist extension or gripping. Recognizing these symptoms is crucial for timely diagnosis and intervention.

Distinguishing lateral epicondylitis from other pathologies is essential for accurate diagnosis and effective treatment. Conditions such as radial tunnel syndrome, cervical radiculopathy, osteoarthritis of the elbow, and ligamentous injuries (radial collateral ligament, lateral ulnar collateral ligament, and annular ligament) may present with similar symptoms.

Ultrasound emerges as a valuable diagnostic tool for lateral elbow pain, not only for its capability to distinguish the pathologies of the common extensor tendons of the wrist but also for its assessment of adjacent neural structures [4]. In this chapter,

---

K.-V. Chang (✉) · W.-T. Wu · S.-Y. Chi · Y.-Y. Tsai
Bei-Hu Branch, National Taiwan University Hospital, Taipei, Taiwan

K.-V. Chang (ed.), *Ultrasonography of Musculoskeletal Pain*,
https://doi.org/10.1007/978-981-96-6787-1_5

we will elaborate on the topographic arrangement of the common extensor tendon as well as some nerve entrapment syndromes pertinent to lateral epicondylitis. We will also shed light on the tips for ultrasound-guided injection for managing lateral elbow pain.

5.2 Regional Anatomy

The lateral epicondyle, situated just above the capitellum, possesses less prominence compared to its medial counterpart. Its morphology can vary significantly among individuals, generally featuring an anterior tubercle, a posterior tubercle, an intertubercular sulcus, and a supercondylar ridge [5] (Fig. 5.1). Additional bony landmarks, such as the superior and inferior tubercles, may be present in certain cases. The visualization of the attachment site of the radial collateral ligament reveals its location in the superior aspect of the intertubercular sulcus. The radial collateral ligament can be traced inferiorly, coursing between the anterior and posterior tubercles before attaching to the annular ligament.

Conversely, the lateral ulnar collateral ligament can be traced from its distal attachment to the ulna's supinator crest, ascending and blending with the annular ligament's fibers. Continuing its course, it merges with the radial collateral ligament's fibers, eventually attaching to the lateral surface of the lateral epicondyle.

On the supracondylar ridge, the extensor carpi radialis longus and brachioradialis muscles attach (Fig. 5.2). The extensor carpi radialis brevis tendon originates from the superior anterior surface of the lateral epicondyle, near or at the anterior tubercle. The attachment points for the extensor digitorum communis and extensor digiti minimi tendons are posterior to the extensor carpi radialis brevis, situated on

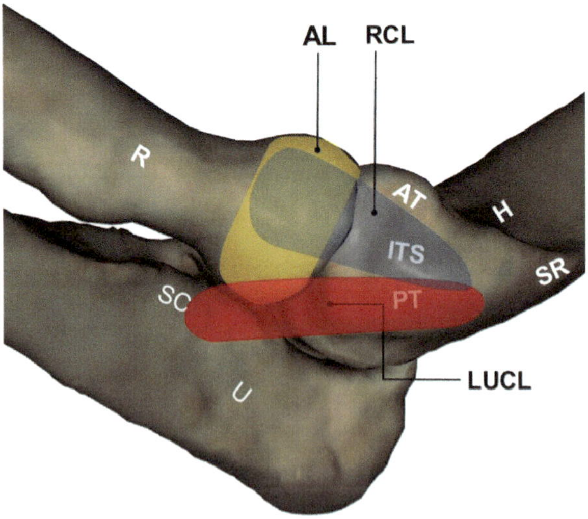

Fig. 5.1 The presentation of a combination of cadaveric reconstruction and schematic drawing, depicts the bony landmarks and ligaments of the lateral elbow. AT anterior tubercle; ITS intertubercular sulcus; PT posterior tubercle; AL annular ligament; RCL radial collateral ligament; LUCL lateral ulnar collateral ligament; SR supracondylar ridge; SC supinator crest; R radius; H humerus; U ulna

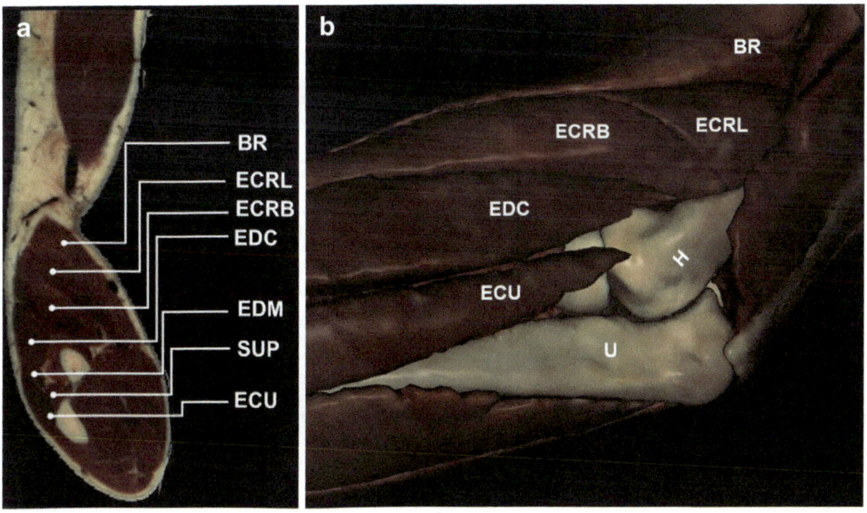

Fig. 5.2 The coronal cross-sectional image of a cadaver (**a**) and corresponding reconstruction image (**b**) depict the muscles over the lateral elbow. BR brachioradialis; ECRL extensor carpi radialis longus; ECRB extensor carpi radialis brevis; EDC extensor digitorum communis; EDM extensor digiti minimi; SUP supinator; ECU extensor carpi ulnaris; U ulna; H humerus

the superior aspect of the lateral epicondyle. Moreover, the extensor carpi ulnaris tendon originates from the posterior inferior surface of the lateral epicondyle. Furthermore, the extensor carpi ulnaris tendon sits on top of the lateral ulnar collateral ligament.

5.3 Sonoanatomy

5.3.1 Common Extensor Tendon of the Wrist

5.3.1.1 Axial Plane-Proximal Radius Level

The topographic arrangement of the common extensor tendon of the wrist can be delineated by positioning the transducer at the level of the proximal radius, where the supinator muscle is readily visible (Fig. 5.3a, b). Atop the supinator, the extensor digitorum communis muscle exhibits a square shape and boasts the largest muscle bulk when compared to the remaining tendinous components of the common extensor tendon of the wrist. Tracing from a caudal to cranial direction, the extensor digiti minimi, characterized by its minimal muscle bulk, is the initial structure to converge into a tendon. Positioned posterior to the extensor digitorum communis, the extensor digiti minimi follows, with the extensor carpi ulnaris situated even further posteriorly. Notably, the extensor carpi radialis brevis, located anterior to the extensor

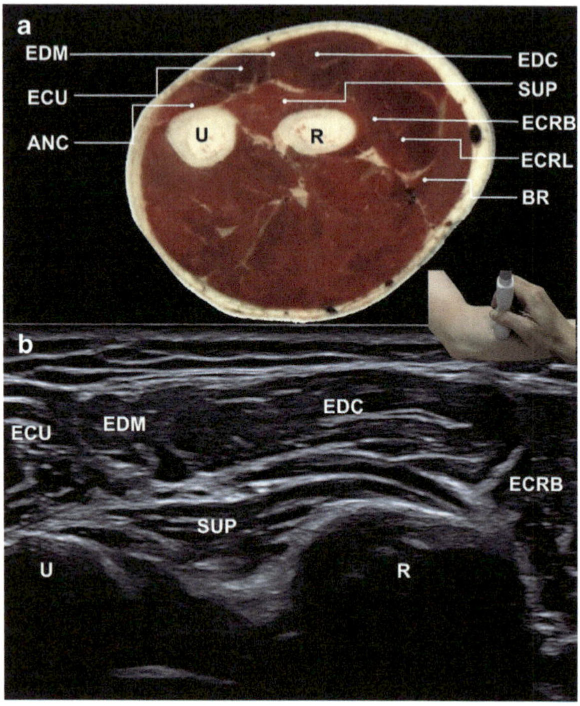

Fig. 5.3 The cadaveric axial cross-sectional image (**a**) and the corresponding sonoanatomy (**b**) depict the common extensor muscles and tendons of the wrist at the proximal one-third of the forearm in axial views. BR brachioradialis; ECRL extensor carpi radialis longus; ECRB extensor carpi radialis brevis; EDC extensor digitorum communis; EDM extensor digiti minimi; ECU extensor carpi ulnaris; ANC anconeus; SUP supinator; R radius; U ulna

digitorum communis, exhibits a distinctive beak-like appearance in its aponeurosis. It is important to note that the extensor carpi radialis longus, positioned anterior to the extensor carpi radialis brevis, does not constitute part of the common extensor tendon of the wrist.

5.3.1.2 Axial Plane-Lateral Epicondyle Level

The transducer is then advanced cranially until it reaches the level of the lateral epicondyle. The most anterior aspect of the lateral epicondyle creates an angulation with the lateral edge of the capitulum fossa, corresponding to the anterior tubercle of the lateral epicondyle. Conversely, the most posterior corner of the lateral epicondyle forms an angulation with the bony plane lateral to the olecranon fossa, aligning with the posterior tubercle of the lateral epicondyle. The concave bony region between these tubercles is identified as the intertubercular sulcus.

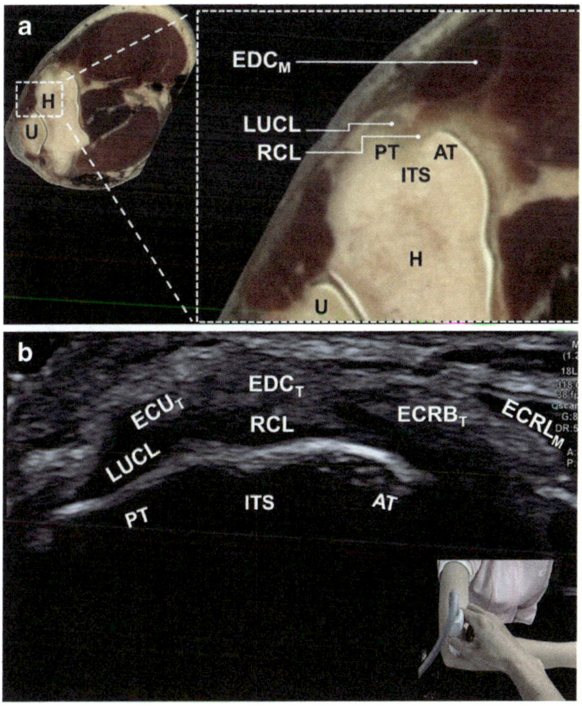

Fig. 5.4 The cadaveric axial cross-sectional image (**a**) and the corresponding sonoanatomy (**b**) depict the common extensor muscles and tendons of the wrist at the lateral epicondyle level in an axial view. AT anterior tubercle; ITS intertubercular sulcus; PT posterior tubercle; RCL radial collateral ligament; LUCL lateral ulnar collateral ligament; $ECRB_T$ extensor carpi radialis brevis tendon; EDC_T extensor digitorum communis tendon; ECU_T extensor carpi ulnaris tendon; $ECRL_M$ extensor carpi radialis longus muscle; U ulna; H humerus

The extensor carpi radialis brevis tendon attaches to the anterior tubercle, while the radial collateral ligament connects to the intertubercular sulcus, and the lateral ulnar collateral ligament attaches to the posterior tubercle (Fig. 5.4a, b). Additionally, the tendons of the extensor digitorum communis, extensor digiti minimi (often indistinguishable from the extensor carpi ulnaris), and extensor carpi ulnaris can be observed sequentially from anterior to posterior, positioned over the radial collateral ligament and lateral ulnar collateral ligament.

5.3.1.3 Long-Axis Plane

Once the topographic arrangement of the common extensor tendon of the wrist is confirmed, the transducer can be rotated 90 degrees to align with the long axis of the forearm [6]. The most anterior component is the extensor carpi radialis brevis, appearing as a single-layered fibrillary structure spanning over the gap between the humerus and radius (Fig. 5.5a, b).

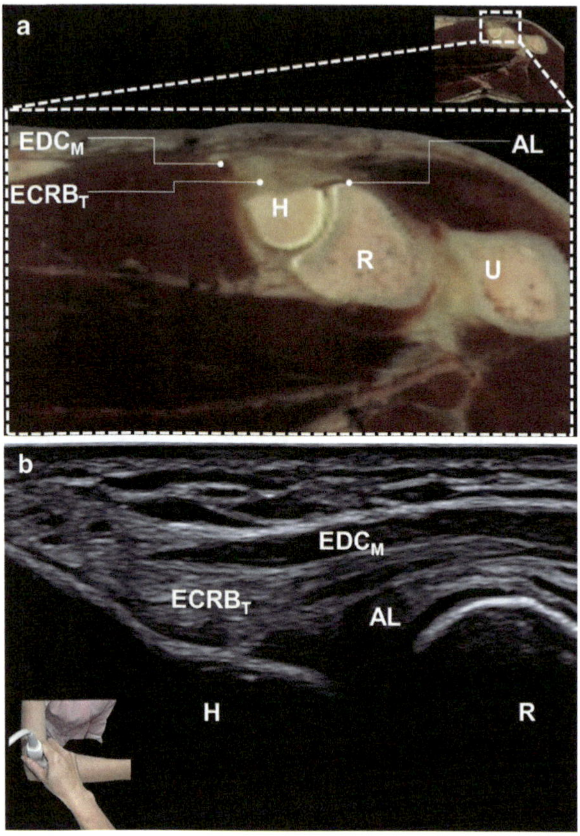

Fig. 5.5 The cadaveric sagittal cross-sectional image (**a**) and the corresponding sonoanatomy (**b**) depict the common extensor tendon of the wrist at the lateral epicondyle in the long axis. AL annular ligament; $ECRB_T$ extensor carpi radialis brevis tendon; EDC_M extensor digitorum communis muscle; H humerus; R radius; U ulna

Maintaining the transducer in the same axis and moving the transducer more posteriorly, a two-layered appearance, with the extensor digitorum communis tendon above and radial collateral ligament below, can be seen. The radial collateral ligament can also be identified as blended with the annular ligament, which encircles the radial head (Fig. 5.6).

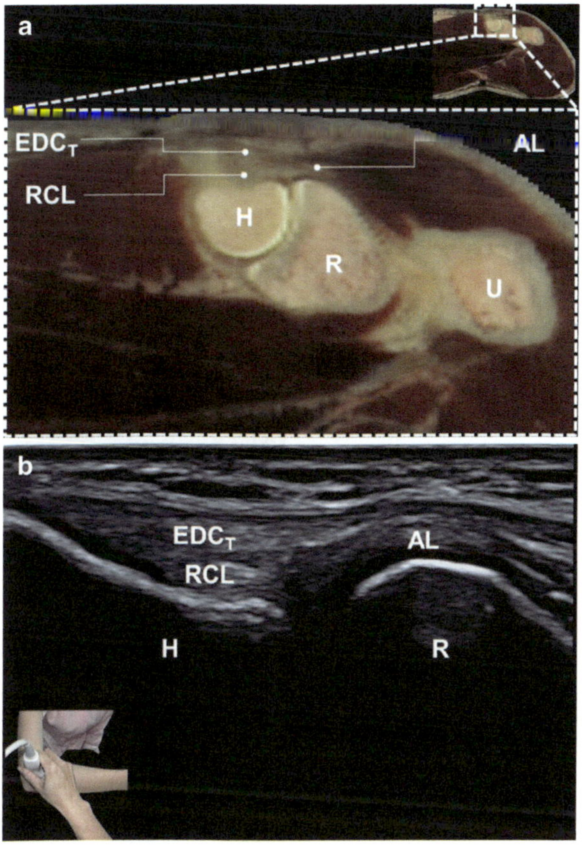

Fig. 5.6 The cadaveric sagittal cross-sectional image (**a**) and the corresponding sonoanatomy (**b**) depict the common extensor tendon of the wrist at the lateral epicondyle in the long axis. EDC$_T$ extensor digitorum communis tendon; AL annular ligament; RCL radial collateral ligament; R radius; U ulna; H humerus

Relocating the transducer more posteriorly, although a two-layered appearance is still seen, the deeper structure transits to the lateral ulnar collateral ligament and the superficial structure transits to the mixture of the extensor digiti minimi and extensor carpi ulnaris tendons (Fig. 5.7a, b). The distal end of the transducer can be pivoted slightly to the supinator crest of the ulna to depict the long axis of the lateral ulnar collateral ligament (Fig. 5.8a, b).

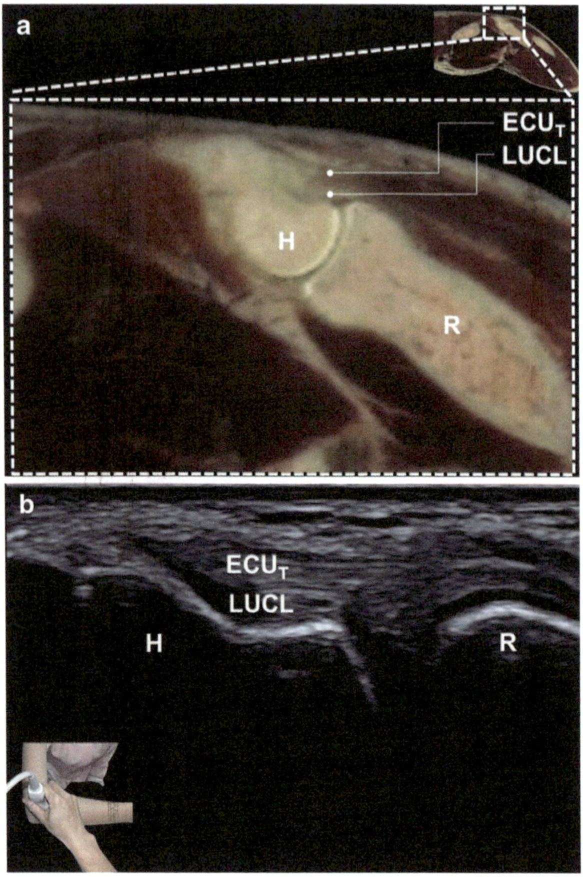

Fig. 5.7 The cadaveric sagittal cross-sectional image (**a**) and the corresponding sonoanatomy (**b**) depict the common extensor tendon of the wrist at the lateral epicondyle in the long axis. ECU$_T$ extensor carpi ulnaris tendon; LUCL lateral ulnar collateral ligament; R radius; H humerus

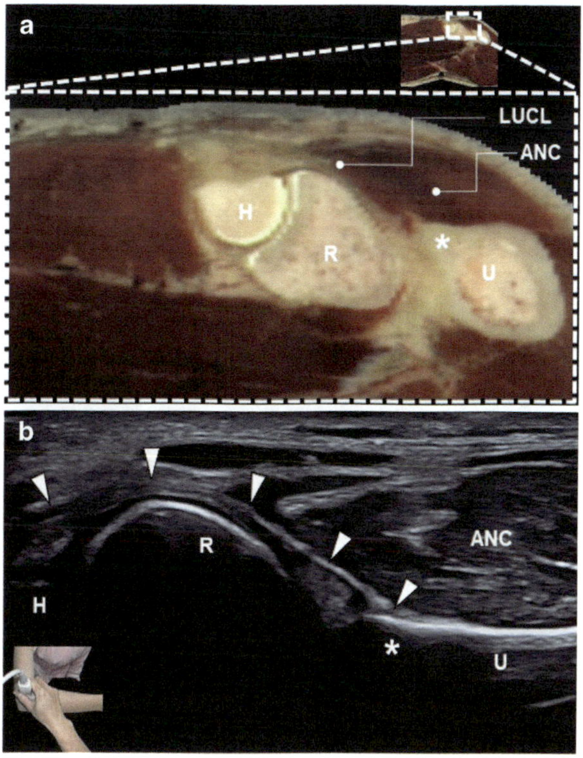

Fig. 5.8 The long-axis depiction presents both the cadaveric image (**a**) and its corresponding sonoanatomy (**b**) of the lateral ulnar collateral ligament (LUCL and white arrowheads). Asterisks: supinator crest of the ulna; ANC anconeus; R radius; U ulna; H humerus

5.3.2 Relevant Neural Structures

5.3.2.1 Posterior Antebrachial Cutaneous Nerve

The posterior antebrachial cutaneous nerve, responsible for innervating the cutaneous region adjacent to the lateral epicondyle, arises from the radial nerve in close proximity to the exit point of the spiral groove (Fig. 5.9a) [7]. When tracing the course of the posterior antebrachial cutaneous nerve in the cranial to caudal direction, it consistently follows its path within the posterior compartment of the arm (Fig. 5.9b), avoiding penetration of the lateral intermuscular septum. In contrast, the main trunk of the radial nerve penetrates the lateral intermuscular septum, reaching the boundary between the brachialis and brachioradialis muscles (Fig. 5.9c). Upon reaching the subcutaneous layer, the posterior antebrachial cutaneous nerve divides into anterior and posterior branches. The posterior branch closely follows the path near the lateral epicondyle, where the common extensor tendon of the wrist attaches (Fig. 5.9d).

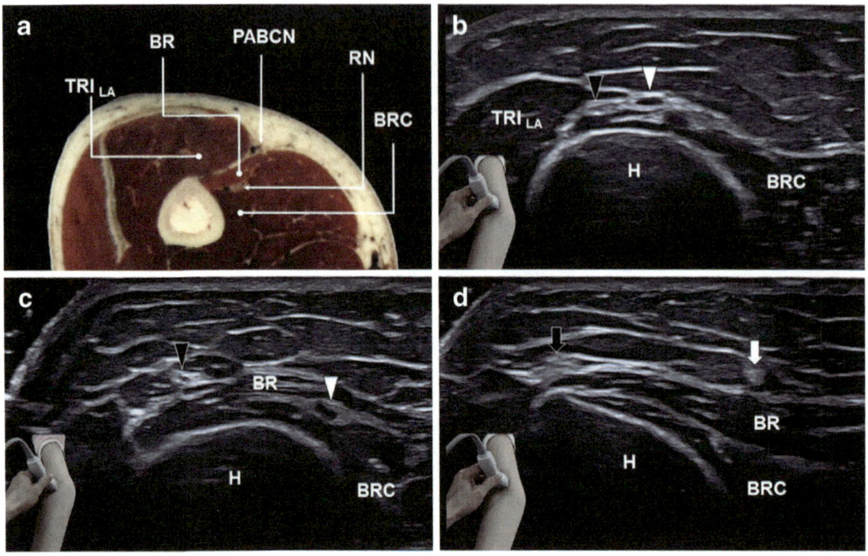

Fig. 5.9 The cadaveric image (**a**) and the corresponding sonoanatomy depict the radial nerve and posterior antebrachial cutaneous nerve in the short axis. At the exit of the spiral groove, the posterior antebrachial cutaneous nerve diverges from the radial nerve (**b**). The radial nerve and the posterior antebrachial cutaneous nerve are distinct from each other from the point where the brachioradialis muscle emerges. The radial nerve pierces the lateral intermuscular septum, while the posterior antebrachial cutaneous nerve remains behind the lateral intermuscular septum and emerges into the subcutaneous tissue, respectively (**c**). The anterior and posterior branches of the posterior antebrachial cutaneous nerve can be identified distally (**d**). RN and white arrowheads: radial nerve; PABCN and black arrowheads: posterior antebrachial cutaneous nerve; white arrow: anterior branch of the posterior antebrachial cutaneous nerve; black arrow: posterior branch of the posterior antebrachial cutaneous nerve; TRI_{LA} lateral head of the triceps brachii; BR brachioradialis muscle; BRC brachialis muscle; H humerus

5.3.2.2 Posterior Interosseous Nerve

Entrapment of the posterior interosseous nerve within the supinator muscle may cause lateral elbow pain, resembling the symptoms of lateral epicondylitis. Identifying the affected nerve segment involves pronating the forearm, which positions the common extensor of the wrist upward. A transducer is used to scan distally from the elbow joint until the supinator muscle (Fig. 5.10a), wrapping around the proximal radius, becomes visible. Before entering the supinator muscle, the posterior interosseous nerve can be observed separate from the superficial radial nerve and located near the recurrent radial artery (Fig. 5.10b). This region is referred to as the “leash of Henry,” a term introduced in the early twentieth century by Dr. Arnold Henry [8], who highlighted the role of the branches of the recurrent radial artery in surgical access to the elbow and proximal forearm.

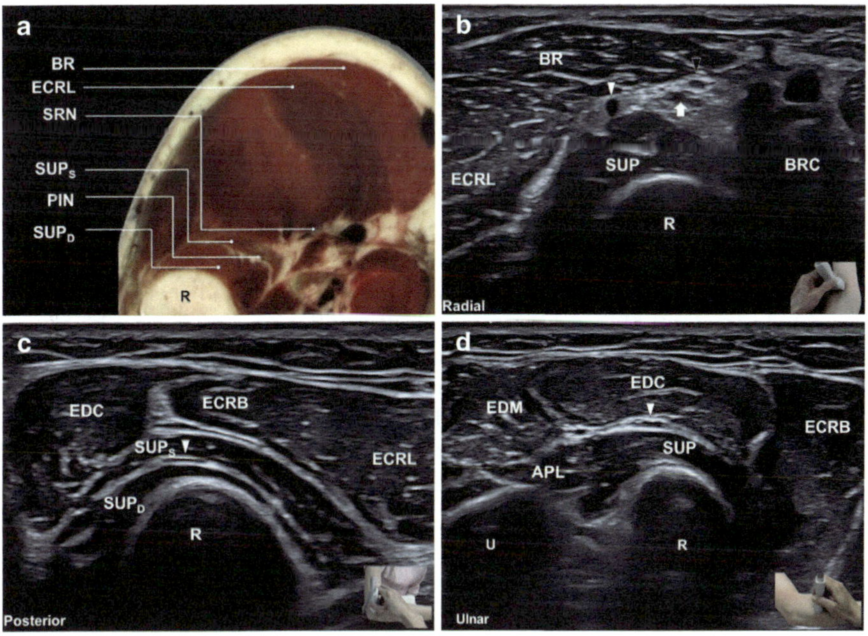

Fig. 5.10 The cadaveric image (**a**) and the corresponding sonoanatomy (**b**) of the posterior interosseous and superficial radial nerves in the short axis at the elbow crease level are shown. The posterior interosseous nerve passes through the supinator tunnel between the superficial and deep heads of the supinator (**c**). The posterior interosseous nerve emerges from the supinator tunnel to innervate the finger extensors (**d**). PIN and white arrowheads: posterior interosseous nerve; SRN and black arrowhead: superficial radial nerve; white arrow: recurrent radial artery; BR brachioradialis; BRC brachialis; ECRB extensor carpi radialis brevis; ECRL extensor carpi radialis longus; EDC extensor digitorum communis; SUP supinator; SUP_D deep head of the supinator; SUP_S superficial head of the supinator; EDM extensor digiti minimi; APL abductor pollicis longus; R radius; U ulna

As the transducer is moved distally, the posterior interosseous nerve passes through the arcade of Frohse [9], a fibrous band forming the proximal border of the superficial head of the supinator muscle. Within this region, the nerve can be identified in a cleavage plane that separates the supinator into superficial and deep components (Fig. 5.10c). After traversing the supinator and exiting it, the nerve divides into multiple branches that innervate the muscles responsible for finger extension (Fig. 5.10d).

5.4 Pathology

When a patient presents with lateral elbow pain, the initial consideration is often lateral epicondylitis, a condition primarily affecting the common extensor tendon of the wrist. While the axial view is more effective in understanding the topographic arrangement of the common extensor, identifying the pathology in the long axis of the common extensor tendon allows for a meticulous distinction of its fibrillary pattern.

The most prevalent pathology in this context is tendinopathy, characterized by a thickened tendon, a blurred fibrillary pattern, focal hypoechoic changes (Fig. 5.11a), increased vascularity (Fig. 5.11b) or calcification (affected side, Fig. 5.12a; normal side, Fig. 5.12b). The identification of a traction spur at the tendon attachment confirms the presence of enthesopathy. Conversely, the presence of an anechoic area devoid of visible fibers within the tendon, without extending through its entire thickness, indicates a partial tear (long axis in the first case, Fig. 5.13a; short axis in the first case, Fig. 5.13b; long axis in the second case, Fig. 5.13c; short axis in the second case, Fig. 5.13d).

Once the lesion is discerned, the transducer can be rotated to visualize the tendon's short axis, allowing for the confirmation of which tendon component contributes to the pathological findings. It is important to recognize that not only the tendon but also the ligament component, such as the radial collateral ligament (affected side, Fig. 5.14a; normal side, Fig. 5.14b), annular ligament (short axis in the affected side, Fig. 5.15a; long axis in the affected side, Fig. 5.15b; short axis in the normal side, Fig. 5.15c; long axis in the normal side, Fig. 5.15d), and lateral ulnar collateral ligament (affected side, Fig. 5.16a; normal side, Fig. 5.16b), may be implicated. In instances where the ligament component is affected, there is a potential compromise of stability in the radiocapitellar joint.

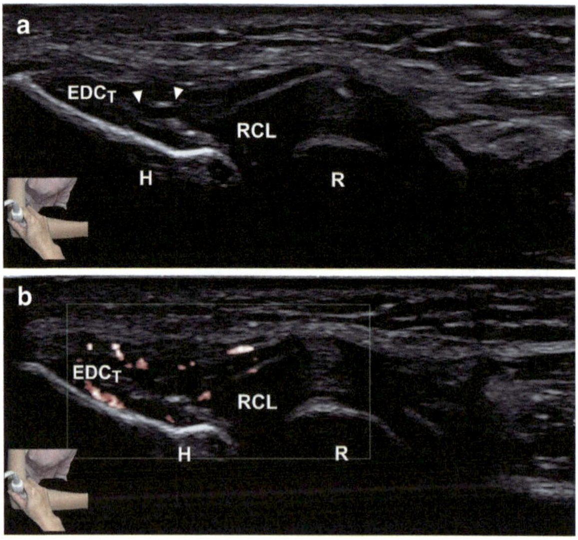

Fig. 5.11 The ultrasonography reveals focal hypoechoic changes (white arrowheads) (**a**) and peritendinous hypervascularity (**b**) in the extensor digitorum communis tendon (EDC$_T$). RCL radial collateral ligament; R radius; H humerus

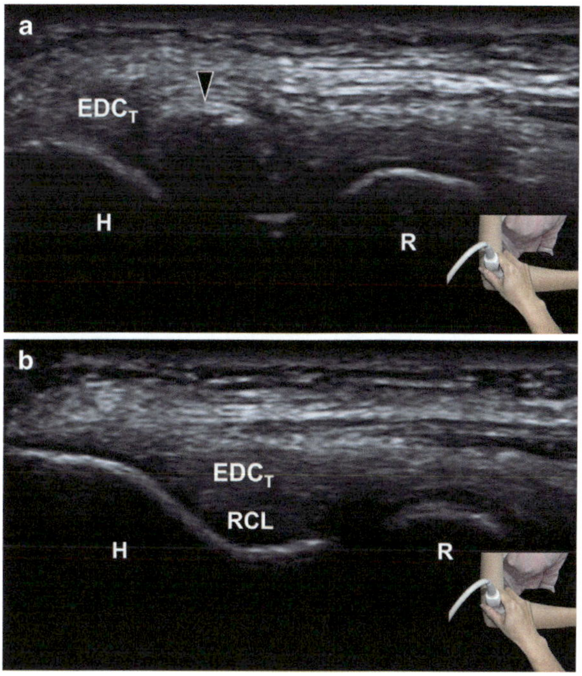

Fig. 5.12 The ultrasonography reveals calcification (black arrowhead) within the extensor digitorum communis tendon (EDC$_T$), accompanied by a notable posterior acoustic shadowing (**a**). Conversely, the contralateral side displays a normal fibrillar pattern of the extensor digitorum communis tendon and the underlying radial collateral ligament (RCL) (**b**). R radius; H humerus

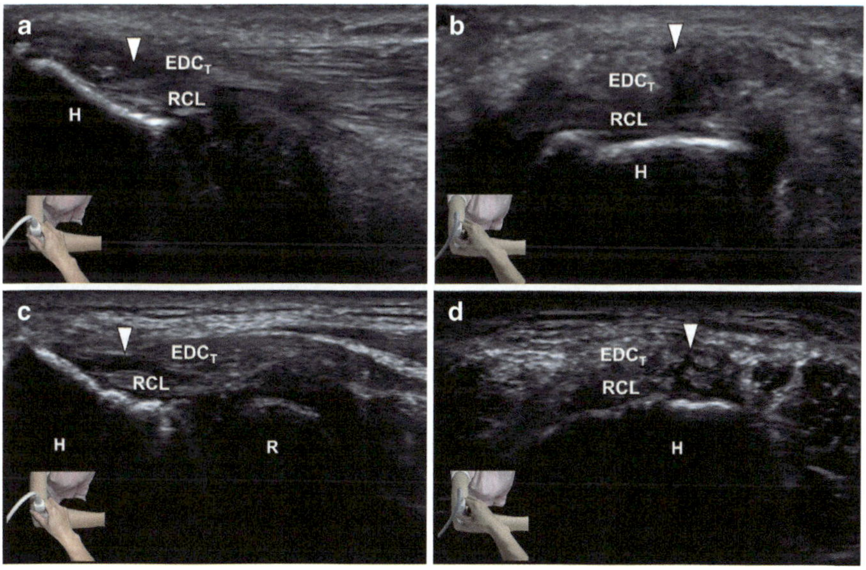

Fig. 5.13 The sonographic images depict a partial tear of the extensor digitorum communis tendon, as indicated by the white arrowheads in both the long-axis (**a**) and short-axis (**b**) views. In another case, the presence of an anechoic area within the tendon suggests a partial thickness tear, visible in both the long-axis (**c**) and short-axis (**d**) views. EDC$_T$ extensor digitorum communis tendon; RCL radial collateral ligament; R radius; H humerus

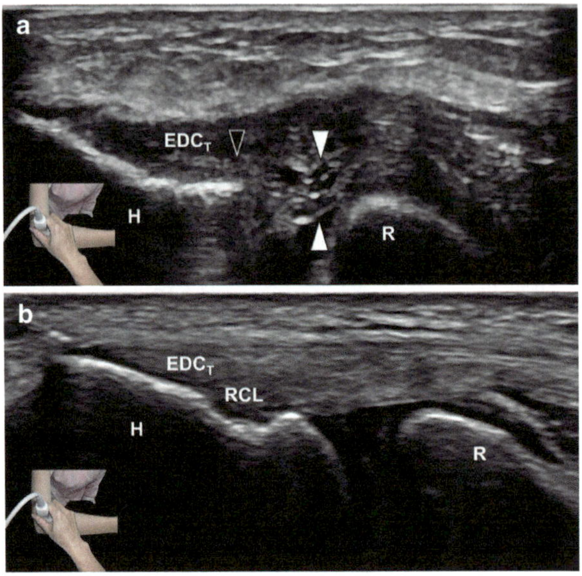

Fig. 5.14 In the long axis view, ultrasonography reveals a partial tear of the radial collateral ligament, as seen in image (**a**), contrasting with a normal appearance depicted in image (**b**). On the pathological side, the proximal radial collateral ligament appears thin (black arrowhead). Notably, the segment of the ligament covering the lateral elbow joint displays multiple anechoic gaps, swelling, loss of fibrillar pattern, and discontinuity in fiber alignment (white arrowheads). RCL radial collateral ligament; EDC$_T$ extensor digitorum communis tendon; R radius; H humerus

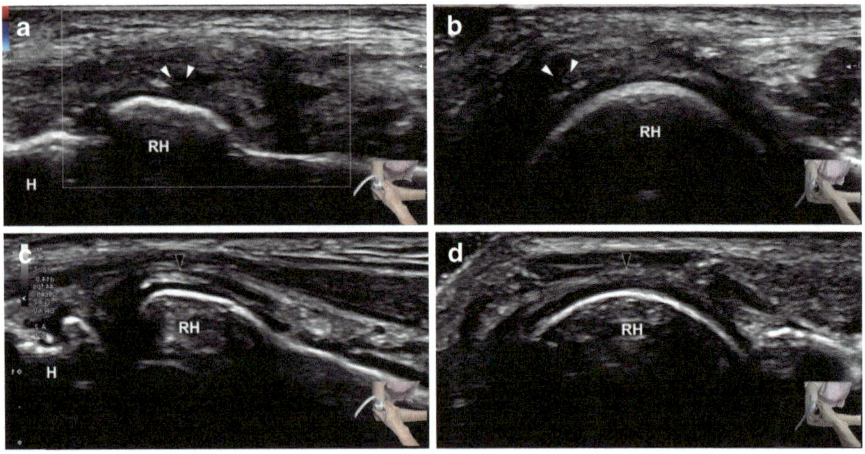

Fig. 5.15 The ultrasonography reveals a partial tear (white arrowheads) of the annular ligament, characterized by a loss of the fibrillar pattern and a well-defined hypoechoic cleft in both the short-axis (**a**) and long-axis (**b**) views of the annular ligament. This is contrasted with the annular ligament (black arrowheads) on the healthy side in both the short-axis (**c**) and long-axis (**d**) views. RH radial head; H humerus

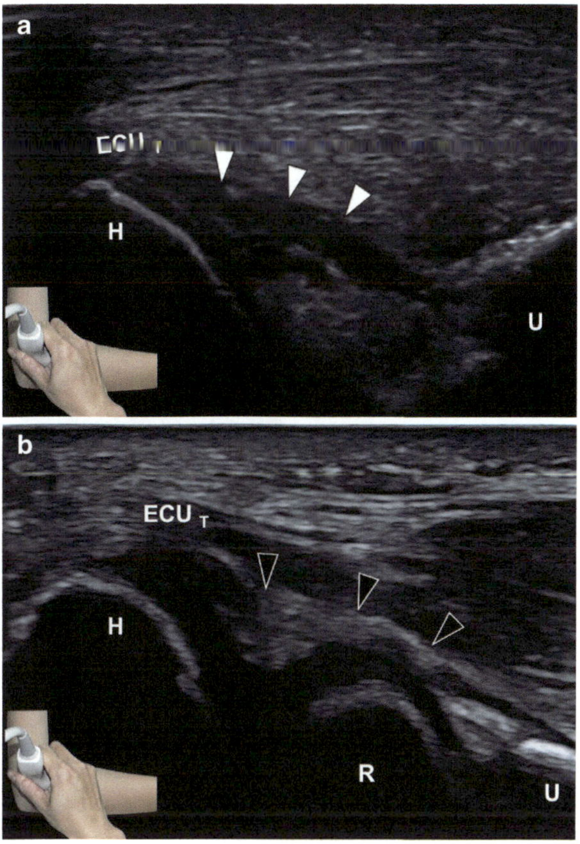

Fig. 5.16 The ultrasonography reveals partial tears (white arrowheads) in the lateral ulnar collateral ligament, characterized by swelling, waviness, and hypoechoic appearance (**a**), in comparison to the healthy side (**b**) where no such abnormalities are observed (black arrowheads). ECU_T extensor carpi ulnairs tendon; R radius; U ulna; H humerus

To assess joint stability, the investigator can measure the distance between the proximal radius and capitellum of the humerus and compare it with the corresponding measurement on the contralateral non-painful side. A significant increase in distance on the painful side indicates joint instability (Fig. 5.17a), whereas a decrease in the joint distance can be seen in patients with osteoarthritis (Fig. 5.17b). When pain originates from the posterior area of the lateral elbow, a careful examination of the anconeus muscle is warranted (normal side, Fig. 5.18a; affected side, Fig. 5.18b, c).

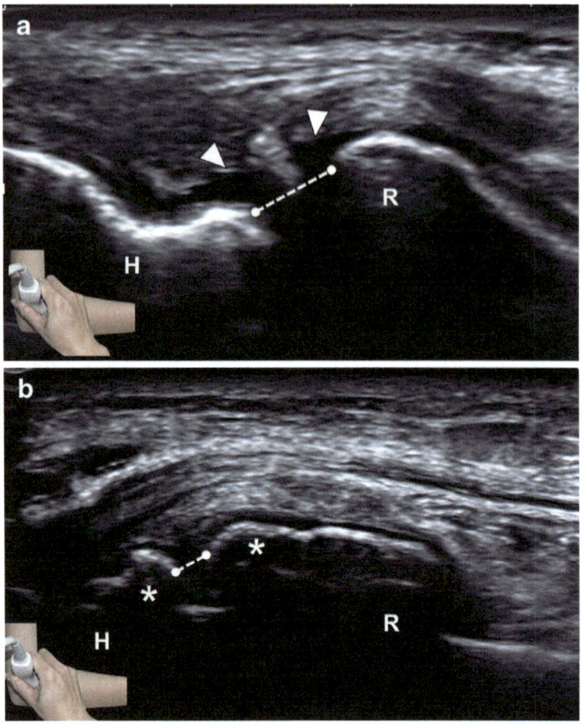

Fig. 5.17 The ultrasonography shows a complete tear of the radial collateral ligament (white arrowheads) and widening of the radiohumeral joint interval (**a**). In contrast, narrowing of the radiohumeral joint interval can be observed in a case of osteoarthritis with evident osteophytes (asterisks) (**b**). Dash lines: radiohumeral joint interval; R radius; H humerus

On the contrary, if the point of maximum pain is not situated at the lateral epicondyle but lies more than one centimeter away from it, consideration should be given to pathologies beyond the lateral epicondyle. A likely scenario involves the entrapment of the posterior interosseous nerve at its entrance to the supinator tunnel (short axis in the affected side, Fig. 5.19a; long axis in the affected side, Fig. 5.19b; short axis in the normal side, Fig. 5.19c; long axis in the normal side, Fig. 5.19d). Since the cutaneous area above the supinator is governed not by the posterior interosseous nerve but by the posterior antebrachial cutaneous nerve or lateral antebrachial cutaneous nerve, the pain may present as diffuse or indistinct. In addition to assessing whether the posterior interosseous nerve is enlarged, the investigator can utilize sonopalpation to verify that the painful region corresponds to the supinator muscle.

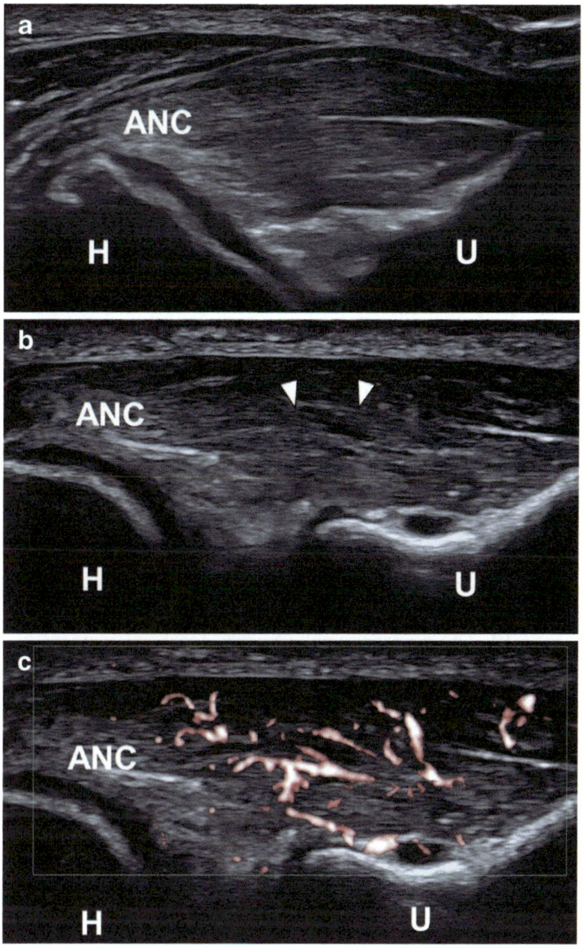

Fig. 5.18 The ultrasonography shows a normal anconeus (ANC) muscle (**a**), alongside a focal loss of fibrillar pattern (white arrowheads) (**b**) and increased vascularity (**c**) in an injured anconeus muscle. U ulna; H humerus

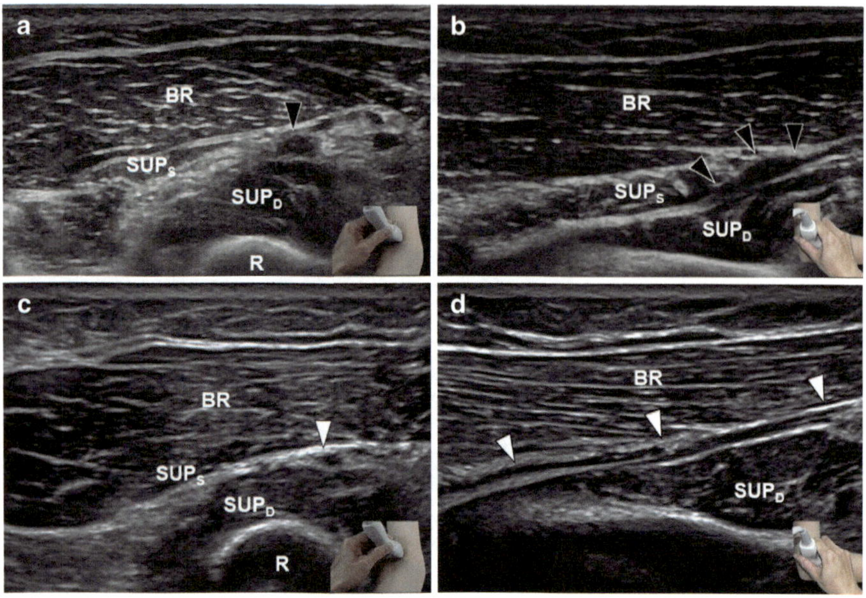

Fig. 5.19 The ultrasonography reveals focal enlargement of the posterior interosseous nerve (black arrowheads) in both the short-axis (**a**) and long-axis (**b**) views, situated between the two heads of the supinator muscle. This is compared to the healthy side (white arrowheads) in both the short-axis (**c**) and long-axis (**d**) views. SUP_S superficial head of the supinator; SUP_D deep head of the supinator; BR brachioradialis; R radius

5.5 Ultrasound-Guided Injection

Various injection regimens are available for treating lateral epicondylitis, including corticosteroid, botulinum toxin, autologous blood products, and platelet-rich plasma. A 2022 network meta-analysis [10] revealed that both corticosteroid and botulinum toxin demonstrated greater efficacy than a placebo in terms of pain reduction. However, corticosteroid was found to be superior to botulinum toxin. Notably, in the third month of treatment, botulinum toxin emerged as the sole intervention surpassing placebo in pain relief. Furthermore, no therapies demonstrated greater efficacy than placebo in the sixth month of treatment.

In ultrasound-guided injections for lateral epicondylitis, it is advised to align the transducer along the long axis of the common extensor tendon of the wrist. The needle should be inserted in a caudal-to-cranial direction, precisely targeting the

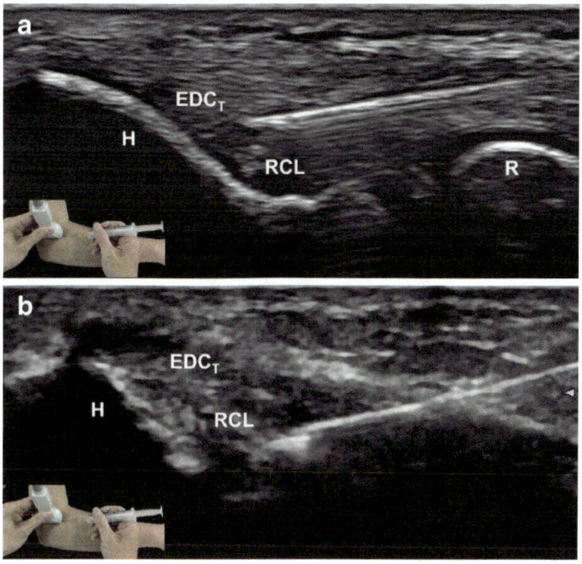

Fig. 5.20 In-plane ultrasound-guided injections are delivered at two key sites: (**a**) the junction between the extensor digitorum communis tendon (EDC$_T$) and radial collateral ligament (RCL), and (**b**) the undersurface of the RCL. R radius; H humerus

lesion if an area devoid of tendon or ligamentous fibers is identified. When the fibers of the common extensor tendon of the wrist are predominantly intact, the injectate can be evenly distributed within the tendon using the peppering injection technique or administered between the undersurface of the extensor digitorum communis and the radial collateral ligament (Fig. 5.20a). Conversely, when the radial collateral ligament is the primary focus, for procedures such as regenerative injections employing platelet-rich plasma or dextrose, the injectate can be directed to the undersurface of the radial collateral ligament (Fig. 5.20b).

Moreover, if there is entrapment of the posterior interosseous nerve, hydro-dissection using regimens such as 5% dextrose can be carried out [11]. Positioning the transducer over the short axis of the forearm enables visualization of both the short-axis of the posterior interosseous nerve and the long axis of the supinator muscle. The needle can be inserted from lateral to medial to hydro-dissect the cleavage plane that separates the superficial and deep heads of the supinator muscle (Fig. 5.21). Finally, in cases resistant to treatment with persistent lateral elbow pain, an ultrasound-guided block using local anesthetics can be performed for the posterior antebrachial cutaneous nerve.

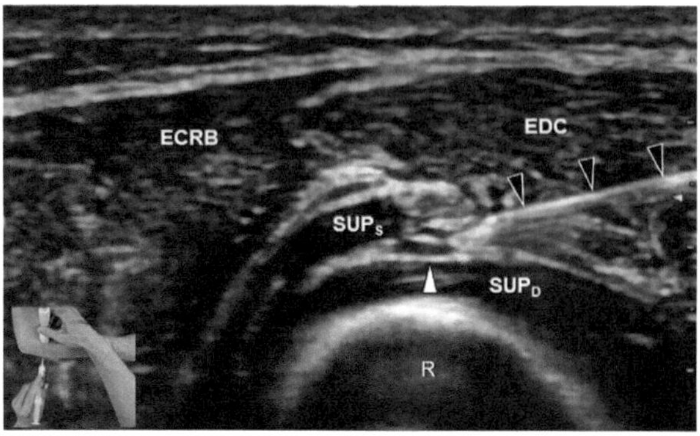

Fig. 5.21 The injection for the posterior interosseous nerve (white arrowhead) is administered via an in-plane ultrasound-guided approach. Black arrowheads: needle; ECRB extensor carpi radialis brevis; EDC extensor digitorum communis; SUP_S superficial head of the supinator; SUP_D deep head of the supinator; R radius

5.6 Conclusion

High-resolution ultrasound can enhance the clarity of the distinct tendinous origins of the common extensor tendon of the wrist, aiding in the precise identification of the lesion and guiding subsequent injections. Posterior interosseous nerve entrapment can produce elbow pain that mimics lateral epicondylitis but can be effectively addressed through ultrasound-guided hydrodissection.

Acknowledgments Images and illustrations adapted from cadaveric images provided by the Visible Human Project® of the National Library of Medicine. Excerpts featured in the VH Dissector are used with permission from Touch of Life Technologies Inc.

References

1. Sanders TL Jr, Maradit Kremers H, Bryan AJ, Ransom JE, Smith J, Morrey BF. The epidemiology and health care burden of tennis elbow: a population-based study. Am J Sports Med. 2015;43(5):1066–71.
2. Park HB, Gwark JY, Im JH, Na JB. Factors associated with lateral epicondylitis of the elbow. Orthop J Sports Med. 2021;9(5):23259671211007734.
3. Kaminsky SB, Baker CL Jr. Lateral epicondylitis of the elbow. Tech Hand Up Extrem Surg. 2003;7(4):179–89.
4. Ricci V, Cocco G, Mezian K, et al. Anatomy and sonographic examination for lateral epicondylitis: EURO-MUSCULUS/USPRM approach. Am J Phys Med Rehabil. 2023;102(4):300–7.
5. Zoner CS, Buck FM, Cardoso FN, et al. Detailed MRI-anatomic study of the lateral epicondyle of the elbow and its tendinous and ligamentous attachments in cadavers. AJR Am J Roentgenol. 2010;195(3):629–36.

6. Wu WT, Chang KV. Letter to editor on "Clinical and ultrasonographic effectiveness of two different splints used for the treatment of lateral epicondylitis: a prospective randomized controlled study". Arch Phys Med Rehabil. 2024;105:1217.
7. García-Martínez J, Miguel-Pérez M, Pérez-Bellmunt A, Ortiz-Miguel S, Viscor G. The course of posterior antebrachial cutaneous nerve: anatomical and sonographic study with a clinical implication. Int J Environ Res Public Health. 2021;18(15)
8. Mohana-Borges AVR, Silva LTSD, Mohana-Borges RS, et al. Neurovascular crossing patterns between leash of Henry and deep branch of radial nerve: implications for neurointervention and diagnostic imaging. Skeletal Radiol. 2024;54:493.
9. Benes M, Kachlik D, Kunc V, Kunc V. The arcade of Frohse: a systematic review and meta-analysis. Surg Radiol Anat. 2021;43(5):703–11.
10. Tavassoli M, Jokar R, Zamani M, Khafri S, Esmaeilnejad-Ganji SM. Clinical efficacy of local injection therapies for lateral epicondylitis: a systematic review and network meta-analysis. Caspian J Intern Med. 2022;13(2):311–25.
11. Lin CP, Chang KV, Huang YK, Wu WT, Özçakar L. Regenerative injections including 5% dextrose and platelet-rich plasma for the treatment of carpal tunnel syndrome: a systematic review and network meta-analysis. Pharmaceuticals (Basel). 2020;13(3)

Chapter 6
Medial Elbow Pain: Golf Elbow and Beyond

Ke-Vin Chang, Wei-Ting Wu, Shao-Yu Chi, and Yuan-Yuan Tsai

6.1 Introduction

Medial elbow pain is less common than its lateral counterpart, as indicated by a population-based study reporting a prevalence of 1.3% for definite lateral epicondylitis compared to 0.4% for medial epicondylitis [1]. Factors such as smoking, obesity, repetitive movements, and forceful activities have demonstrated independent associations with medial epicondylitis [2]. Those involved in overhead throwing and heavy lifting professions face an elevated risk of developing medial elbow pain. In the pediatric context, little league elbow, encompassing various injuries to the medial side of the elbow in adolescent pitchers, is a potential diagnosis [3].

For adults, a thorough consideration of multiple pathologies is essential. This may encompass ulnar nerve neuropathy with or without nerve dislocation, as well as potential entrapment of the medial antebrachial cutaneous nerve [4]. Moreover, medial epicondylitis, involving the attachment of the common flexor of the wrist, is the predominant concern.

Utilizing ultrasound imaging proves invaluable for diagnosing these conditions. Microtears or chronic tendinosis of the common flexor origin are detectable pathologies through ultrasound, which is also effective in evaluating issues with the ulnar collateral ligament and relevant neuropathy. Going beyond mere diagnosis, this chapter also seeks to illuminate the application of ultrasound-guided injections in the treatment of medial elbow disorders.

K.-V. Chang (✉) · W.-T. Wu · S.-Y. Chi · Y.-Y. Tsai
Bei-Hu Branch, National Taiwan University Hospital, Taipei, Taiwan

K.-V. Chang (ed.), *Ultrasonography of Musculoskeletal Pain*,
https://doi.org/10.1007/978-981-96-6787-1_6

6.2 Regional Anatomy

6.2.1 Common Flexor of the Wrist

The medial epicondyle of the humerus is a noticeable projection situated at the distal end of the medial supracondylar ridge. Significantly more prominent than its lateral counterpart, this bony prominence on the inner side of the elbow serves as a crucial anatomical landmark. Within the medial epicondyle, a groove accommodating the ulnar nerve is present.

Multiple muscles attach to the medial epicondyle, collectively forming the common flexor tendon. These muscles consist of the humeral head of the pronator teres, flexor carpi radialis, palmaris longus, flexor carpi ulnaris, and flexor digitorum superficialis (Fig. 6.1). The attachment of the humeral head of the pronator teres is positioned more cranially than the remainder of the common flexor and is closely aligned with the medial supracondylar ridge [5].

The arrangement of the flexor carpi radialis, palmaris longus, and flexor carpi ulnaris progresses from the radial to the ulnar aspect, caudal to the attachment of the humeroulnar head of the pronator teres. The humeral head of the flexor digitorum superficialis originates distal to the attachment points of these three muscles (Fig. 6.2). On the other hand, the flexor digitorum profundus does not originate from the medial epicondyle of the humerus, but rather from the proximal three-quarters of the anterior and medial surfaces of the ulna and the interosseous membrane.

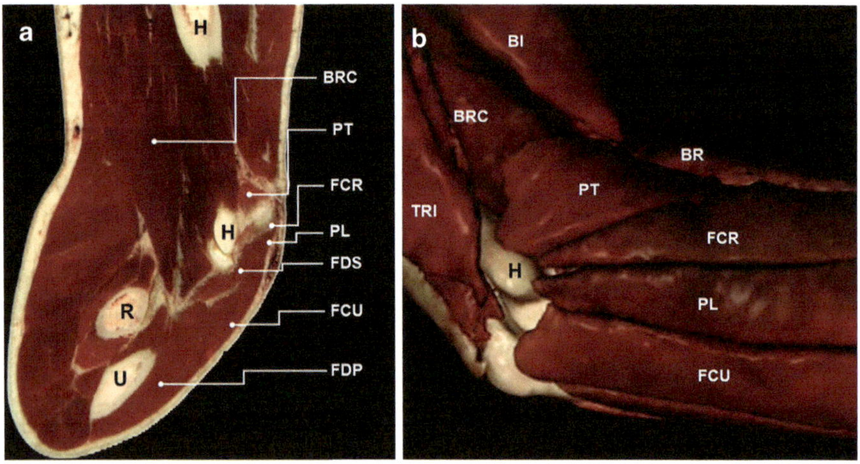

Fig. 6.1 Sagittal cross-section of the elbow musculature around the medial epicondyle (**a**) and its gross anatomy (**b**). BRC Brachialis; BI biceps brachii; TRI triceps brachii; BR brachioradialis; FCR flexor carpi radialis; FCU flexor carpi ulnaris; FDS flexor digitorum superficialis; FDP flexor digitorum profundus; PL palmaris longus; PT pronator teres; R radius; U ulna; H humerus

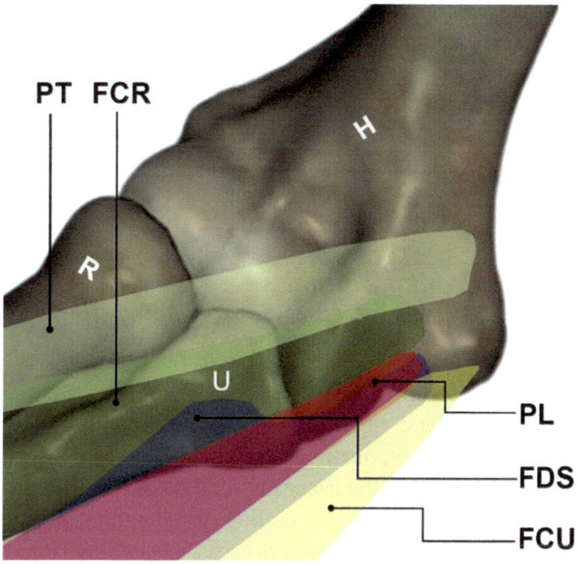

Fig. 6.2 The illustration shows the muscles attaching to the medial epicondyle, layer by layer, forming the common flexor tendon. FCR flexor carpi radialis; FCU flexor carpi ulnaris; FDS humeroulnar head of the flexor digitorum superficialis; PL palmaris longus; PT pronator teres; R radius; U ulna; H humerus

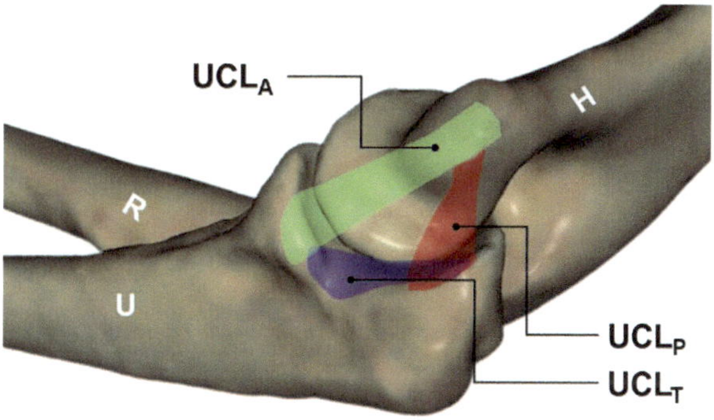

Fig. 6.3 Illustration of the three bundles of the ulnar collateral ligament over the medial epicondyle. UCL_A anterior bundle of the ulnar collateral ligament; UCL_P posterior bundle of the ulnar collateral ligament; UCL_T transverse bundle of the ulnar collateral ligament; R radius; U ulna; H humerus

6.2.2 Ulnar Collateral Ligament

Beneath the common flexor tendon of the wrist lies the ulnar collateral ligament, a crucial structure divides into distinct components: the anterior bundle, posterior bundle, and transverse bundle [6]. The anterior bundle emerges from the anteroinferior surface of the medial epicondyle, securing its attachment to the sublime tubercle of the ulna. Functioning as the primary stabilizer during valgus stress, it plays a pivotal role in maintaining elbow stability (Fig. 6.3).

Conversely, the posterior bundle also originates from the medial epicondyle, with its footprint positioned posteriorly to that of the anterior bundle. This bundle attaches to the medial wall of the olecranon, concurrently serving as the floor of the cubital tunnel. Notably, the posterior bundle contributes significantly to stability, particularly when the elbow is in a flexed position.

Bridging the anterior and posterior bundles is the transverse bundle, originating from the olecranon process and inserting onto the coronoid process. Although present, the transverse bundle makes a minimal contribution to overall elbow stability. In this intricate network, the ulnar collateral ligament collectively ensures the structural integrity of the elbow joint, with each component playing a distinct role in maintaining its function and resilience.

6.2.3 Cubital Tunnel

The ulnar nerve descends within the anterior muscular compartment of the arm, eventually piercing the medial intermuscular septum and transitioning into the posterior muscular compartment [7]. Continuing its course, it passes beneath the arcade of Struthers, an aponeurotic band connecting the medial intermuscular septum to the medial head of the triceps brachii. Osborne's ligament, also known as the cubital retinaculum, serves as the ceiling of the cubital tunnel. Extending from the medial epicondyle to the olecranon process, it seamlessly connects with the fascia linking the humeral and ulnar heads of the flexor carpi ulnaris. The tunnel's floor comprises the posterior bundle of the ulnar collateral ligament. After its posterior passage beyond the medial epicondyle, the ulnar nerve proceeds into the forearm, navigating between the two heads of the flexor carpi ulnaris, also known as the arcuate ligament (Fig. 6.4) [8].

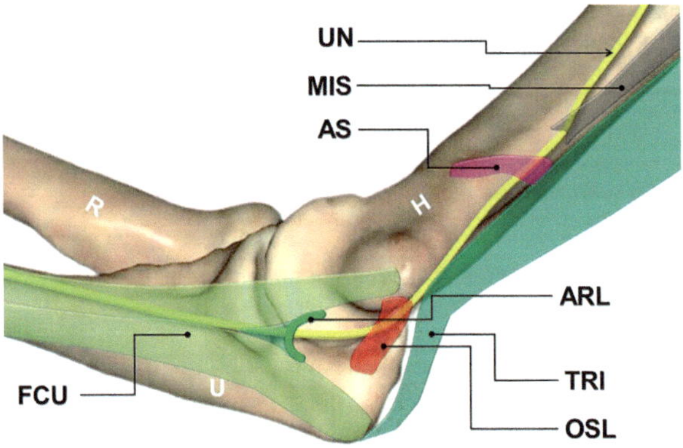

Fig. 6.4 The illustration depicts the course of the ulnar nerve and the nearby structures that can cause nerve entrapment at various levels. UN ulnar nerve; MIS medial intermuscular septum of the arm; AS arcade of Struthers; OSL Osborne's ligament; ARL arcuate ligament; FCU flexor carpi ulnaris; TRI triceps brachii; R radius; U ulna; H humerus

6.3 Sonoanatomy

The transducer is initially positioned in the axial plane over the proximal volar forearm. Successively, the pronator teres, flexor carpi radialis, palmaris longus, humeroulnar head of the flexor digitorum superficialis and flexor carpi ulnaris can be visualized from the radial to the ulnar aspect (Fig. 6.5a, b). Subsequently, the transducer is advanced more cranially, and the tendons, starting from the most ulnar side (flexor carpi ulnaris), converge on the medial epicondyle first. The humeral head of the pronator teres is the last to attach to the medial epicondyle, with its attachment point situated more cranially than the remaining part of the common flexor tendon of the wrist (near the elbow crease, Fig. 6.6a, c; at the medial epicondyle, Fig. 6.6b, d).

To visualize the anterior bundle of the ulnar collateral ligament, participants are instructed to supinate the forearm and flex the elbow. This posture optimally straightens the anterior bundle, enhancing the visualization of its origin from the

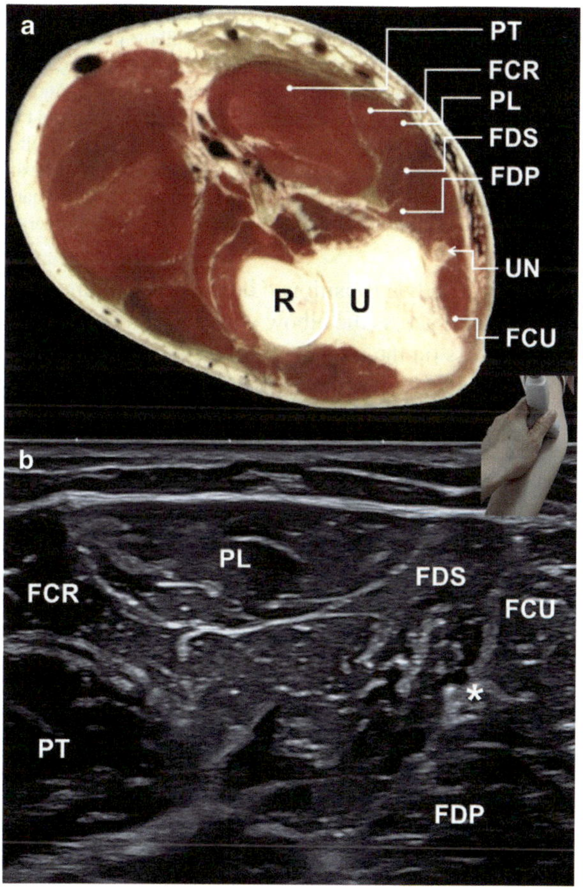

Fig. 6.5 The cadaveric image (**a**) and the corresponding sonoanatomy (**b**) show the flexor muscles of the wrist and hand at the proximal forearm level in an axial view. Asterisk and UN: ulnar nerve; FCR flexor carpi radialis; FCU flexor carpi ulnaris; FDS flexor digitorum superficialis; FDP flexor digitorum profundus; PL palmaris longus; PT pronator teres; R radius; U ulna

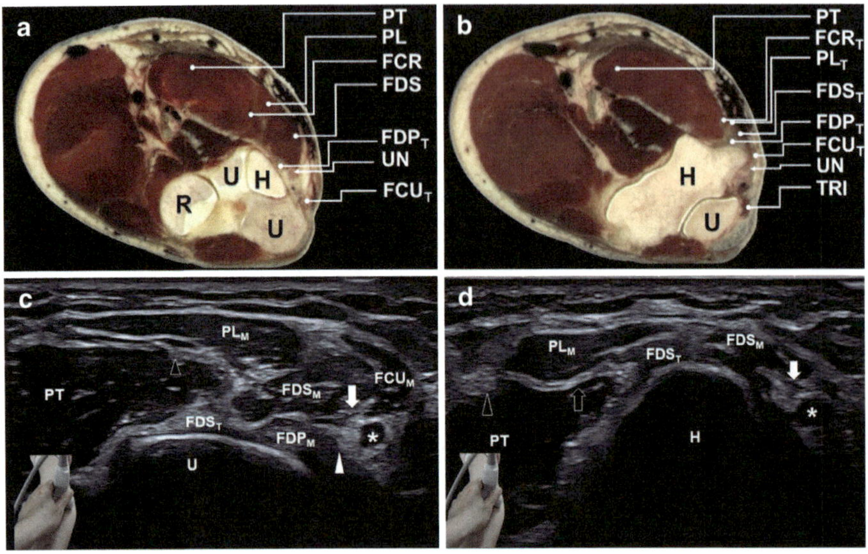

Fig. 6.6 The cadaveric images ((**a**) near the elbow crease; (**b**) at the medial epicondyle level) and the corresponding sonoanatomy ((**c**) near the elbow crease; (**d**) at the medial epicondyle level) show the common flexor muscles and tendons of the wrist and hand in an axial view. Asterisks and UN: ulnar nerve; black arrowheads: tendon of the flexor carpi radialis; white arrows: tendon of the flexor carpi ulnaris; white arrowhead: tendon of the flexor digitorum profundus; black arrow: tendon of the palmaris longus; FCR flexor carpi radialis; FCU flexor carpi ulnaris; FDS flexor digitorum superficialis; FDP flexor digitorum profundus; PL palmaris longus; PT pronator teres; TRI triceps brachii; $_M$ muscle; $_T$ tendon; R radius; U ulna; H humerus

medial epicondyle (positioned deep to the common flexor tendon of the wrist). The bundle spans across the elbow joint and attaches to the sublime tubercle of the coronoid process on the ulna (Fig. 6.7a, b). The long axis of the common flexor tendon is seen overlying the anterior bundle of the ulnar collateral ligament.

To visualize the posterior bundle, the proximal end of the transducer should remain fixed on the medial epicondyle, with the distal end pivoted toward the olecranon (Fig. 6.8a, b). The posterior bundle is situated over the floor of the cubital tunnel, positioned beneath the ulnar nerve and the medial head of the triceps brachii muscle.

Observation of the transverse bundle can be achieved by sliding the proximal end of the transducer to the olecranon process and pivoting the distal end toward the sublime tubercle. The transverse bundle appears as a thin fiber crossing a bony pit on the proximal ulna. (Fig. 6.9a, b).

The initial axial view of the ulnar nerve is acquired at the medial epicondyle level, where it closely aligns with the posterior wall of the medial epicondyle (Fig. 6.10a, b). Progressing distally with the transducer, the ulnar nerve becomes discernible between the humeral and ulnar heads of the flexor carpi ulnaris (Fig. 6.11a, b). Shifting the transducer cranially reveals the ulnar nerve situated atop the medial head of the triceps muscle within the posterior compartment of the arm. Subsequently, it traverses the medial intermuscular septum, entering the anterior compartment and positioning itself posterior to the axillary artery.

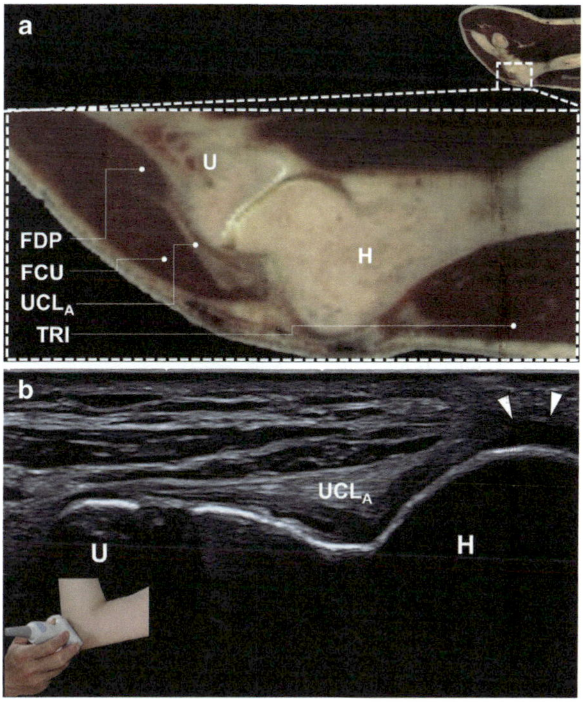

Fig. 6.7 The cadaveric image (**a**) and corresponding sonoanatomy (**b**) of the anterior bundle of the ulnar collateral ligament. White arrowheads: common flexor tendon; UCL_A anterior bundle of the ulnar collateral ligament; FCU flexor carpi ulnaris; FDP flcxor digitorum profundus; TRI triceps brachii; U ulna; H humerus

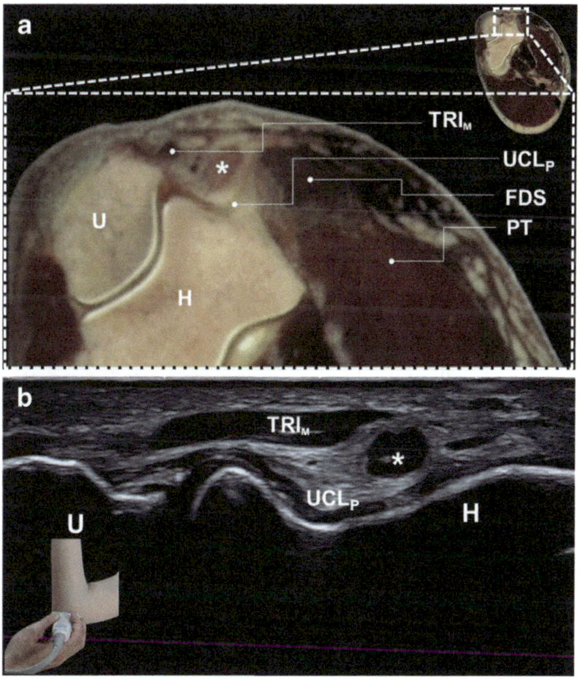

Fig. 6.8 The cadaveric image (**a**) and the corresponding sonoanatomy (**b**) of the posterior bundle of the ulnar collateral ligament in an axial view. Asterisk: ulnar nerve; UCL_P posterior bundle of the ulnar collateral ligament; FDS flexor digitorum superficialis; PT pronator teres; TRI_M medial head of the triceps brachii muscle; U ulna; H humerus

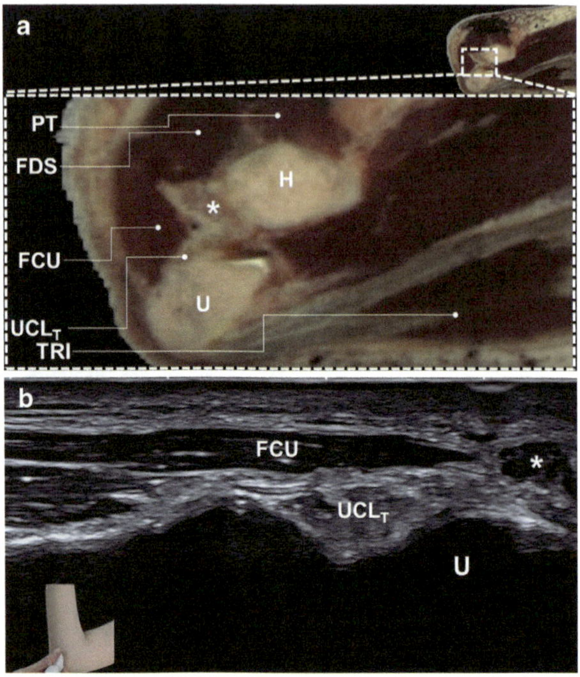

Fig. 6.9 The cadaveric image (**a**) and the corresponding sonoanatomy (**b**) of the transverse bundle of the ulnar collateral ligament. Asterisk: ulnar nerve; UCL_T transverse bundle of the ulnar collateral ligament; FCU flexor carpi ulnaris; FDS flexor digitorum superficialis; PT pronator teres; TRI triceps brachii; U ulna; H humerus

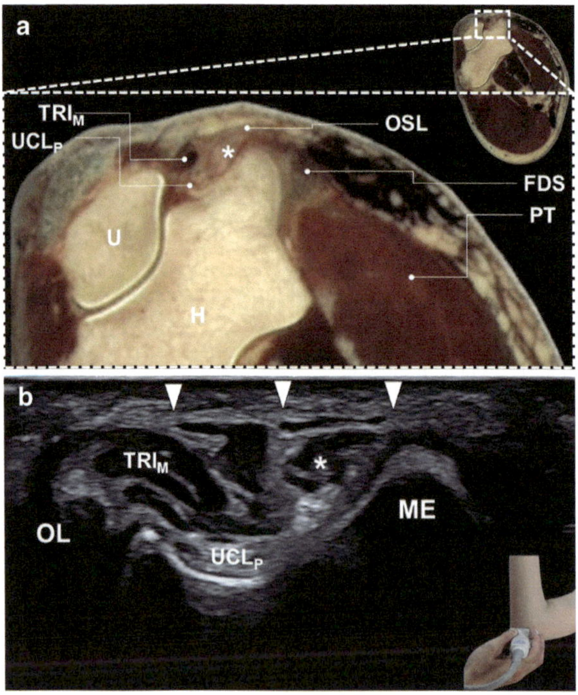

Fig. 6.10 The cadaveric image (**a**) and the corresponding sonoanatomy (**b**) of the ulnar nerve at the medial epicondyle (ME) of the humerus. Asterisks: ulnar nerve; white arrowheads and OSL: Osborne's ligament; FDS flexor digitorum superficialis; PT pronator teres; TRI_M medial head of the triceps brachii muscle; UCL_P posterior bundle of the ulnar collateral ligament; OL olecranon of the ulna; U ulna; H humerus

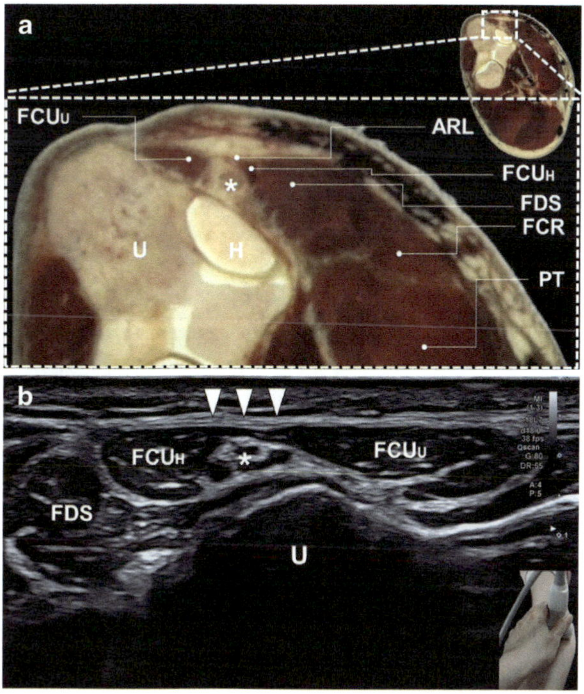

Fig. 6.11 The cadaveric image (**a**) and the corresponding sonoanatomy (**b**) of the ulnar nerve at the level of both heads of the flexor carpi ulnaris muscle. Asterisk: ulnar nerve; white arrowheads and ARL: arcuate ligament; FCR flexor carpi radialis; FCU_H humeral head of the flexor carpi ulnaris; FCU_U ulnar head of the flexor carpi ulnaris; FDS flexor digitorum superficialis; PT pronator teres; U ulna; H humerus

6.4 Pathology

Typical ultrasound findings in cases of medial epicondylitis reveal localized areas with reduced echogenicity. Noteworthy markers include tendon thickening (affected side, Fig. 6.12a; normal side, Fig. 6.12b), irregularities in the cortical structure (Fig. 6.13a), loss of fibrillary pattern (Fig. 6.13b), intratendinous calcifications, and heightened vascularity. When intratendinous hypoechogenicity is observed, applying light compression allows the investigator to assess if adjacent tissues herniate into the hypoechoic area, strongly suggesting at least a partial tear. Severe cases, such as complete tears, may exhibit retraction of the tendon fibers. A 2008 ultrasound study, using clinical symptoms as the reference standard, demonstrated a sensitivity of 95.2%, specificity of 92%, accuracy of 93.5%, positive predictive value of 90.9%, and negative predictive value of 95.8% for clinical medial epicondylitis [9]. The predominant pathological diagnosis in the study was tendinopathy, followed by partial thickness tear.

It is essential to recognize that injuries to the anterior bundle of the ulnar collateral ligament can either simulate or coexist with medial epicondylitis. In a 2014 ultrasound study that included 368 asymptomatic professional baseball pitchers [10], the researchers identified 12 players with ulnar collateral ligament injuries. These individuals exhibited calcifications (long axis, Fig. 6.14a; short axis, Fig. 6.14b), nonsignificant increases in baseline ligament thickness, ulnohumeral

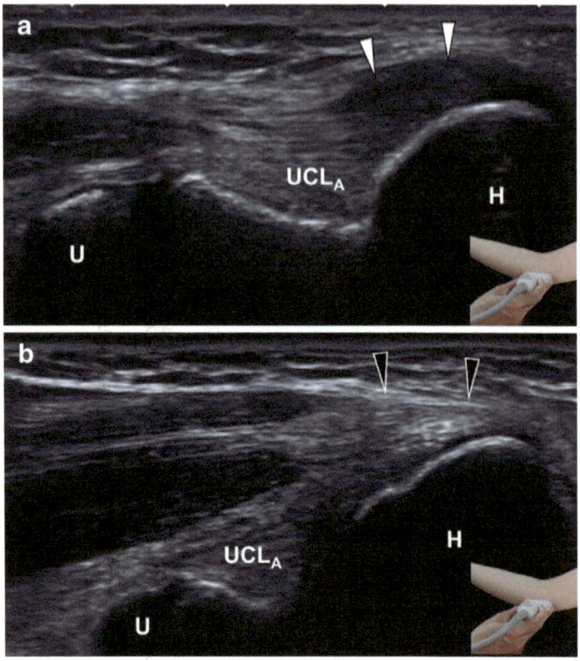

Fig. 6.12 The ultrasonography reveals tendon thickening and hypoechogenicity (white arrowheads) in the common flexor tendon (**a**), in comparison with the tendon (black arrowheads) in the normal side (**b**). UCL$_A$ anterior bundle of the ulnar collateral ligament; U ulna; H humerus

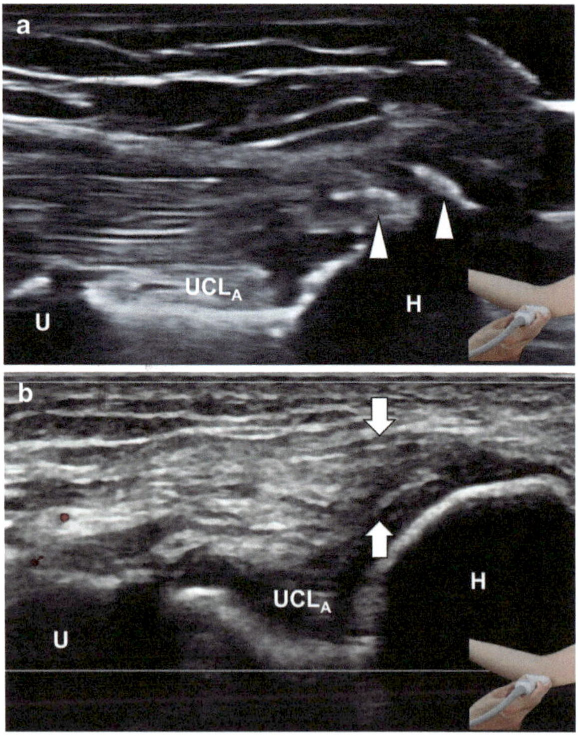

Fig. 6.13 The ultrasonography reveals irregularities (white arrowheads) on the medial epicondyle of the humerus (**a**) and a loss of the fibrillar pattern (white arrows) in the common flexor tendon (**b**). UCL$_A$ anterior bundle of the ulnar collateral ligament; U ulna; H humerus

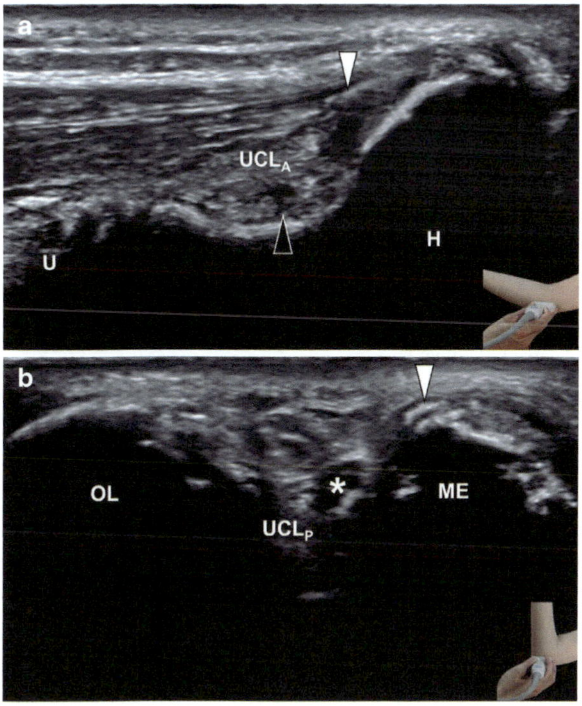

Fig. 6.14 An ultrasound image in the long-axis view (**a**) shows calcification (white arrowheads) in the anterior bundle of the ulnar collateral ligament. A concomitant small partial tear is identified (black arrowhead). The calcification can be more clearly seen by redirecting the transducer to bridge the medial epicondyle and olecranon (**b**). Note: The figures are not from the original study [10] but are similar cases from our databank. Asterisk: ulnar nerve; UCL$_A$ anterior bundle of the ulnar collateral ligament; UCL$_P$ posterior bundle of the ulnar collateral ligament; ME medial epicondyle of the humerus; OL olecranon of the ulna; U ulna; H humerus

joint space gapping under stress (at the static position, Fig. 6.15a; during stress, Fig. 6.15b), as well as the presence of hypoechoic foci on the affected side. A 2022 review has emphasized that employing stress ultrasound imaging can unveil abnormal ulnohumeral joint laxity in cases of ulnar collateral ligament injury [11]. An abnormality is indicated by a distance difference of 2.4 mm before and after the stress test in an injured elbow, and a difference of 1 mm under stress between the involved and non-involved elbows, signifying abnormal ulnohumeral joint laxity. Besides the sonographic findings described in the study, hypervascularity can be observed in the ulnar collateral ligament (Fig. 6.16). Additionally, partial- or full-thickness tears of the ulnar collateral ligament (affected side, Fig. 6.17a; normal side, Fig. 6.17b) or common flexor tendon (partial-thickness tear, Fig. 6.18a; full-thickness tear, Fig. 6.18b) can be present in certain cases.

Excessive stress on the developing skeleton of young athletes can result in elbow injuries collectively referred to as “Little League elbow.” This condition includes both medial epicondylar fragmentation and osteochondritis dissecans (OCD) of the capitellum. In a 2006 ultrasound study involving 153 players from youth baseball teams, sonography revealed that 33 subjects had medial epicondylar fragmentation, while two exhibited early-stage osteochondritis dissecans of the capitellum [12]. Medial epicondylar fragmentation is characterized by a discontinuity in the medial

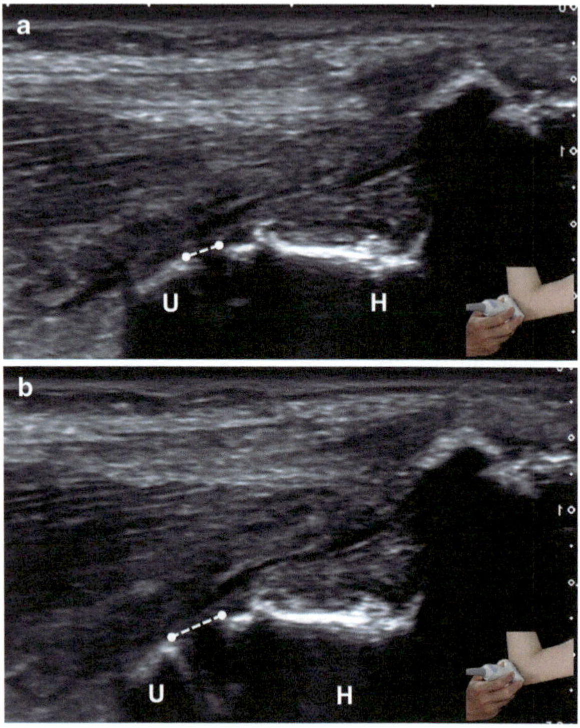

Fig. 6.15 Ultrasonography in the static position (**a**) and during the valgus stress examination (**b**) in a case with an antecedent ulnar collateral ligament injury shows widening of the ulnohumeral joint interval under the valgus stress (dashed line). Note: The figures are not from the original study [10] but are similar cases from our databank. U ulna; H humerus

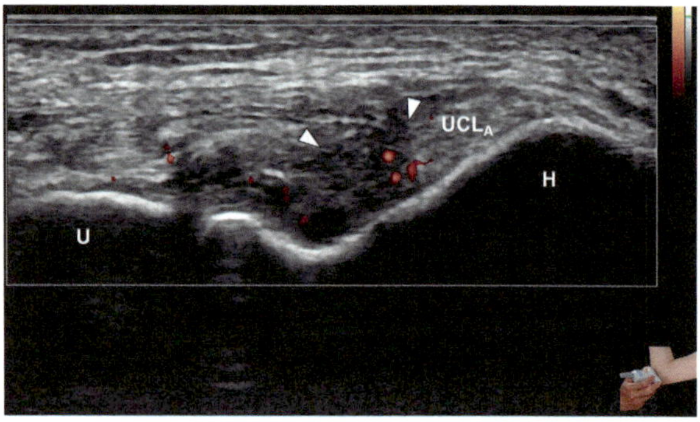

Fig. 6.16 The ultrasonography reveals hypervascularity (white arrowheads) over the anterior bundle of the ulnar collateral ligament (UCL_A). U ulna; H humerus

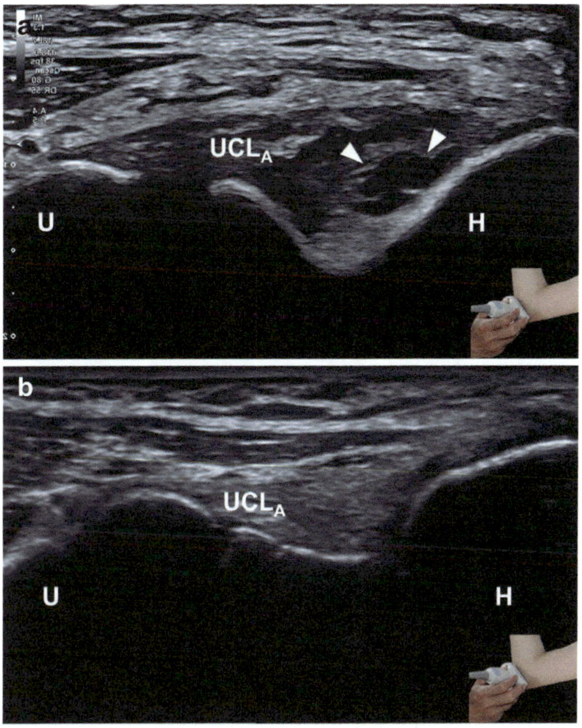

Fig. 6.17 The ultrasonography of the anterior bundle of the ulnar collateral ligament (UCL$_A$) in a case of full-thickness tear (white arrowheads) (**a**) in comparison with the normal side (**b**). U ulna; H humerus

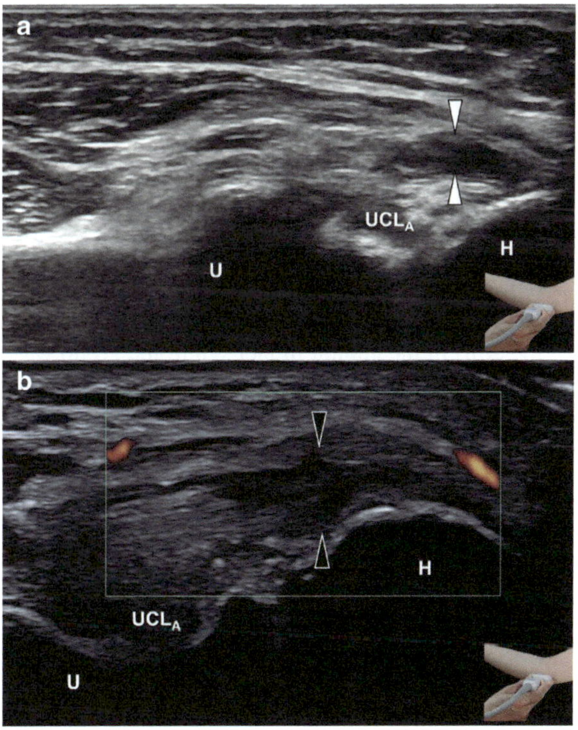

Fig. 6.18 The ultrasonography in the long-axis view of the common flexor tendon reveals a partial thickness tear (white arrowheads) (**a**) and a full-thickness tear (black arrowheads) (**b**). UCL$_A$ anterior bundle of the ulnar collateral ligament; U ulna; H humerus

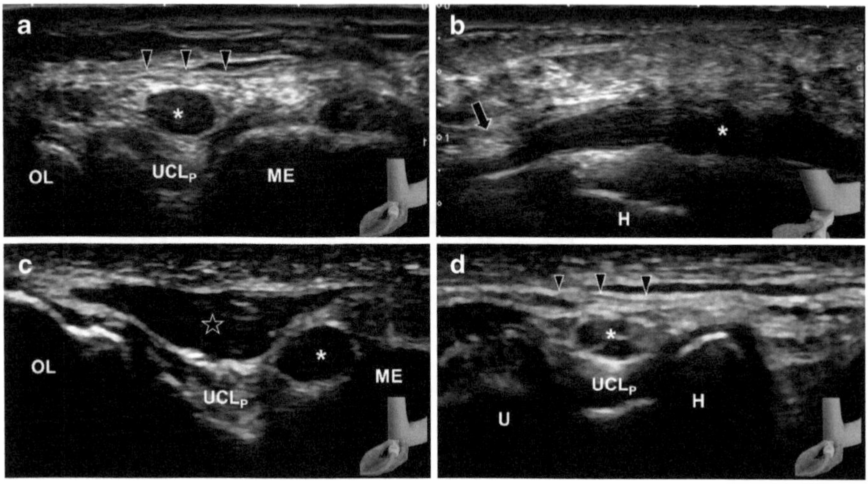

Fig. 6.19 Ultrasonography of cubital tunnel syndrome shows nerve swelling and loss of the fascicular pattern of the ulnar nerve (asterisks) in both the short-axis (**a**) and long-axis (**b**) views. In another case, the ulnar nerve is seen to be entrapped by the anconeus epitrochlearis (star) muscle (**c**), as compared to a normal image (**d**). Black arrowheads: Osborne's ligament; black arrow: arcuate ligament; ME medial epicondyle of the humerus; OL olecranon of the ulna; UCL_P posterior bundle of the ulnar collateral ligament; U ulna; H humerus

epicondyle. On the other hand, OCD of the capitellum with a nondisplaced fragment can be visualized as double-high echogenic contours in the capitellar subchondral bone. Meanwhile, OCD of the capitellum with a displaced fragment may present with an observable osteochondral defect.

Ultrasound has demonstrated its capability in diagnosing cubital tunnel syndrome (short axis, Fig. 6.19a; long axis, Fig. 6.19b), as evidenced by a 2018 meta-analysis [13]. In patients with cubital tunnel syndrome, the cross-sectional area (CSA) was found to be largest at the medial epicondyle level, with a pooled difference of 6 mm^2 between the asymptomatic and symptomatic sides. Using a cutoff point of 10 mm^2 at the medial epicondyle level, the sensitivities and specificities were 0.85 and 0.91, respectively. A subsequent meta-analysis in 2019 [14] revealed that the pooled nerve swelling ratio (such as the maximal CSA divided by the CSA of the arm) in the cubital tunnel syndrome group was significantly larger than that of the controls, potentially serving as a complementary diagnostic parameter. Moreover, entrapment of the ulnar nerve can occur due to the presence of an aberrant muscle, such as the anconeus epitrochlearis (affected side, Fig. 6.19c; non-affected side, Fig. 6.19d). Likewise, a ganglion cyst at the ulnohumeral joint may compress the ulnar nerve, leading to cubital tunnel syndrome (short axis, Fig. 6.20a; long axis, Fig. 6.20b).

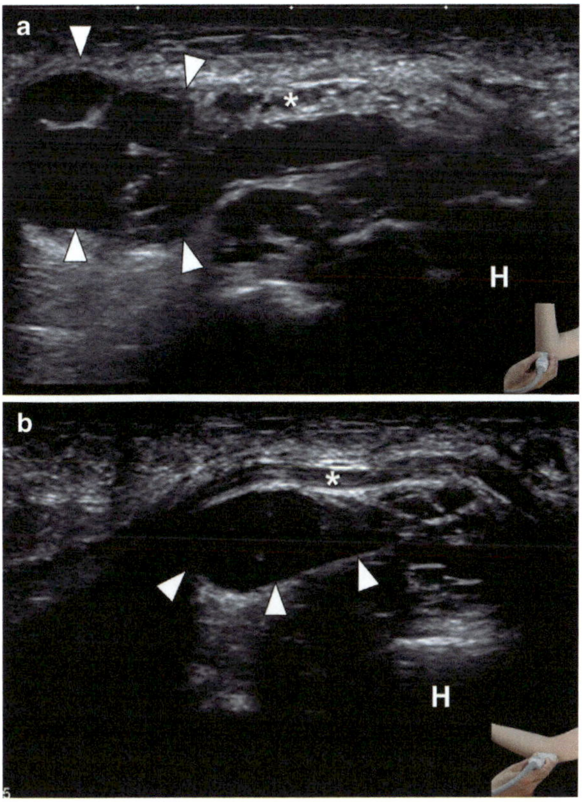

Fig. 6.20 The ultrasound image reveals entrapment of the ulnar nerve (asterisks) due to a nearby ganglion cyst (white arrowheads), shown in both the short-axis (**a**) and long-axis (**b**) views of the ulnar nerve. H humerus

In addition to static ultrasound, dynamic ultrasound proves useful in diagnosing ulnar nerve subluxation. During the examination, the elbow is initially positioned in an extended position with the transducer bridging between the olecranon and medial epicondyle. As the elbow is gradually flexed, individuals with ulnar nerve instability may exhibit subluxation of the ulnar nerve to the anterior aspect of the medial epicondyle (during elbow extension, Fig. 6.21a; during elbow flexion, Fig. 6.21b). In some cases, the medial head of the triceps brachii can also be observed following the ulnar nerve, subluxing to the anterior aspect of the medial epicondyle.

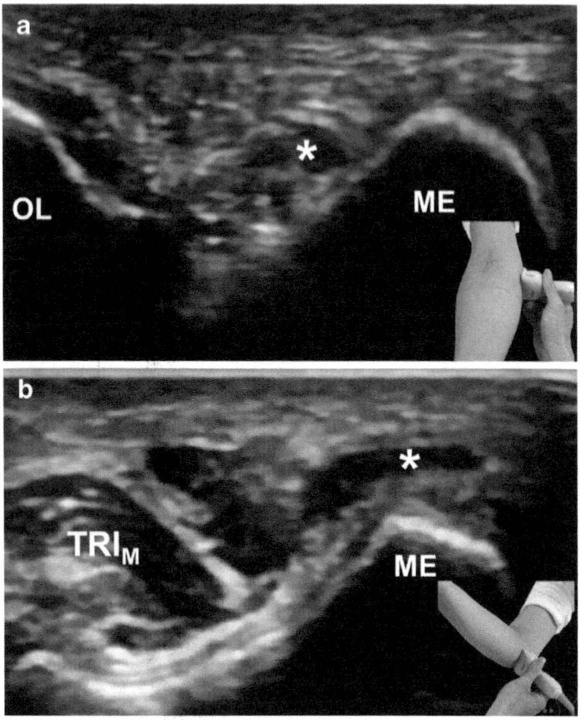

Fig. 6.21 The ultrasonography images in the elbow extension position (**a**) and flexion position (**b**) demonstrate subluxation of the ulnar nerve (asterisk) during elbow flexion. ME medial epicondyle of the humerus; OL olecranon of the ulna; TRI_M medial head of the triceps brachii muscle

6.5 Ultrasound-Guided Intervention

In contrast to studies on lateral epicondylitis, there is a dearth of research investigating the efficacy of various injectables in the treatment of medial epicondylitis. Following a similar approach to the treatment of lateral epicondylitis, options such as corticosteroid, dextrose, platelet-rich plasma, and botulinum toxin can be considered for injecting medial epicondylitis. However, a precautionary step involves assessing the presence of a tear in the common flexor tendon of the wrist or ulnar collateral ligament. If a tear is identified, the use of corticosteroids should be avoided due to their potential adverse effects on connective tissue healing.

When conducting an ultrasound-guided injection for the common flexor tendon of the wrist or the anterior band of the ulnar collateral ligament, it is recommended that the patient lie supine with the arm abducted, elbow flexed, and forearm supinated. In this position, the transducer is aligned along the long axis of the common flexor tendon, and the needle is inserted from caudal to cranial aspects using the in-plane approach (Fig. 6.22). This approach facilitates clear visualization of the tendon and ligament fibers during the injection.

Alternatively, if the patient is seated with the elbow flexed and forearm supinated on the examination table, the transducer can be positioned in the short-axis view of the common flexor tendon of the wrist. While introducing the needle from the

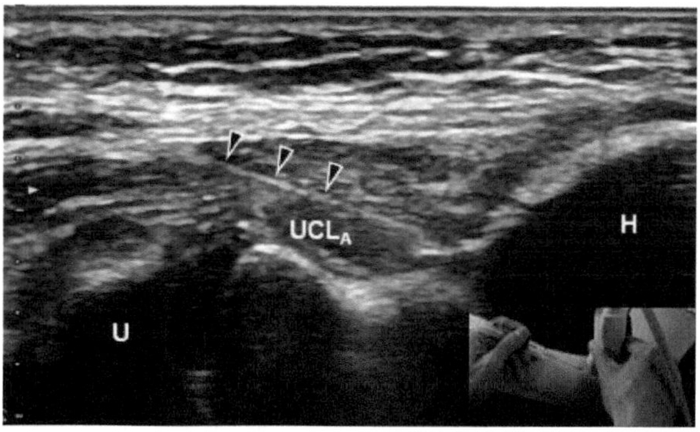

Fig. 6.22 The ultrasound-guided injection is administered to the anterior bundle of the ulnar collateral ligament (UCL_A) using the in-plane approach. Black arrowhead: needle; U ulna; H humerus

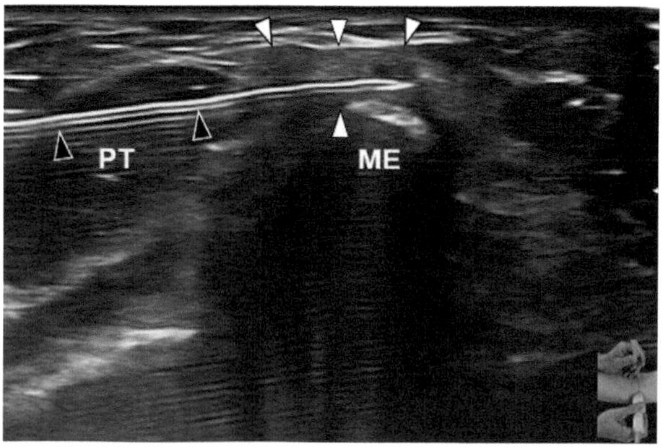

Fig. 6.23 The ultrasound-guided injection is administered to the common flexor tendon (white arrowheads) using the in-plane approach in the short-axis view. Black arrowheads: needle; ME medial epicondyle of the humerus; PT pronator teres

ventral to dorsal aspect is feasible in this view, it is important to note that the view may not provide a distinct demarcation between the common flexor tendon and ulnar collateral ligament due to anisotropy affecting the underlying ulnar collateral ligament (Fig. 6.23). Caution should be exercised, as the medial antebrachial cutaneous nerve may traverse the subcutaneous layer along the needle trajectory.

For injecting the ulnar nerve in patients with cubital tunnel syndrome, both 5% dextrose and corticosteroid have been reported to provide symptomatic relief. If the injection site is chosen at the medial epicondyle, the patient can be seated with the hand resting on the examination table, and the forearm should be pronated to expose the medial aspect of the elbow. Placing one end of the transducer on the medial epicondyle and the other slightly away from the olecranon process (creating an injection window), the needle can be introduced from the olecranon side to the medial epicondyle side (Fig. 6.24).

However, according to a 2018 meta-analysis [13], the most swollen part of the ulnar nerve in cubital tunnel syndrome is at the medial epicondyle. This suggests that the most compressive part should be more distal, such as the area between both heads of the flexor carpi ulnaris, which should be prioritized as the site for nerve hydrodissection. In this case, the patient can lie supine with the elbow flexed and

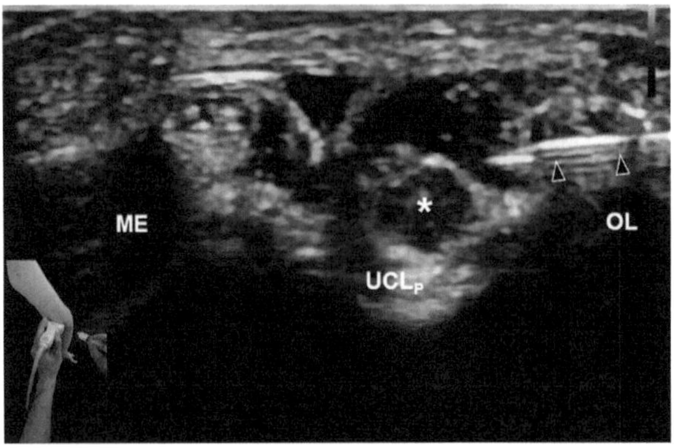

Fig. 6.24 The ultrasound-guided injection is administered to the ulnar nerve (asterisk) at the level of the medial epicondyle of the humerus using the in-plane approach. Black arrowheads: needle; OL olecranon of the ulna; ME medial epicondyle of the humerus; UCL_P posterior bundle of the ulnar collateral ligament

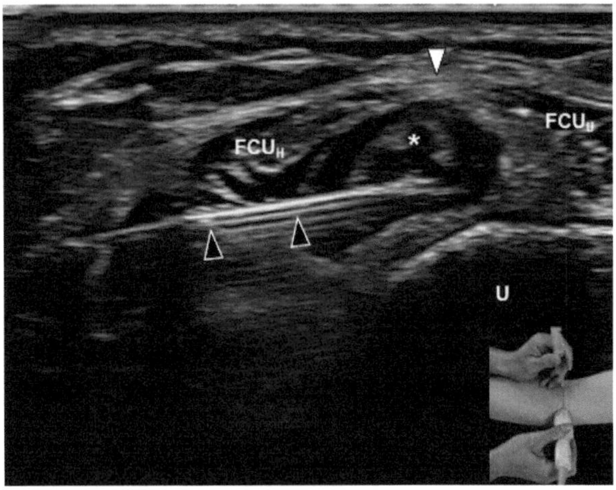

Fig. 6.25 The ultrasound-guided injection is administered to the ulnar nerve (asterisk) between the two heads of the flexor carpi ulnaris using the in-plane approach. Black arrowheads: needle; white arrowhead: arcuate ligament; FCU_H humeral head of the flexor carpi ulnaris; FCU_U ulnar head of the flexor carpi ulnaris; U ulna

forearm supinated. The transducer is then positioned to visualize the ulnar nerve underneath the conjunction of both heads of the flexor carpi ulnaris. The needle can be introduced from the humeral head of the flexor carpi ulnaris to its ulnar head to perform hydrodissection of the ulnar nerve (Fig. 6.25). Moreover, at the cubital tunnel, an anastomosis occurs between the superior ulnar collateral artery and the posterior ulnar recurrent artery (at the medial epicondyle, Fig. 6.26a, b; at both heads of the flexor carpi ulnaris, Fig. 6.26c, d). It is advisable to activate power Doppler before proceeding with the injection.

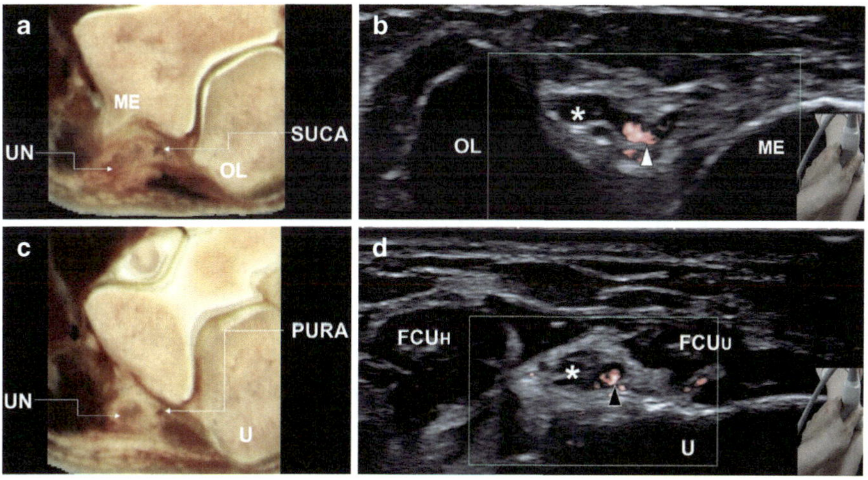

Fig. 6.26 The cadaveric image (**a**) and the corresponding sonoanatomy (**b**) depict the superior ulnar collateral artery (SUCA and white arrowhead) at the cubital tunnel. Distal to the cubital tunnel, the cadaveric image (**c**) and the corresponding sonoanatomy (**d**) show the posterior ulnar recurrent artery (PURA and black arrowhead) between the two heads of the flexor carpi ulnaris. UN and asterisks: ulnar nerve; ME medial epicondyle of the humerus; FCU_H humeral head of the flexor carpi ulnaris; FCU_U ulnar head of the flexor carpi ulnaris; U ulna

6.6 Conclusion

Static ultrasound imaging is well-suited for assessing pathologies of the common flexor tendon of the wrist, ulnar collateral ligament, and ulnar nerve at the elbow level. Dynamic ultrasound proves beneficial in evaluating abnormal ulnohumeral joint laxity and the presence of ulnar nerve subluxation. The patient's positioning is crucial when administering injections over the structures of the medial elbow to establish a suitable window for needle introduction.

Acknowledgment Images and illustrations adapted from cadaveric images provided by the Visible Human Project® of the National Library of Medicine. Excerpts featured in the VH Dissector are used with permission from Touch of Life Technologies Inc.

References

1. Shiri R, Viikari-Juntura E, Varonen H, Heliövaara M. Prevalence and determinants of lateral and medial epicondylitis: a population study. Am J Epidemiol. 2006;164(11):1065–74.
2. Descatha A, Leclerc A, Chastang JF, Roquelaure Y. Medial epicondylitis in occupational settings: prevalence, incidence and associated risk factors. J Occup Environ Med. 2003;45(9):993–1001.
3. Barco R, Antuña SA. Medial elbow pain. EFORT Open Rev. 2017;2(8):362–71.

4. Chang KV, Mezian K, Naňka O, et al. Ultrasound imaging for the cutaneous nerves of the extremities and relevant entrapment syndromes: from anatomy to clinical implications. J Clin Med. 2018;7(11)
5. Luxenburg D, Rizzo MG. Anatomy, shoulder and upper limb, pronator teres. In: StatPearls. Treasure Island (FL) ineligible companies. Disclosure: Michael Rizzo declares no relevant financial relationships with ineligible companies.: StatPearls Publishing Copyright © 2024, StatPearls Publishing LLC.; 2024.
6. Labott JR, Aibinder WR, Dines JS, Camp CL. Understanding the medial ulnar collateral ligament of the elbow: review of native ligament anatomy and function. World J Orthop. 2018;9(6):78–84.
7. Wu CH, Chang KV, Özçakar L, et al. Sonographic tracking of the upper limb peripheral nerves: a pictorial essay and video demonstration. Am J Phys Med Rehabil. 2015;94(9):740–7.
8. Green JR Jr, Rayan GM. The cubital tunnel: anatomic, histologic, and biomechanical study. J Shoulder Elb Surg. 1999;8(5):466–70.
9. Park G-Y, Lee S-M, Lee MY. Diagnostic value of ultrasonography for clinical medial epicondylitis. Arch Phys Med Rehabil. 2008;89(4):738–42.
10. Ciccotti MG, Atanda A Jr, Nazarian LN, Dodson CC, Holmes L, Cohen SB. Stress sonography of the ulnar collateral ligament of the elbow in professional baseball pitchers: a 10-year study. Am J Sports Med. 2014;42(3):544–51.
11. Sutterer BJ, Boettcher BJ, Payne JM, Camp CL, Sellon JL. The role of ultrasound in the evaluation of elbow medial ulnar collateral ligament injuries in throwing athletes. Curr Rev Musculoskelet Med. 2022;15(6):535–46.
12. Harada M, Takahara M, Sasaki J, Mura N, Ito T, Ogino T. Using sonography for the early detection of elbow injuries among young baseball players. AJR Am J Roentgenol. 2006;187(6):1436–41.
13. Chang KV, Wu WT, Han DS, Özçakar L. Ulnar nerve cross-sectional area for the diagnosis of cubital tunnel syndrome: a meta-analysis of ultrasonographic measurements. Arch Phys Med Rehabil. 2018;99(4):743–57.
14. Chen IJ, Chang KV, Wu WT, Özçakar L. Ultrasound parameters other than the direct measurement of ulnar nerve size for diagnosing cubital tunnel syndrome: a systemic review and meta-analysis. Arch Phys Med Rehabil. 2019;100(6):1114–30.

Chapter 7
Posterior Elbow Pain Unveiled: Elaborating the Triceps Brachii Distal Tendon

Ke-Vin Chang, Wei-Ting Wu, and Yuan-Yuan Tsai

7.1 Introduction

In a magnetic resonance imaging study, Koplas et al. [1] analyzed 801 consecutive elbow examinations, offering a thorough overview of clinical findings. From this extensive review, the researchers identified 28 patients with a total of 30 triceps brachii tendon injuries, distinguishing between partial and complete tears. The prevalence of triceps brachii tendon injuries in this study was 3.8%. Among this cohort, partial tears emerged as the most prevalent injury, with pain standing out as the predominant symptom. Notably, athletic-related factors, particularly in weightlifting, were identified as the primary cause of injuries. The study also shed light on significant associations, revealing six cases where tendon tears were complications of infection and three cases linked to steroid use.

Furthermore, the investigation uncovered an increased incidence of distal triceps brachii tendon injuries, attributing this trend to the growing popularity of weight training [2]. This noteworthy finding challenges conventional perceptions that typically associate weightlifter's elbow with triceps brachii tendon inflammation or degeneration, highlighting the substantial impact on the triceps brachii tendon located at the posterior aspect of the elbow.

Building upon these pivotal insights, the subsequent chapter will intricately explore the anatomy of the triceps myotendinous complex. It aims to elucidate the application of ultrasound for scrutinizing the triceps brachii tendon, provide a comprehensive discussion on common pathologies, and offer valuable tips for conducting ultrasound-guided injections. This scientific thesis endeavors to contribute to a broader understanding of triceps brachii tendon injuries and their clinical management.

K.-V. Chang (✉) · W.-T. Wu · Y.-Y. Tsai
Bei-Hu Branch, National Taiwan University Hospital, Taipei, Taiwan

K.-V. Chang (ed.), *Ultrasonography of Musculoskeletal Pain*,
https://doi.org/10.1007/978-981-96-6787-1_7

7.2 Regional Anatomy

The long head of the triceps brachii arises from the infraglenoid tubercle of the scapula, establishing a point of attachment that facilitates not only elbow extension but also exerts a modest influence on the glenohumeral joint [3]. When the arm is adducted, the triceps brachii muscle aids in maintaining the head of the humerus within the glenoid cavity, preventing displacement. Additionally, the long head plays a role in the extension and adduction of the arm at the shoulder joint. In contrast, the medial head stems from the dorsal humerus, inferior to the radial groove, and connects to the medial intermuscular septum (Fig. 7.1). Lacking an attachment to the scapula, the medial head does not influence the glenohumeral joint regarding stabilization or movement. Nevertheless, it engages during forearm extension at the elbow joint, especially when the forearm is in a supinated or pronated position. Similar to the medial head, the lateral head arises from the dorsal humerus but is cranial to the spiral groove, fusing with the lateral intermuscular septum. Recognized as the strongest among the three heads, the lateral head is also active during forearm extension at the elbow joint, particularly in supinated or pronated forearm positions.

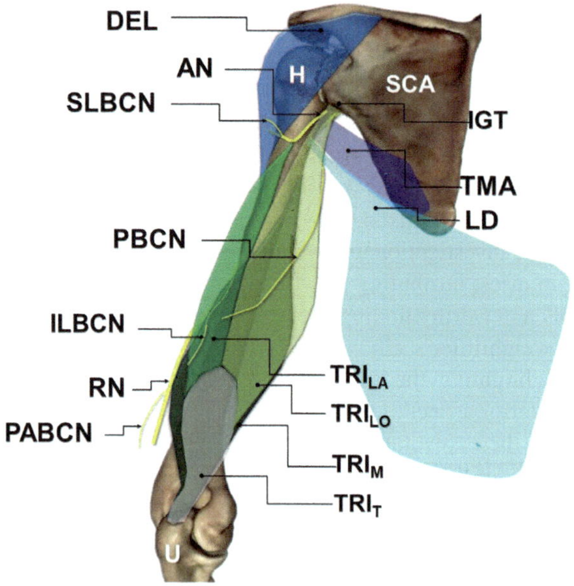

Fig. 7.1 The illustration depicts the three heads of the triceps brachii (long head, lateral head, and medial head), the courses of the peripheral nerves in the posterior arm as they travel between the surrounding muscles, and their relation with the humerus (H), scapula (SCA) and ulna (U). TMA teres major; LD latissimus dorsi; TRI_{LA} lateral head of the triceps brachii; TRI_{LO} long head of the triceps brachii; TRI_M medial head of the triceps brachii; TRI_T tendon of the triceps brachii; PBCN posterior brachial cutaneous nerve; ILBCN inferior lateral brachial cutaneous nerve; PABCN posterior antebrachial cutaneous nerve; RN radial nerve; AN axillary nerve; SLBCN superior lateral brachial cutaneous nerve; DEL deltoid; IGT infraglenoid tubercle

The radial nerve supplies nerves to the triceps brachii. However, findings from a cadaveric study conducted by Athlani et al. [4] suggest that the medial head of the triceps brachii may receive innervation from the ulnar nerve. Additionally, further research indicates that the long head of the triceps brachii can also be innervated by the axillary nerve. On the contrary, the radial nerve branches into various cutaneous nerves, including the posterior brachial cutaneous nerve (for the back of the arm), the inferior lateral brachial cutaneous nerve (for the lower lateral part of the arm), and the posterior antebrachial cutaneous nerve (for the skin on the lower half of the arm and the posterior lateral aspect of the forearm). As for the proximal region of the long head of the triceps brachii and the posterior lateral deltoid muscle, they receive innervation from the superior lateral brachial cutaneous nerve (also known as the superior lateral cutaneous nerve of the arm), a branch stemming from the axillary nerve, which supplies the aforementioned skin areas (Fig. 7.2).

Beletani [5] and colleagues conducted a cadaveric investigation to describe the normal magnetic resonance anatomy of the triceps brachii tendon insertion. Twelve cadaveric elbows were utilized following institutional guidelines. T1-weighted spin-echo magnetic resonance images were acquired, and the findings from imaging were compared with data from anatomic and histologic studies. On the magnetic resonance images, the triceps brachii tendon exhibited a bipartite appearance upon insertion into the olecranon in all specimens. The insertion of the medial head was deeper compared to the long and lateral heads, primarily demonstrating a muscular connection at its insertion, with a minor portion of the tendon blending with the muscle distally. Histopathological analysis revealed a common insertion of the three heads of the triceps brachii on the olecranon. Interestingly, the bipartite aspect observed in the images was absent in the histologic examination, indicating a fusion of the medial and common tendons just prior to their insertion into the bone.

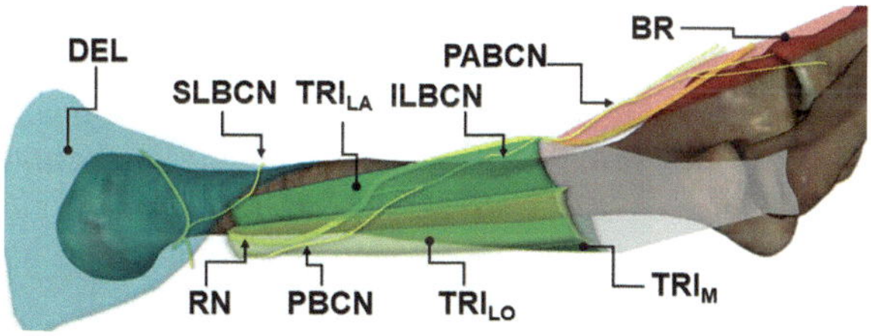

Fig. 7.2 The illustration delineates the trajectories of the terminal branches of radial and axillary nerves in the posterior arm along with the pertinent structures. SLBCN superior lateral brachial cutaneous nerve; PBCN posterior brachial cutaneous nerve; ILBCN inferior lateral brachial cutaneous nerve; RN radial nerve; PABCN posterior antebrachial cutaneous nerve; DEL deltoid; TRI$_{LO}$ long head of the triceps brachii; TRI$_{LA}$ lateral head of triceps brachii; TRI$_{M}$ medial head of the triceps brachii; BR brachioradialis

7.3 Sonoanatomy

The examinee can position the hand being examined over the table, with the elbow flexed and the olecranon facing toward the examiner. The scanning begins at the olecranon in the axial plane, where the triceps brachii tendon, primarily originating from the convergence of the lateral and long heads of the triceps brachii muscle, attaches. By moving the transducer cranially, the short axis of the triceps brachii distal tendon can be visualized (Fig. 7.3a, b). By shifting the transducer to the ulnar aspect, the medial head of the triceps brachii muscle and the ulnar nerve can be visualized (Fig. 7.4a, b). Beneath the distal triceps brachii tendon lies the muscle of the medial head of the triceps brachii, and the olecranon fossa, normally filled with fat, is seen deep to this muscle (Fig. 7.5a, b).

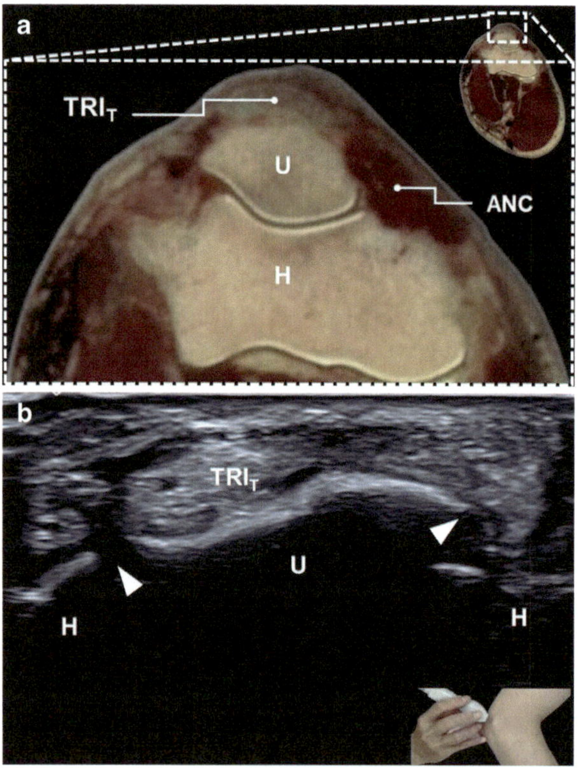

Fig. 7.3 The cadaveric image (**a**) and corresponding sonoanatomy (**b**) display the triceps brachii tendon in the axial view at the level of the ulnohumeral joint (white arrowheads). TRI$_T$ triceps brachii tendon; ANC anconeus; U ulna; H humerus

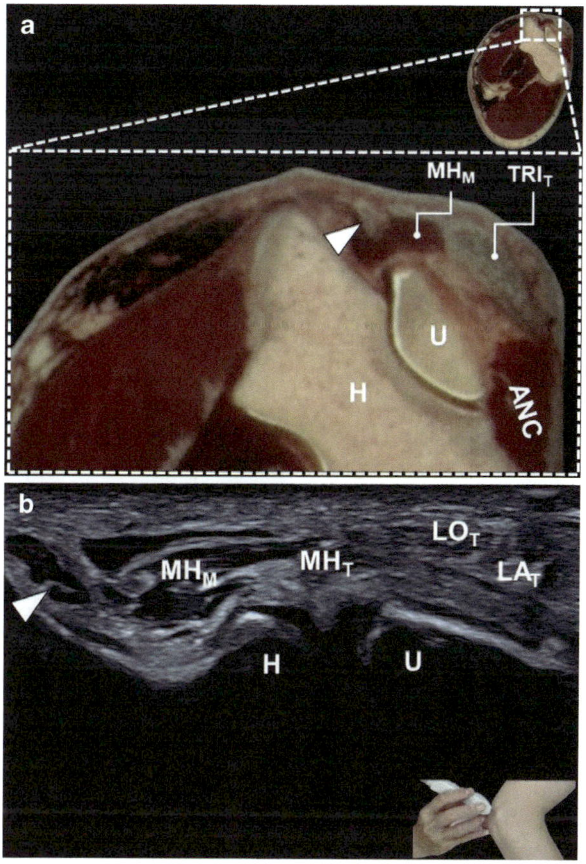

Fig. 7.4 The cadaveric image (**a**) and corresponding sonoanatomy in the axial view (**b**) depict the medial head of the triceps brachii muscle at the level of the ulnohumeral joint. White arrowheads: ulnar nerve; MH$_M$ medial head muscle of the triceps brachii; TRI$_T$ triceps brachii tendon; MH$_T$ medial head tendon of the triceps brachii; LO$_T$ long head tendon of the triceps brachii; LA$_T$ lateral head tendon of the triceps brachii; U ulna; H humerus

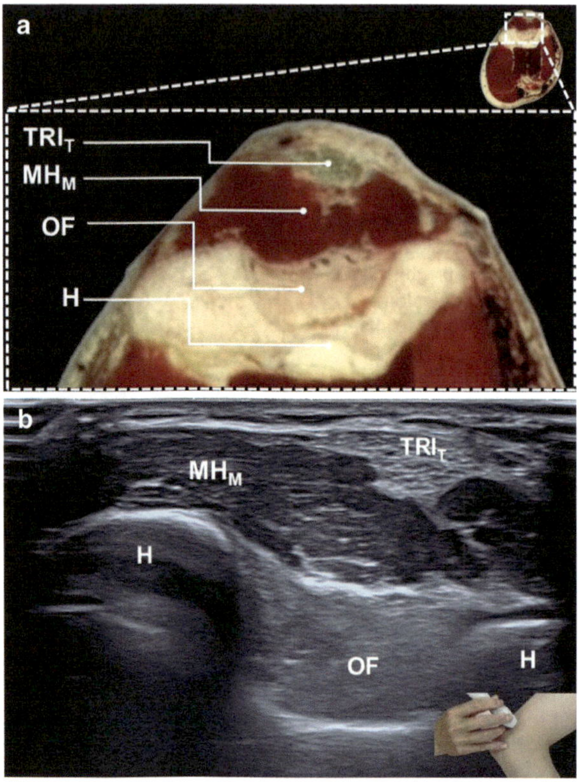

Fig. 7.5 The cadaveric image (**a**) and corresponding sonoanatomy (**b**), shown in the axial view, depict the triceps brachii tendon at the level of the olecranon fossa. TRI$_T$ triceps brachii tendon; MH$_M$ medial head muscle of the triceps brachii; OF olecranon fossa; H humerus

In the axial view at the cranial end of the olecranon fossa, the medial head of the triceps brachii muscle encircles the majority of the posterior humeral shaft (Fig. 7.6a, b). Further cranial movement of the transducer reveals an increase in the muscle bulk of the long and lateral heads of the triceps brachii, while the muscle bulk of the medial head of the triceps brachii decreases (Fig. 7.7a, b). More cranially, the radial nerve is first observed at the spiral groove between the medial and lateral heads of the triceps brachii muscle. As the muscle volume of the medial head of the triceps brachii diminishes, the origin of the medial head becomes clearly demarcated in the

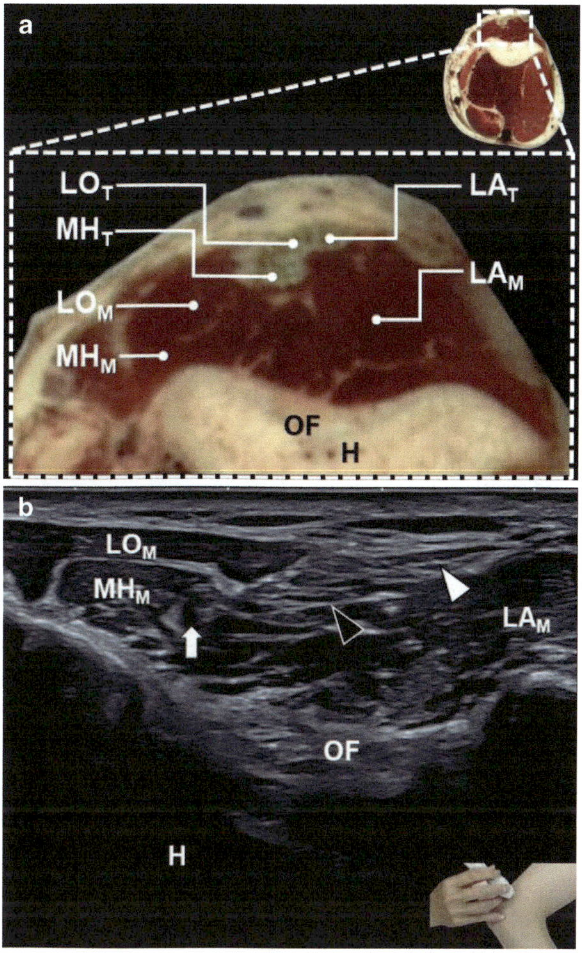

Fig. 7.6 The cadaveric image (**a**) and corresponding sonoanatomy (**b**) in the axial view depict the three heads of the triceps brachii muscle at the cranial end of the olecranon fossa. LA_T and white arrowhead: lateral head tendon of the triceps brachii; LO_T and black arrowhead: long head tendon of the triceps brachii; MH_T and white arrow: medial head tendon of the triceps brachii; MH_M medial head muscle of the triceps brachii; LO_M long head muscle of the triceps brachii; LA_M lateral head muscle of the triceps brachii; OF olecranon fossa; H humerus

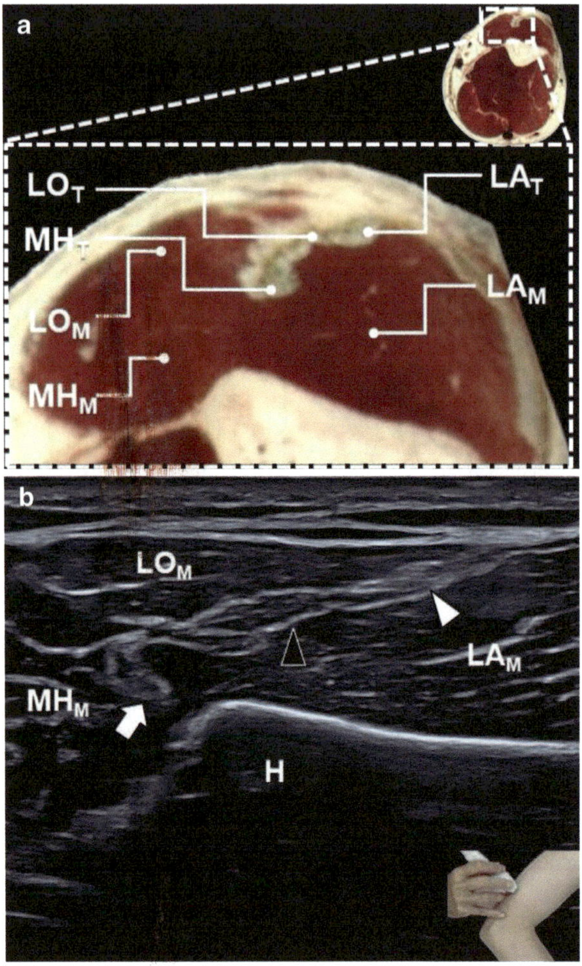

Fig. 7.7 The cadaveric image (**a**) and corresponding sonoanatomy (**b**) in the axial view depict the three heads of the triceps brachii muscle and their tendons in the lower third of the arm. LA_T and white arrowhead: lateral head tendon of the triceps brachii; LO_T and black arrowhead: long head tendon of the triceps brachii; MH_T and white arrow: medial head tendon of the triceps brachii; MH_M medial head muscle of the triceps brachii; LO_M long head muscle of the triceps brachii; LA_M lateral head muscle of the triceps brachii; H humerus

axial (Fig. 7.8a, b) and longitudinal views (Fig. 7.8b, d). On the other hand, the origin of the lateral head of the triceps muscle can be identified in its axial (Fig. 7.9a, c) and longitudinal views (Fig. 7.9b, d), just caudal to the attachment of the teres minor muscle on the posterior lateral humerus. Finally, the transducer can be moved cranially to the level of the infraglenoid tubercle of the scapulae, where the origin of the long head of the triceps muscle can be depicted in both axial (Fig. 7.10a, c) and longitudinal views (Fig. 7.10b, d).

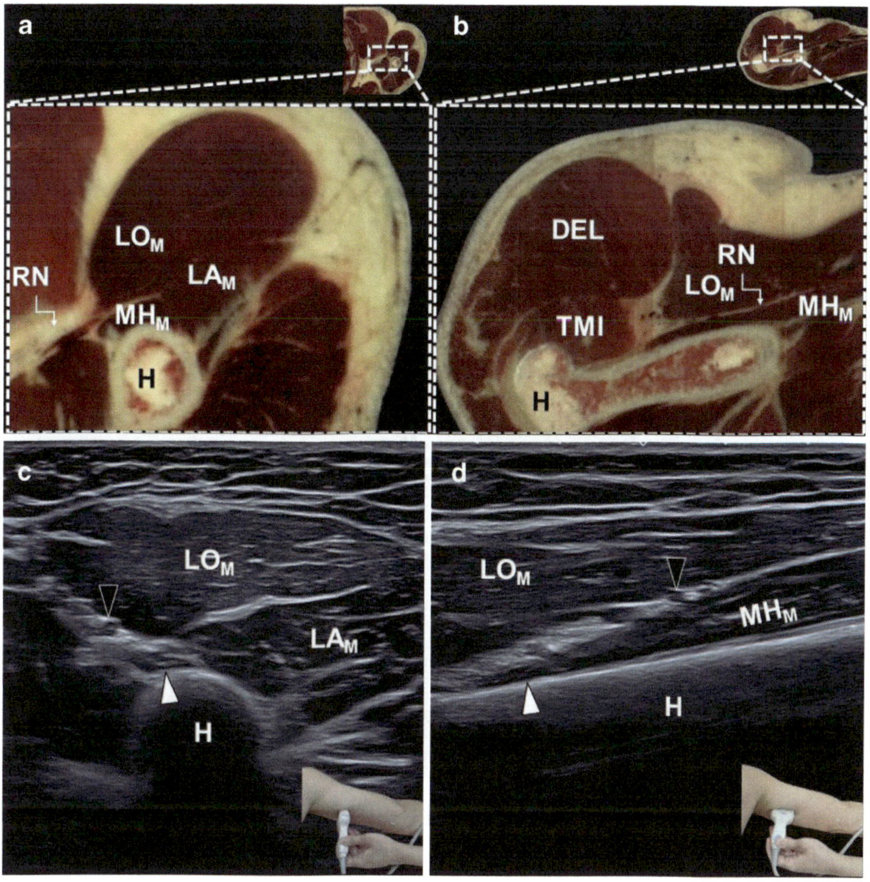

Fig. 7.8 The cadaveric images and corresponding sonoanatomy in the axial (**a**, **c**) and longitudinal (**b**, **d**) views illustrate the origin of the medial head of the triceps brachii muscle and its associated structures. RN and black arrowheads: radial nerve; white arrowhead: medial head origin of the triceps brachii; MH_M medial head muscle of the triceps brachii; LO_M long head muscle of triceps brachii; LA_M lateral head muscle of triceps brachii; TMI teres minor; DEL deltoid; H humerus

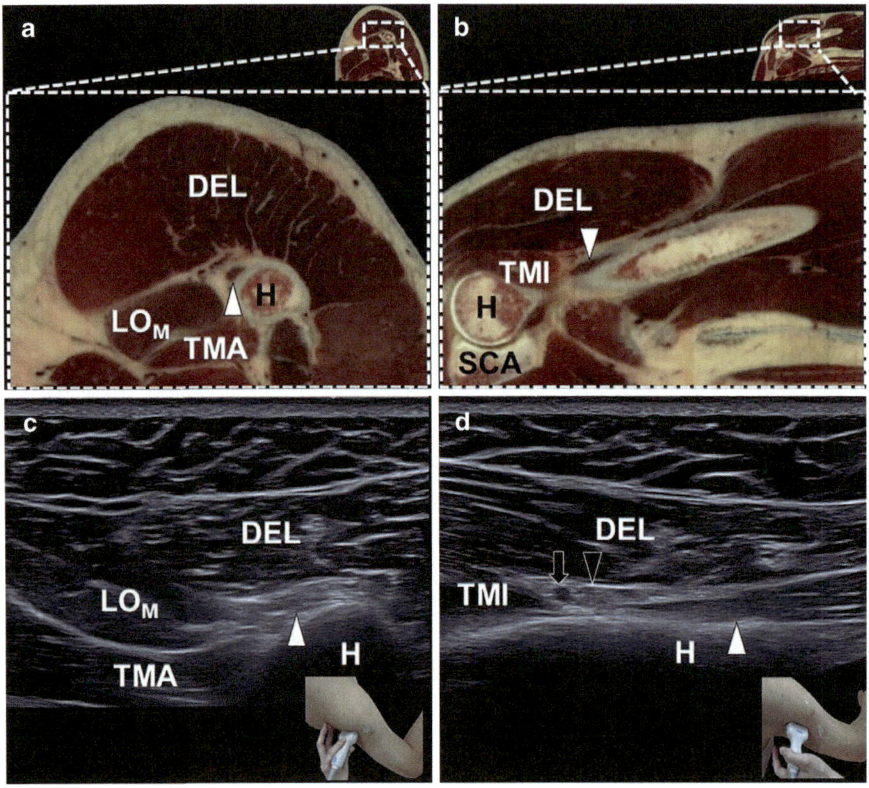

Fig. 7.9 The cadaveric images and corresponding sonoanatomy in the axial (**a**, **c**) and longitudinal (**b**, **d**) views depict the origin of the lateral head of the triceps brachii muscle and its associated structures. White arrowheads: lateral head origin of the triceps brachii; black arrowhead: axillary nerve; black arrow: posterior humeral circumflex artery; DEL deltoid; LO_M long head muscle of the triceps brachii; TMA teres major; TMI teres minor; SCA scapula; H humerus

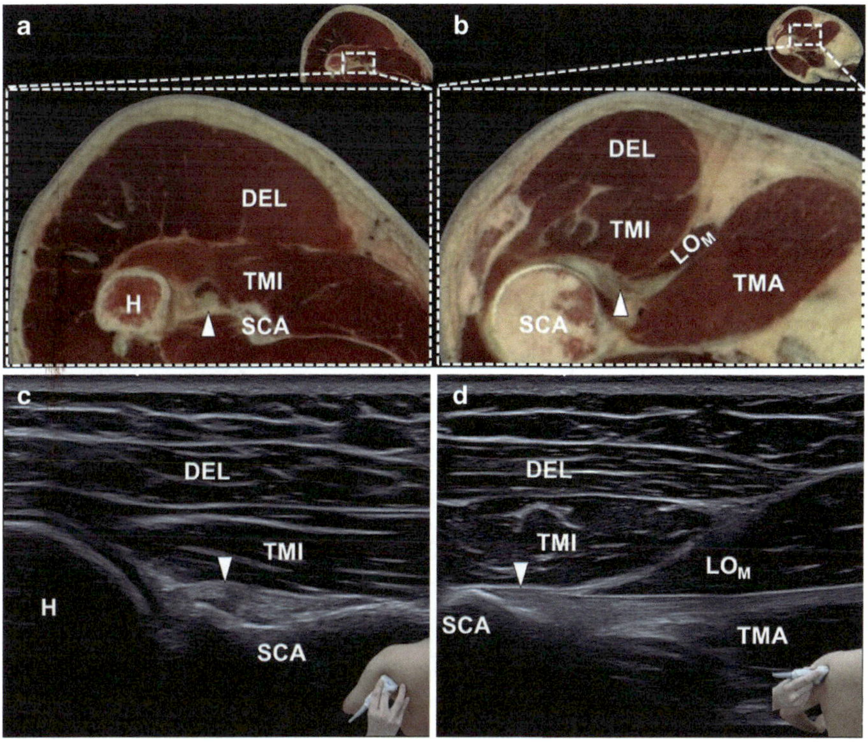

Fig. 7.10 The cadaveric image and the corresponding sonoanatomy in the axial (**a**, **c**) and longitudinal (**b**, **d**) views illustrate the origin of the long head of the triceps brachii muscle and the relevant structures. White arrowheads: long head origin of the triceps brachii; LO_M long head muscle of the triceps brachii; DEL deltoid; TMI teres minor; TMA teres major; SCA scapula; H humerus

After investigating the reciprocal relationship of the three heads of the triceps brachii muscle in the axial view, the transducer can be rotated 90 degrees to observe the distal tendon, which displays a hyperechoic fibrillary pattern attaching to the proximal tip of the olecranon. The scanning sequence begins along the long axis of the lateral head (Fig. 7.11a, b), proceeds to the junction between the lateral and long heads (Fig. 7.12a, b), and concludes at the long axis of the medial head (Fig. 7.13a, b).

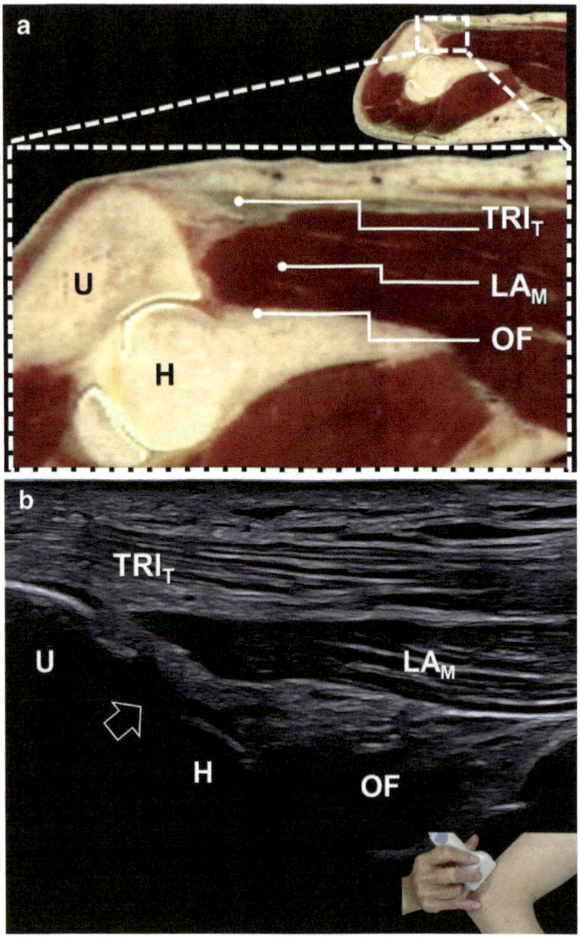

Fig. 7.11 The cadaveric image (**a**) and corresponding sonoanatomy (**b**) depict the triceps brachii tendon along the long axis of the lateral head muscle of the triceps brachii. TRI_T triceps brachii tendon; black arrow: ulnohumeral joint; LA_M lateral head muscle of triceps brachii; OF olecranon fossa; U ulna; H humerus

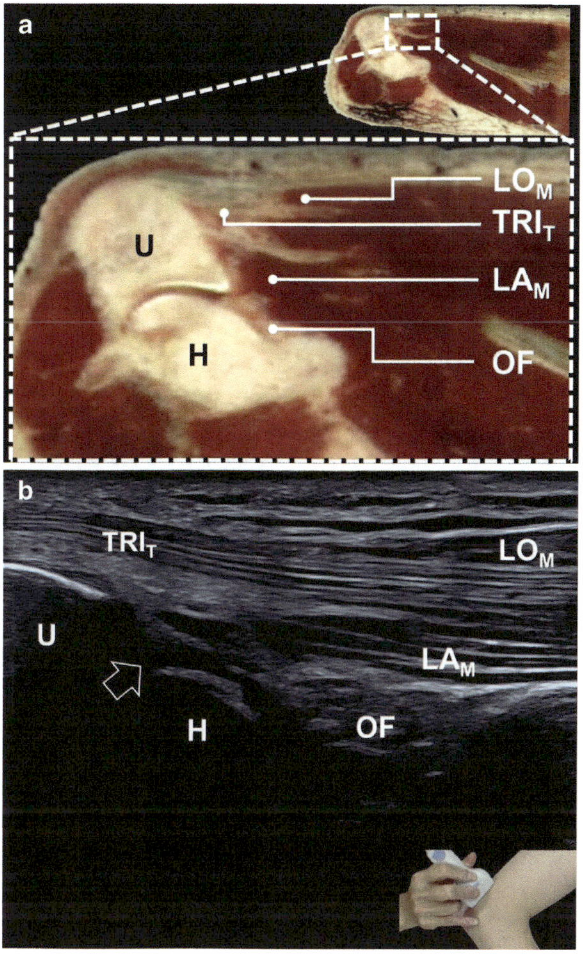

Fig. 7.12 The cadaveric image (**a**) and corresponding sonoanatomy (**b**) depict the triceps brachii tendon at the junction between the lateral and long heads of the triceps brachii muscle. TRI_T: triceps brachii tendon; black arrow: ulnohumeral joint; LA_M lateral head muscle of the triceps brachii; LO_M long head muscle of the triceps brachii; OF olecranon fossa; U ulna; H humerus

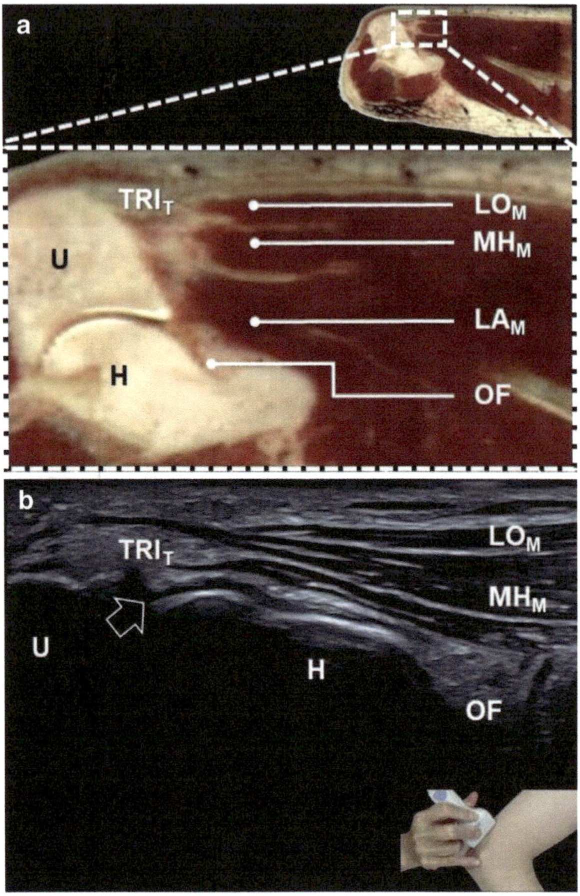

Fig. 7.13 The cadaveric image (**a**) and corresponding sonoanatomy (**b**) depict the triceps brachii tendon along the medial head of the triceps brachii. Black arrow: ulnohumeral joint; TRI$_T$ triceps brachii tendon; LA$_M$ lateral head muscle of the triceps brachii; LO$_M$ long head muscle of the triceps brachii; MH$_M$ medial head muscle of the triceps brachii; OF olecranon fossa; U ulna; H humerus

There are many cutaneous nerves relevant to the posterior arm extending to the elbow. After exiting the quadrilateral space, the axillary nerve divides into an anterior branch, which innervates the deltoid muscle, and a posterior branch, which innervates both the deltoid and teres minor muscles. The posterior branch also gives rise to the superior lateral brachial cutaneous nerve, supplying sensation to the superolateral aspect of the arm (short axis, Fig. 7.14a, b; long axis, Fig. 7.14c).

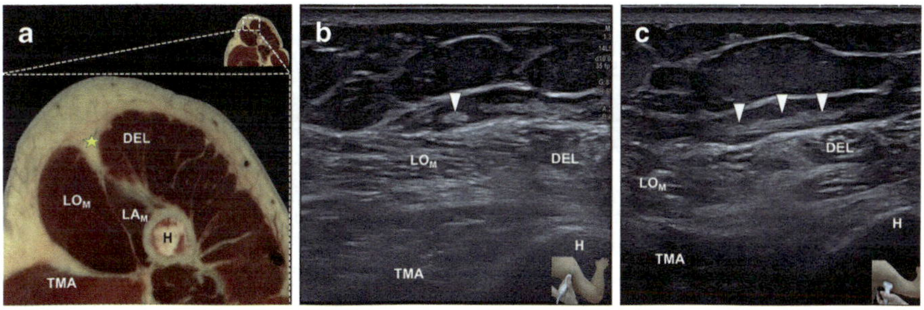

Fig. 7.14 The cadaveric image in the axial plane (**a**) and corresponding sonoanatomy in the short axis (**b**) and long axis (**c**) illustrate the superior lateral brachial cutaneous nerve (star and white arrowheads) and its relevant structures. DEL deltoid; LA_M lateral head muscle of triceps brachii; LO_M long head muscle of triceps brachii; TMA teres major; H humerus

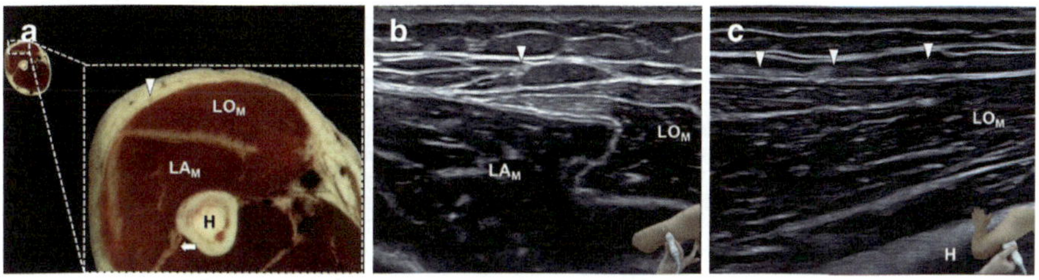

Fig. 7.15 The cadaveric image (**a**) and the corresponding sonoanatomy depict the posterior brachial cutaneous nerve in the short axis (**b**) and the long axis (**c**). White arrow: radial nerve; white arrowheads: posterior brachial cutaneous nerve; LO_M long head muscle of the triceps brachii; LA_M lateral head muscle of the triceps brachii; H humerus

The superior lateral brachial cutaneous nerve may anastomose with the posterior brachial cutaneous nerve, also known as the posterior cutaneous nerve of the arm. As the first branch of the radial nerve, the posterior brachial cutaneous nerve penetrates the long head of the triceps brachii before entering the spiral groove. It then pierces the brachial fascia superficially and courses laterally between the long and lateral heads of the triceps brachii muscle (short axis, Fig. 7.15a, b; long axis, Fig. 7.15c).

During its course in the spiral groove, the radial nerve gives rise to the inferior lateral brachial cutaneous nerve, also known as the inferior lateral cutaneous nerve of the arm, which penetrates the lateral head of the triceps brachii muscle and into the brachial fascia (short axis, Fig. 7.16a, c; long axis, Fig. 7.16b, d). Finally, the posterior antebrachial cutaneous nerve separates from the main trunk of the radial nerve upon exiting the spiral groove [6]. It emerges to the subcutaneous layer between the brachioradialis and triceps brachii, bypassing the lateral intermuscular septum unlike the main trunk of the radial nerve (short axis, Fig. 7.17a, b; long axis,

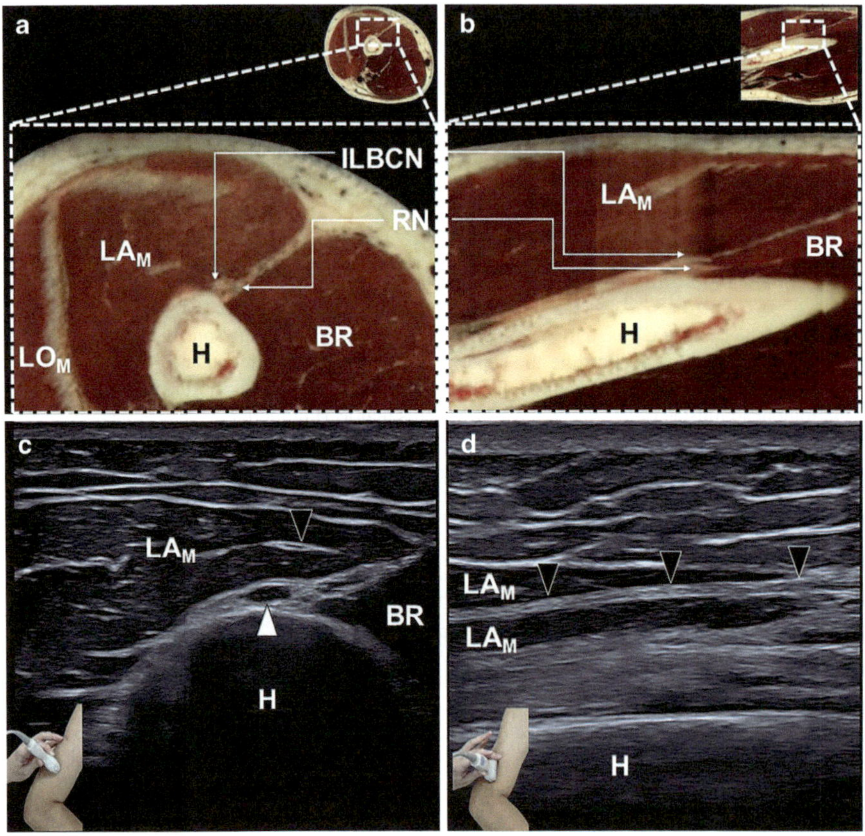

Fig. 7.16 The cadaveric images and corresponding sonoanatomy in the short-axis (**a**, **c**) and long-axis (**b**, **d**) views depict the inferior lateral brachial cutaneous nerve and the associated muscles. White arrowhead: radial nerve; black arrowheads: inferior lateral brachial cutaneous nerve; LO_M long head muscle of the triceps brachii; LA_M lateral head muscle of the triceps brachii; BR brachioradialis muscle; H humerus

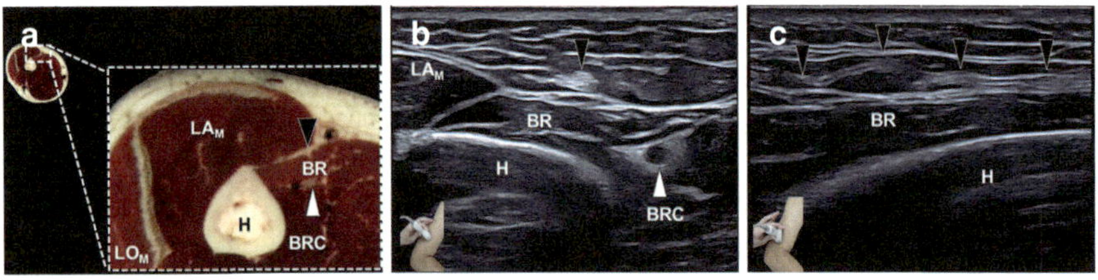

Fig. 7.17 The cadaveric image (**a**) and the corresponding sonoanatomy depict the posterior antebrachial cutaneous nerve in the short-axis (**b**) and long-axis (**c**) views. White arrowheads: radial nerve; black arrowheads: posterior antebrachial cutaneous nerve; LO_M long head muscle of the triceps brachii; LA_M lateral head muscle of triceps brachii; BR brachioradialis; BRC brachialis; H humerus

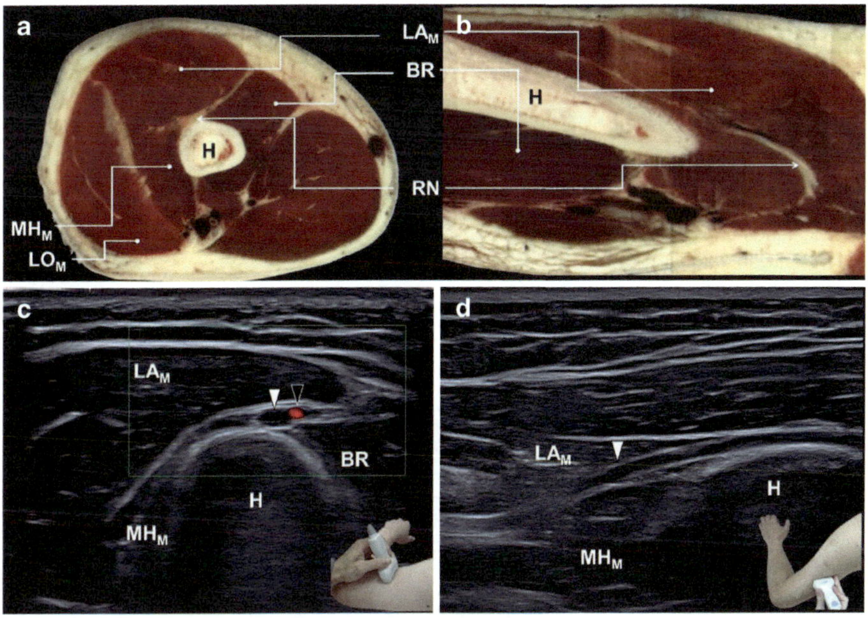

Fig. 7.18 The cadaveric images and corresponding sonoanatomy in the axial (**a**, **c**) and sagittal (**b**, **d**) planes illustrate the anatomical relationships of the radial nerve, profunda brachii artery, and associated muscles. White arrowheads and RN: radial nerve; black arrowhead: profunda brachii artery; MH_M medial head muscle of the triceps brachii; LO_M long head muscle of triceps brachii; LA_M lateral head muscle of triceps brachii; BR brachioradialis; H humerus

Fig. 7.17c). Notably, the profunda brachii artery accompanies the main trunk of the radial nerve (short axis, Fig. 7.18a, c; long axis, Fig. 7.18b, d). Power Doppler ultrasound is useful in differentiating between the anechoic, circular structures of the nerve and the artery.

Laterally to the olecranon process, the oblique-oriented anconeus muscle becomes visible (Fig. 7.19a, b). The lateral edge of the transducer should be pivoted towards the lateral epicondyle to mark the cranial origin of the muscle. The muscle's caudal attachment encompasses the olecranon process and the superior part of the posterior ulna.

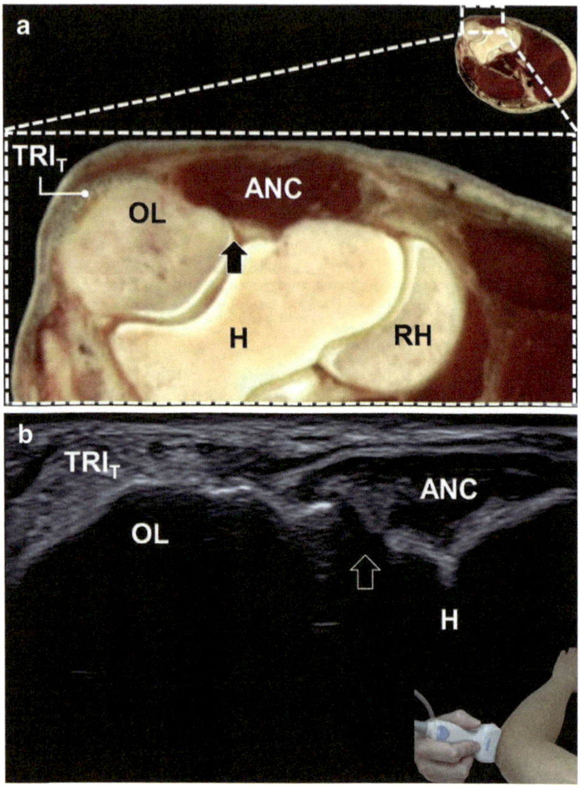

Fig. 7.19 The cadaveric image in the axial plane (**a**) and the corresponding sonoanatomy (**b**) depict the anconeus muscle. Black arrows: ulnohumeral joint; TRI$_T$ triceps brachii tendon; ANC anconeus; OL olecranon process of ulna; RH head of the radius; H humerus

7.4 Pathologies

The evaluation of the distal triceps brachii tendon should span from its origin at the myotendinous junction to its insertion on the olecranon. Employing flexion-extension and medio-lateral movements can assist in discerning tendinous components, particularly those associated with the deep medial and superficial long/lateral heads of the triceps brachii. Triceps tendinopathy can present along a spectrum ranging from tendinosis to complete triceps tendon rupture. In instances of tendinopathy, the triceps tendon insertion exhibits thickening and hypoechoic characteristics, potentially accompanied by a few flecks of calcification (Fig. 7.20a) as well as intra-tendinous hypervascularity (long axis, Fig. 7.20b; short axis, Fig. 7.20c).

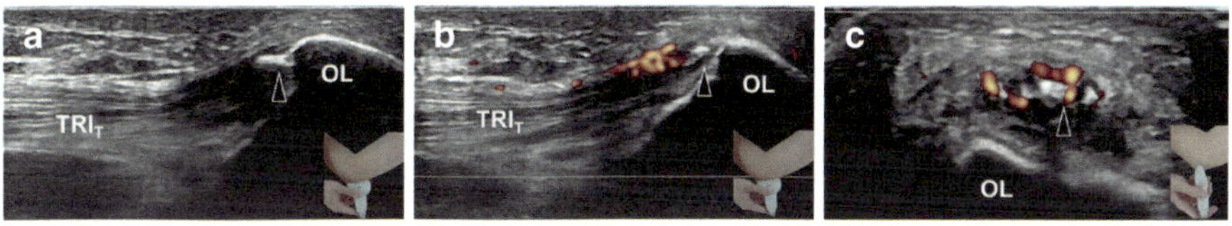

Fig. 7.20 The ultrasonography reveals a hyperechoic deposit (black arrowheads), indicating calcified tendinosis (**a**). Power Doppler shows hypervascularity, indicating inflammation in both the long-axis (**b**) and short-axis (**c**) views. Black arrowheads: calcification; TRI$_T$ tendon of the triceps brachii; OL olecranon of the ulna

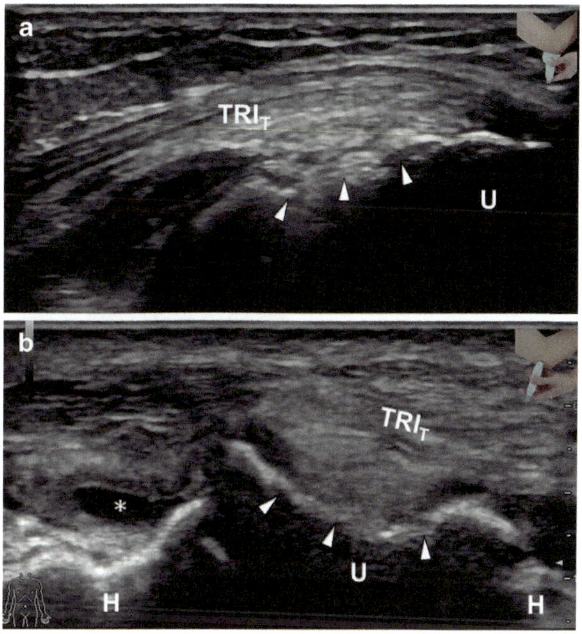

Fig. 7.21 The ultrasonography depicts enthesitis along the long axis of the distal triceps brachii tendon (**a**) in one case of rheumatoid arthritis, while in another case, enthesitis is evident in the axial view of the same tendon (**b**). White arrowheads: irregularity of the bony cortex; asterisk: effusion; TRI$_T$ tendon of the triceps brachii; U ulna; H humerus

In patients with spondyloarthritis or rheumatoid arthritis, enthesitis of the distal triceps tendon can be clearly depicted on ultrasound imaging, presenting as increased thickness, hypoechogenicity of the enthesis, enthesophytes, erosions, and cortical irregularities (long axis, Fig. 7.21a; short axis, Fig. 7.21b). Color Doppler imaging may reveal neovascularity within the tendon or involving the underlying fat pad (long axis, Fig. 7.22a; short axis, Fig. 7.22b).

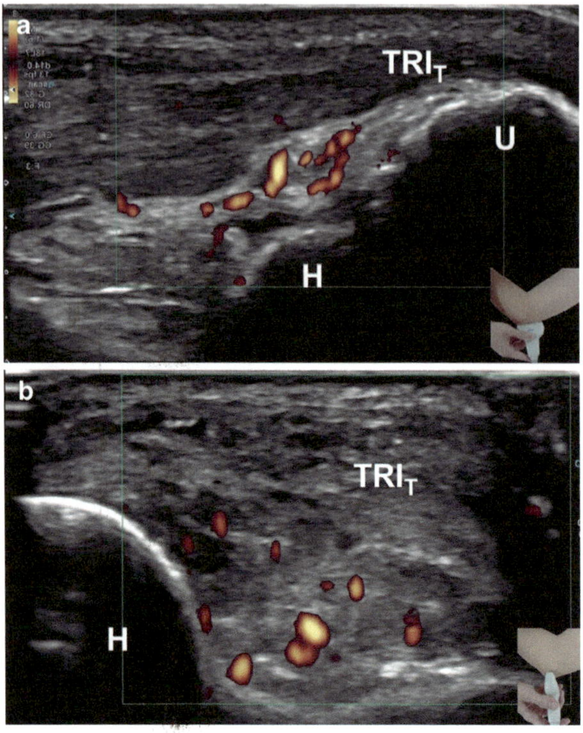

Fig. 7.22 The ultrasonography reveals neovascularity involving the underlying fat pad in both the long-axis (**a**) and the short-axis (**b**) views. TRI_T tendon of the triceps brachii; U ulna; H humerus

In cases of partial rupture involving the distal triceps brachii, the torn tendon may exhibit several hypoechoic clefts and partial retraction of the tendon fibers (short axis, Fig. 7.23a; long axis, Fig. 7.23b). Even after the torn tendon has healed, the normal fibrillary pattern might be absent, with disorganized tendon fibers interspersed with some hyperechoic calcific plaques (long axis, Fig. 7.24a; short axis, Fig. 7.24b). Adjusting the transducer medially and distally facilitates the demonstration of the normal insertion of the medial head of the triceps brachii on the olecranon (if present). Regarding a complete tear, a long-axis ultrasound scan reveals the proximal stump of the triceps brachii tendon, displaying a wavy aspect and the presence of fluid collection.

In cases of olecranon bursitis, inflammation affects the bursa covering the olecranon process at the proximal aspect of the ulna. Bursal inflammation can be

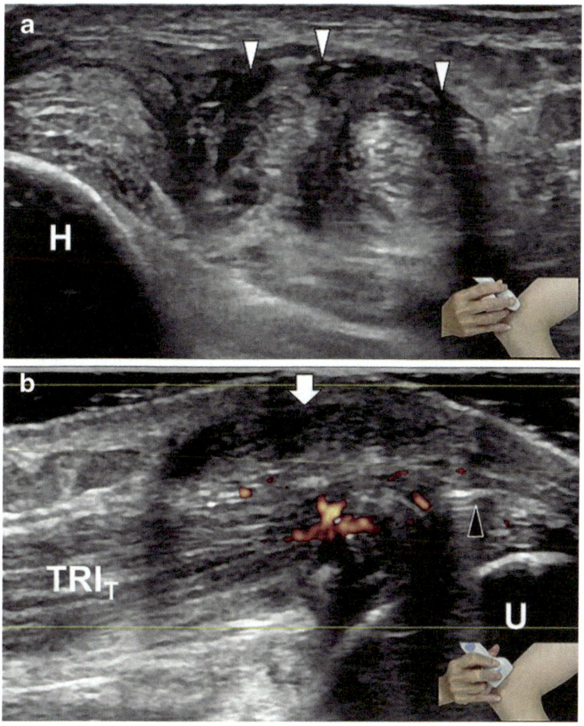

Fig. 7.23 The ultrasonography reveals the hypoechoic clefts (white arrowheads), indicating partial-thickness tears of the triceps brachii tendon in short axis (**a**) in a case of the olecranon fracture. In the same case, hypervascularity on power Doppler, hypertrophy of the olecranon bursa (white arrow), and a pin (black arrowhead) can be identified in the long axis of the triceps brachii tendon (**b**). TRI_T tendon of the triceps brachii; U ulna; H humerus

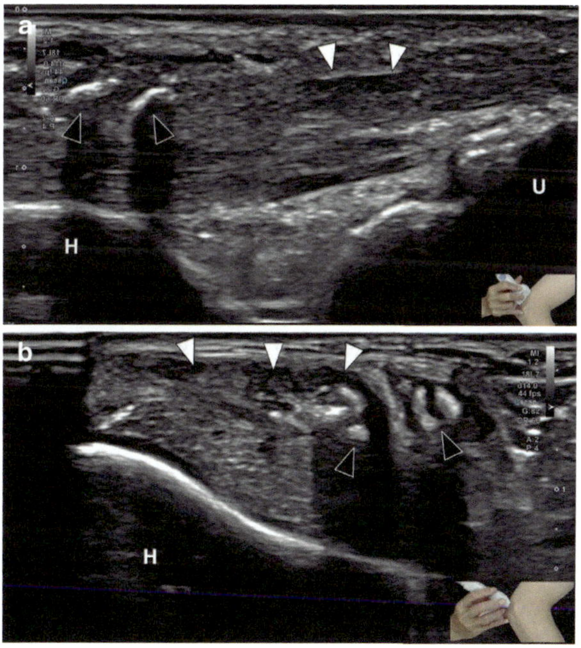

Fig. 7.24 The ultrasonography of the healed distal triceps brachii tendon reveals the absence of fibrillary tendon fibers (white arrowheads) and the presence of intra-tendinous calcifications (black arrowheads) in both the long-axis (**a**) and the short-axis (**b**) views. U ulna; H humerus

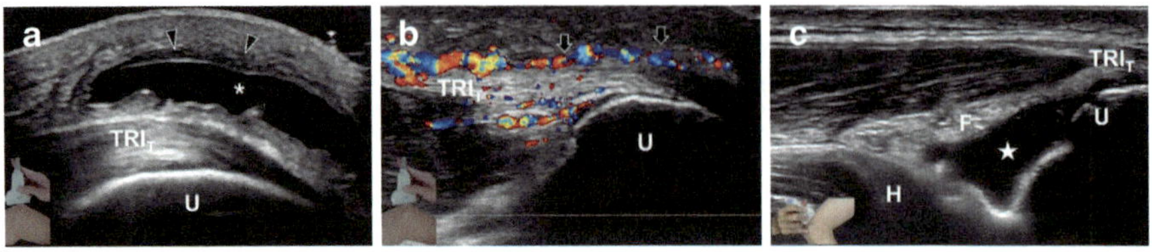

Fig. 7.25 Ultrasonography reveals effusion (asterisk) inside the olecranon bursa with thickening (black arrowheads) of the bursal wall (**a**). In another case, ultrasonography reveals neovascularity involving the olecranon bursa (black arrows) and peritendinous area (**b**). In a third case, ultrasonography reveals effusion (star) in the olecranon fossa with displacement of the fat pad (F) from the bottom of the fossa (**c**). TRI_T tendon of the triceps brachii; U ulna; H humerus

triggered by various factors, making it prone to inflammation due to acute or repetitive trauma, given its superficial location. Less commonly, inflammation may be linked to infection, rheumatoid arthritis, gout, and pseudogout. Ultrasound examinations demonstrate bursal effusion accompanied by thickening of the bursal wall, possibly containing a small amount of fluid and solid material (Fig. 7.25a). Longitudinal ultrasound imaging of the posterior aspect of the elbow reveals mixed echogenicity, fluid, and debris within the olecranon bursa. Additional observations include a proliferating synovium of the olecranon bursa. Gouty tophi may be found in the olecranon bursa, appearing as a single hyperechoic, heterogeneous nodule or multiple grouped hypoechoic heterogeneous nodules. A perilesional hypoechoic halo may also be evident, indicating a perilesional inflammatory reaction. In patients with posterior elbow pain, hypervascularity near the distal triceps brachii tendon, along with involvement of the olecranon bursa (Fig. 7.25b), might be observed. In such cases, there may be no effusion inside the bursa, and the ultrasound image may resemble paratendonitis. A more common pathology in the posterior elbow is effusion inside the olecranon fossa, which displaces the normally occupied fat pad from the fossa (Fig. 7.25c).

Hypertrophic synovium with increased vascularity can be observed within the olecranon fossa (Fig. 7.26a), while osteophytes may be present in patients who also have ulnohumeral osteoarthritis (Fig. 7.26b). In cases of olecranon fractures, ultrasound imaging is useful for evaluating the post-operative condition. It can help identify irritation of the distal triceps brachii tendon caused by the fixation screw. Additionally, ultrasound can monitor the proper union of the separated bony compartments (plain radiograph, Fig. 7.27a; long axis, Fig. 7.27b; short axis, Fig. 7.27c).

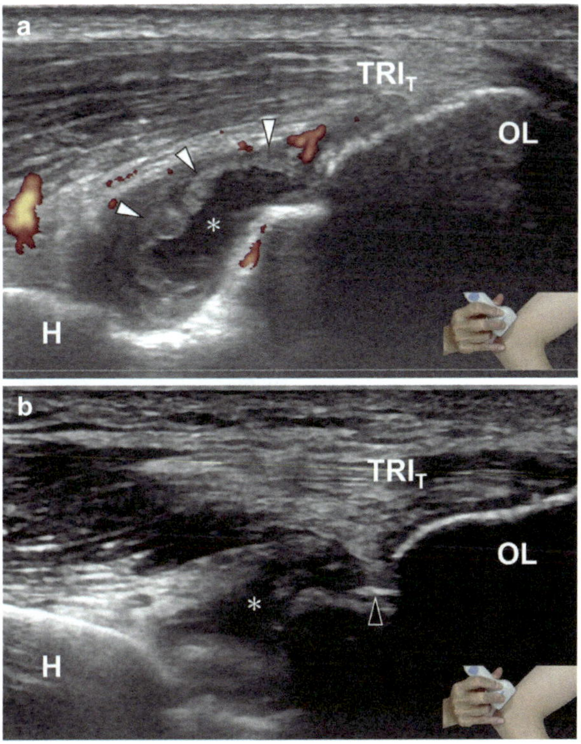

Fig. 7.26 The ultrasonography reveals hypertrophic synovium (white arrowheads) with hypervascularity and effusion (asterisk) in the olecranon fossa (**a**). In another case, the osteophyte (black arrowhead) can be observed in the posterior ulnohumeral joint, indicating osteoarthritis (**b**). TRI$_T$ tendon of the triceps brachii; OL olecranon process of the ulna; H humerus

In patients experiencing dull pain in the posterior lateral distal arm, radial nerve entrapment in the spiral groove is a possible cause. The nerve's cross-sectional area proximal to the compression site (Fig. 7.28a) is typically larger than its normal distal segment (Fig. 7.28b). To locate the entrapment site, pivoting the transducer along the nerve's long axis is helpful (Fig. 7.28c). Additionally, in patients with a metal implant in the humerus following a fracture, radial nerve entrapment (short axis, Fig. 7.29a, b; long axis, Fig. 7.29c) by the implant (plain radiograph, Fig. 7.29d) is not uncommon, and removal of the implant may be necessary to alleviate symptoms.

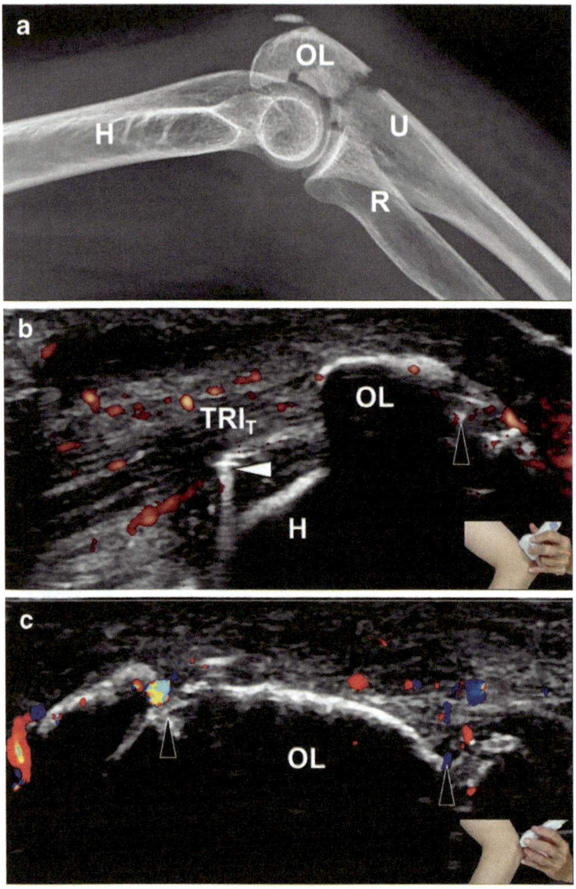

Fig. 7.27 In a case with an olecranon fracture (**a**), ultrasonography reveals improper union of the olecranon process (black arrowheads) and a screw (white arrowhead) likely irritating the distal triceps brachii tendon in the tendon's longitudinal (**b**) and axial (**c**) views. TRI$_T$ tendon of the triceps brachii; OL olecranon process of the ulna; U ulna; R radius; H humerus

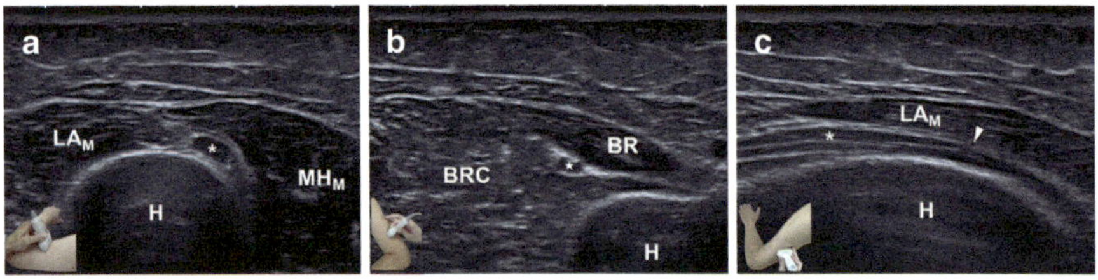

Fig. 7.28 The ultrasound image shows swelling of the radial nerve (asterisks) at the spiral groove (**a**), compared to its normal distal segment (star) (**b**). Viewing the nerve along its long axis helps in identifying the entrapment site (white arrowhead) (**c**). LA$_M$ lateral head muscle of the triceps brachii; MH$_M$ medial head muscle of the triceps brachii; BR brachioradialis; BRC brachialis; H humerus

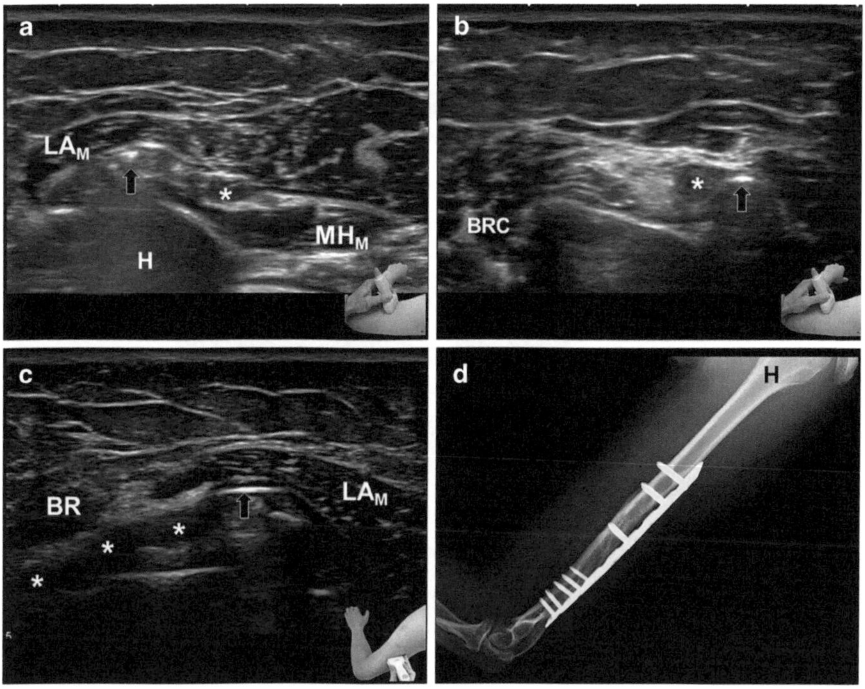

Fig. 7.29 The ultrasonography reveals swelling of the radial nerve (asterisks) both proximal (**a**) and distal (**b**) to the plate (black arrows) in short axis as well as the nerve's long axis (**c**). The corresponding radiograph illustrates the location of the plate used for the fixation of the humerus (**d**). LA_M lateral head muscle of the triceps brachii; MH_M medial head muscle of the triceps brachii; BRC brachialis; BR brachioradialis; H humerus

7.5 Ultrasound-Guided Injection

During the injection procedure for the triceps brachii tendon or olecranon bursa, the patient's elbow can be flexed with the hand resting on the examination table. The transducer is positioned along the long axis of the triceps brachii tendon. When targeting the distal triceps brachii tendon, the needle is introduced using an in-plane approach from caudal to cranial, aspirating the dilated olecranon bursa (Fig. 7.30a) or injecting the tendon and its distal attachment (Fig. 7.30b).

When aspirating olecranon bursitis, it is recommended to position the transducer in proximity to the distal triceps tendon without applying heavy compression to the skin. This precaution helps prevent the collapse of the bursa. The needle can be

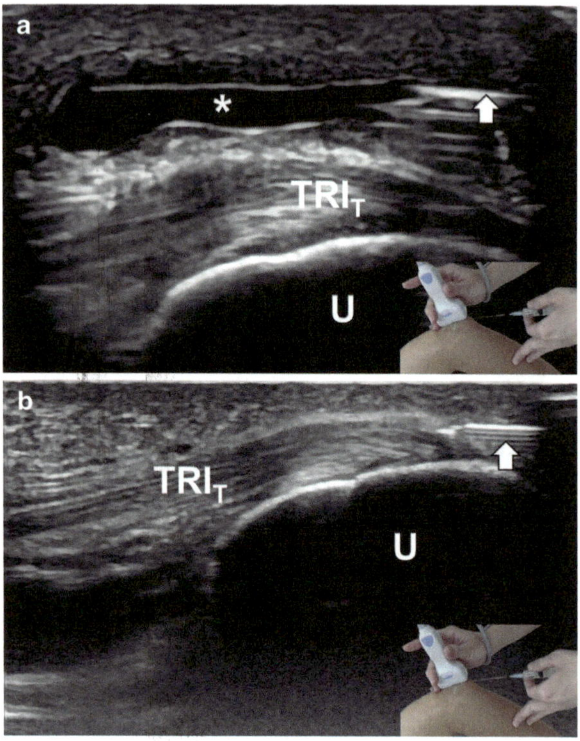

Fig. 7.30 The ultrasound-guided aspiration of the olecranon bursa effusion (asterisk) is performed using an in-plane approach (**a**). Similarly, the ultrasound-guided injection into the distal triceps brachii tendon is administered using an in-plane approach (**b**). White arrows: needle; TRI_T tendon of the triceps brachii; U ulna

inserted from lateral to medial or caudal to cranial until it is inside the anechoic bursa, ready for aspiration. When the pain is located slightly proximal, an injection into the myotendinous junction through the short axis of the distal triceps brachii tendon would be helpful (Fig. 7.31). If the goal is the olecranon fossa (or the posterior elbow joint), the injection can be administered in the same way, though the target will be deeper than the tendon (Fig. 7.32). Similarly, when the pain can be palpated from the posterior elbow joint space, the in-plane injection can be performed using a similar approach, targeting the space between the olecranon process of the ulna and the distal humerus (Fig. 7.33).

Finally, various nerve entrapment syndromes may occur at the posterior lateral elbow, where ultrasound helps detect the entrapment site, as described in the pathology section [7]. Once the compression point is identified, ultrasound-guided hydrodissection along the nerve's short axis is preferable, ensuring adequate dilatation of the perineural space both above and below the nerve. The targets can range from the main trunk, such as the radial nerve at the spiral groove (Fig. 7.34), to certain cutaneous branches, like the posterior brachial cutaneous nerve (Fig. 7.35), the posterior ante brachial cutaneous nerve (Fig. 7.36), and the superior lateral brachial cutaneous nerve (Fig. 7.37). The choice of injectate depends on the disease stage and the status of perineural inflammation, as elaborated in previous studies and reviews [7–9].

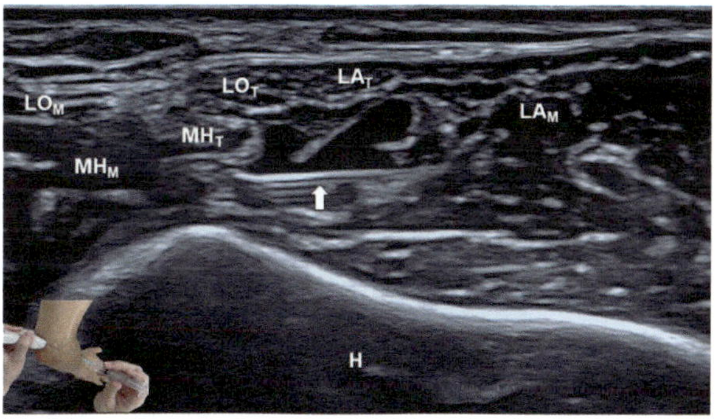

Fig. 7.31 The ultrasound-guided in-plane injection is administered to the distal myotendinous junction of the triceps brachii muscle in its short axis. White arrow: needle; LA_M lateral head muscle of the triceps brachii; MH_M medial head muscle of the triceps brachii; LO_M long head muscle of the triceps brachii; MH_T medial head tendon of the triceps brachii; LO_T long head tendon of the triceps brachii; LA_T lateral head tendon of the triceps brachii muscle; H humerus

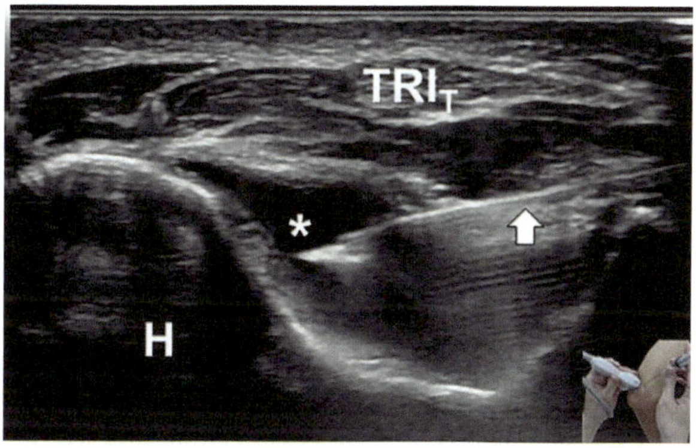

Fig. 7.32 The ultrasound-guided aspiration for effusion (asterisk) inside the olecranon fossa is performed using an in-plane approach along the short axis view of the distal triceps brachii tendon. White arrow: needle; TRI_T tendon of the triceps brachii; H humerus

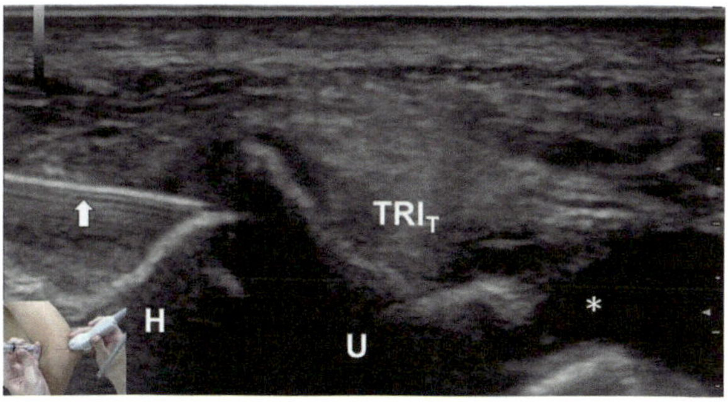

Fig. 7.33 The ultrasound-guided injection is administered to the posterior elbow joint using an in-plane approach from the lateral to medial direction. The injectate can be observed flowing to the opposite side of the joint effusion. Asterisk: injectate; white arrow: needle; TRI_T tendon of the triceps brachii; U ulna; H humerus

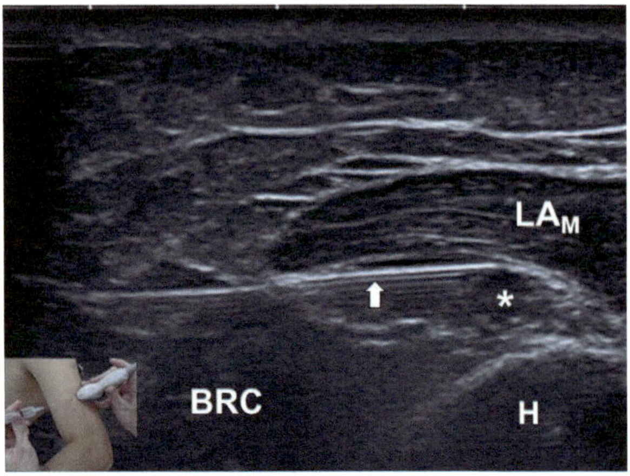

Fig. 7.34 The ultrasound-guided hydrodissection is performed on the radial nerve at the exit of the spiral groove. Asterisk: radial nerve; white arrow: needle; LA$_M$ lateral head muscle of the triceps brachii; BRC brachialis; H humerus

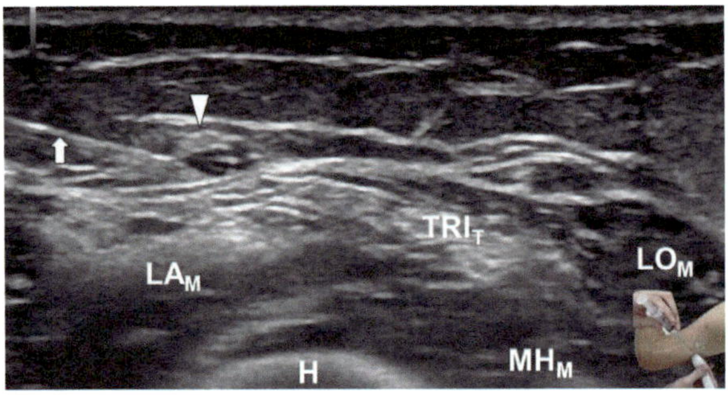

Fig. 7.35 The ultrasound-guided hydrodissection is administered to the posterior brachial cutaneous nerve (white arrowhead) from a lateral-to-medial direction using an in-plane approach. White arrow: needle; TRI$_T$ tendon of the triceps brachii; LA$_M$ lateral head muscle of the triceps brachii; MH$_M$ medial head muscle of the triceps brachii; LO$_M$ long head muscle of the triceps brachii; H humerus

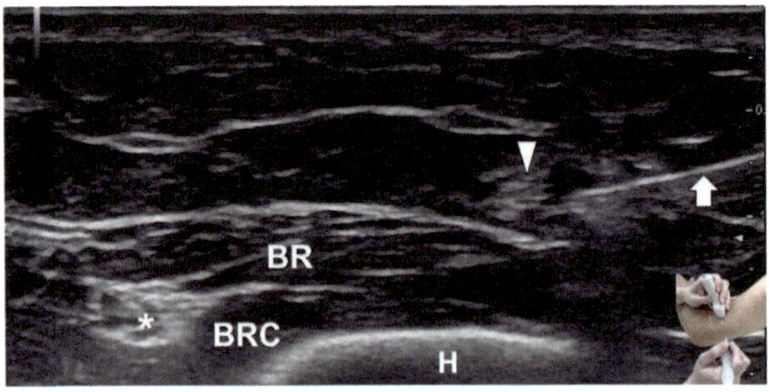

Fig. 7.36 The ultrasound-guided hydrodissection is performed on the posterior antebrachial cutaneous nerve (white arrowhead) superficial to the brachioradialis from a lateral-to-medial direction using an in-plane approach. White arrow: needle; asterisk: radial nerve; BR brachioradialis; BRC brachialis; H humerus

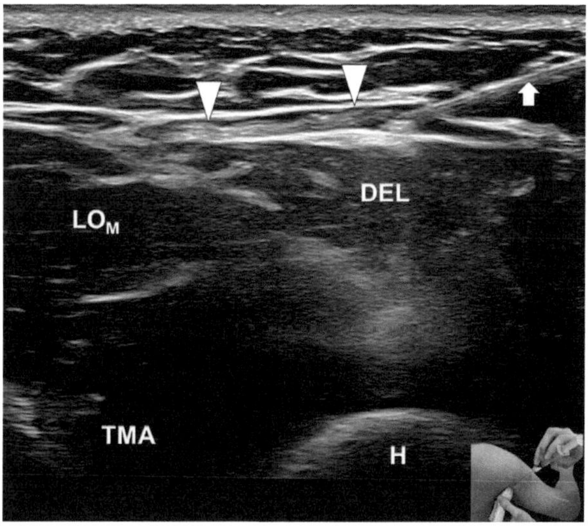

Fig. 7.37 The ultrasound-guided injection is administered to the superior lateral brachial cutaneous nerve (white arrowheads) using an in-plane approach along the nerve's long axis. White arrow: needle; LO_M long head muscle of the triceps brachii; TMA teres major; DEL deltoid; H humerus

7.6 Conclusion

In summary, the triceps brachii, characterized by distinct heads, plays a pivotal role in elbow and shoulder dynamics. The long head facilitates elbow extension and provides modest glenohumeral support, while the medial and lateral heads contribute to forearm extension. Nerve supply, primarily radial, may involve the ulnar and axillary nerves. The sonoanatomy of the triceps brachii tendon reveals a bipartite appearance on imaging, validated by histologic examination. Crucial for diagnosis, pathologies like tendinopathy and olecranon bursitis can be effectively managed through ultrasound-guided injections.

Acknowledgments Images and illustrations adapted from cadaveric images provided by the Visible Human Project® of the National Library of Medicine. Excerpts featured in the VH Dissector are used with permission from Touch of Life Technologies Inc.

References

1. Koplas MC, Schneider E, Sundaram M. Prevalence of triceps tendon tears on MRI of the elbow and clinical correlation. Skeletal Radiol. 2011;40(5):587–94.
2. Sollender JL, Rayan GM, Barden GA. Triceps tendon rupture in weight lifters. J Shoulder Elb Surg. 1998;7(2):151–3.
3. Tiwana MS, Sinkler MA, Bordoni B. Anatomy, shoulder and upper limb, triceps muscle. In: StatPearls. Treasure Island (FL) ineligible companies. Disclosure: Margaret Sinkler declares no relevant financial relationships with ineligible companies. Disclosure: Bruno Bordoni declares no relevant financial relationships with ineligible companies.: StatPearls Publishing. Copyright © 2024, StatPearls Publishing LLC; 2024.

4. Athlani L, Delgove A, Dautel G, Casoli V. Anatomy of the ulnar nerve in the posterior compartment of the upper arm: relationships with the triceps brachii muscle. Morphologie. 2020;104(345):85–90.
5. Belentani C, Pastore D, Wangwinyuvirat M, et al. Triceps brachii tendon: anatomic-MR imaging study in cadavers with histologic correlation. Skeletal Radiol. 2009;38(2):171–5.
6. Chang KV, Mezian K, Nanka O, et al. Ultrasound imaging for the cutaneous nerves of the extremities and relevant entrapment syndromes: from anatomy to clinical implications. J Clin Med. 2018;7(11)
7. Chang KV, Wu WT, Ozcakar L. Ultrasound imaging and guidance in peripheral nerve entrapment: hydrodissection highlighted. Pain Manag. 2020;10(2):97–106.
8. Wang JC, Hsu PC, Wang KA, Chang KV. Response: "commentary: ultrasound-guided triamcinolone acetonide hydrodissection for carpal tunnel syndrome: a randomized controlled trial". Front Med (Lausanne). 2022;9:841609.
9. Lin CP, Chang KV, Huang YK, Wu WT, Ozcakar L. Regenerative injections including 5% dextrose and platelet-rich plasma for the treatment of carpal tunnel syndrome: a systematic review and network meta-analysis. Pharmaceuticals (Basel). 2020;13(3)

Chapter 8
Anterior Elbow Pain: Distal Biceps Brachii Tendon Reviewed

Ke-Vin Chang, Wei-Ting Wu, and Shao-Yu Chi

8.1 Introduction

The biceps brachii tendon consists of two heads originating from the coracoid process (short head) and the supraglenoid tubercle of the scapula (long head), attaching to the radial tuberosity. It functions as a robust supinator of the forearm and serves as a comparatively less powerful elbow flexor. In cases of distal biceps rupture, symptoms such as ecchymosis, swelling, and tenderness may appear in the antecubital fossa. If the lacertus fibrosus is involved, the muscle may retract to the upper arm, and a noticeable defect in the distal tendon may be evident.

Clinically, the rupture of the distal biceps brachii tendon can be assessed using the biceps squeeze test, conducted with elbow flexion and forearm pronation. A positive test is indicated by the absence of forearm or wrist supination. In a study by Safran and colleagues [1], 15 patients with complete distal biceps brachii tendon injuries were evaluated, with the dominant extremity affected in 86% of cases. The research identified excessive eccentric tension as a common injury mechanism, and smokers faced a 7.5 times higher risk of distal biceps tendon rupture, as revealed by Poisson regression analysis. The incidence of such ruptures is 1.2 per 100,000 patients, predominantly occurring in the dominant elbow of middle-aged male smokers.

Regarding distal biceps brachii tendon pathologies, ultrasound proves useful for scrutiny. Various ultrasound scanning views exist, each with strengths and weaknesses for diagnosis or intervention. Additionally, ultrasound imaging can detect collateral involvement of the lateral antebrachial cutaneous nerve in patients with biceps brachii tendon pathologies. The subsequent chapter will delve into ultrasound imaging and guided injections for distal biceps brachii tendon disorders.

K.-V. Chang (✉) · W.-T. Wu · S.-Y. Chi
Bei-Hu Branch, National Taiwan University Hospital, Taipei, Taiwan

K.-V. Chang (ed.), *Ultrasonography of Musculoskeletal Pain*,
https://doi.org/10.1007/978-981-96-6787-1_8

8.2 Regional Anatomy

8.2.1 Distal Biceps Brachii Tendon

In the investigation carried out by Rajiv et al. [2], involving the examination of 74 cadaveric elbows, it was identified that the distal biceps brachii tendon follows a predictable spiral pattern on the radial tuberosity. The anteromedial fibers, originating from the short head, pursue a direct course for distal attachment, while the posterolateral fibers from the long head coil beneath the medial fibers, attaching cranially on the radial tuberosity (Fig. 8.1). Athwal et al.'s study [3] reported that the short-head tendon insertion on the radial tuberosity averaged 12 mm in length, 7 mm in width, and 60 mm^2 in area, whereas the long-head tendon insertion averaged 9 mm in length, 7 mm in width, and 48 mm^2 in area. The attachment of the distal biceps brachii tendon extends to the radial tuberosity and adjacent regions. Mazzocca et al. [4] classified three types of radial tuberosities: bifid ridge type, featuring prominent medial and lateral ridges with a trough in between; smooth type, lacking ridges; and single-ridge type, having only one ridge on the radial tuberosity.

Observations in individuals with non-fused biceps brachii muscle bellies revealed unfused distal biceps brachii tendons capable of independent gliding. The distal tendon is characterized as a paratenon-covered extrasynovial tendon with three blood supply zones: a proximal zone supplied by the brachial artery, a distal zone receiving branches from the posterior interosseous recurrent artery, and a middle zone covered by a thinner paratenon receiving vessels from both arteries.

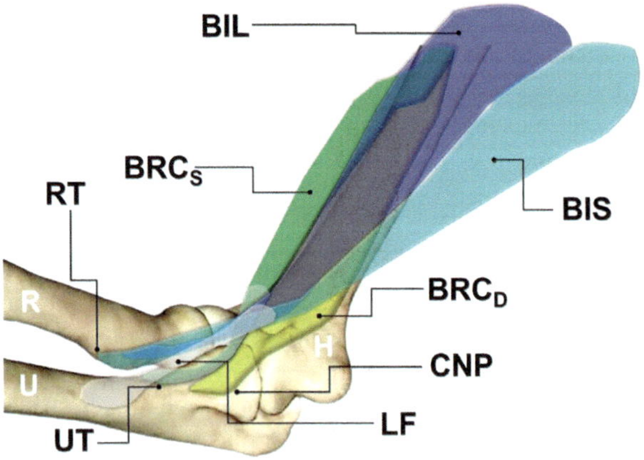

Fig. 8.1 The illustration of the distal biceps brachii, the brachialis, and their respective tendinous insertions. BIL long head of the biceps brachii; BIS short head of the biceps brachii; BRC$_D$ deep head of the brachialis; BRC$_S$ superficial head of the brachialis; CNP coronoid process of the ulna; LF lacertus fibrosus; R radius; RT radial tuberosity; U ulna; UT ulnar tuberosity; H humerus

8.2.2 Lacertus Fibrosus

Concerning the lacertus fibrosus (biceps aponeurosis), a slender fibrous structure, it radiates in an ulnar direction before merging with the superficial fascia on the ulnar side of the forearm (Fig. 8.1), just prior to the anterior passage of the distal biceps brachii tendon over the elbow joint. This aponeurosis is acknowledged for safeguarding the neurovascular bundle in the antecubital fossa (Fig. 8.2). The lacertus fibrosus has a broad insertion and plays a significant role in the forearm, encircling the flexors, establishing robust connections with the antebrachial fascia, particularly over the ulnar flexors, and traversing the median nerve and biceps brachii tendon.

8.2.3 Bicipitoradial Bursa

The distal biceps brachii tendon's attachment is enveloped by the bicipitoradial bursa, a teardrop-shaped structure, positioned between the brachialis muscle and the distal tendons (Fig. 8.3). During pronation, the radial tuberosity rotates posteriorly, exerting pressure on the bicipitoradial bursa situated between the biceps' tendon and the radial cortex. This rotation is expected to increase the pressure within the bursa and between the proximal radius and biceps tendon.

In a cadaveric study conducted by Skaf et al. [5], the bicipitoradial bursa was examined in the axial plane, revealing a wide base along the superficial aspect of the radius with an average dimension of 2.8 cm. In the sagittal oblique plane, the biceps brachii tendon was partially enclosed by the bicipitoradial bursa for an average length of 4.1 cm proximal to the radial tuberosity. Additionally, the study reported that the mean volume of contrast material that could be injected into the bursa without encountering resistance was 4.1 ml.

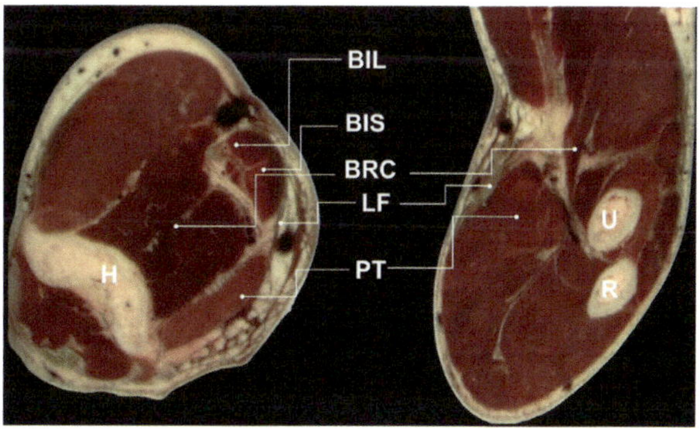

Fig. 8.2 Lacertus fibrosus (LF) of the elbow in transverse and coronal cross-sectional views. BIL long head of the biceps brachii; BIS short head of the biceps brachii; BRC brachialis; PT pronator teres; U ulna; R radius; H humerus

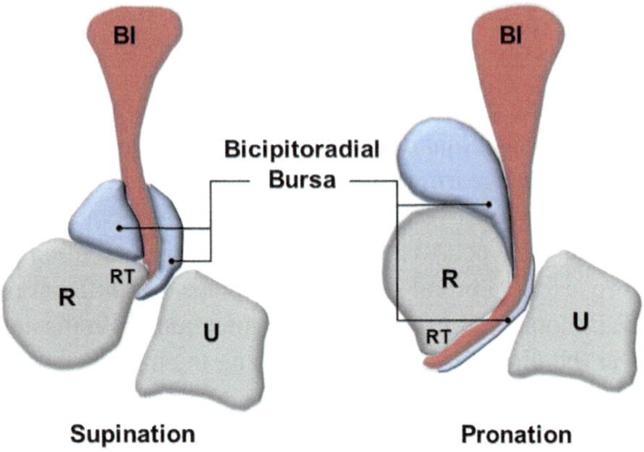

Fig. 8.3 The illustration of the bicipitoradial bursa during forearm supination and pronation. BI biceps brachii tendon; R radius; RT radial tuberosity; U ulna

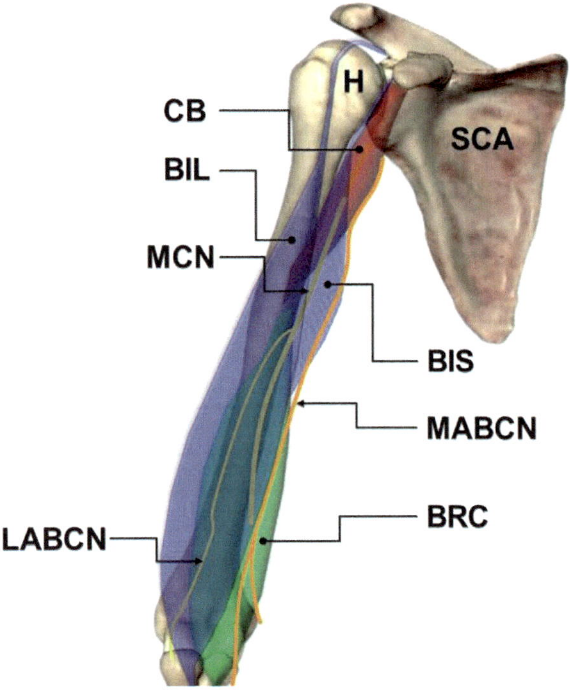

Fig. 8.4 The illustration shows the pathways of the lateral antebrachial cutaneous nerve and the medial antebrachial cutaneous nerve in the anterior forearm. BIL long head of the biceps brachii; BIS short head of the biceps brachii; BRC brachialis; CB coracobrachialis; LABCN lateral antebrachial cutaneous nerve; MABCN medial antebrachial cutaneous nerve; MCN musculocutaneous nerve; SCA scapula; H humerus

8.2.4 Lateral Antebrachial Cutaneous Nerve

The lateral antebrachial cutaneous nerve serves as the concluding branch of the musculocutaneous nerve, comprising exclusively sensory fibers [6] (Fig. 8.4). It emerges from beneath the lateral aspect of the biceps brachii muscle, specifically within the region of the interepicondylar line of the humerus. As it courses through the subcutaneous fat proximal to the crossover of the abductor pollicis longus and extensor pollicis brevis over the extensor carpi radialis longus and extensor carpi radialis brevis, the cephalic vein closely mirrors the path of the lateral antebrachial cutaneous nerve. Following its passage over the muscle bellies of the abductor pollicis longus and extensor pollicis brevis, the lateral antebrachial cutaneous nerve, along with the superficial radial nerve, often branches out intricately and diverges along with the cephalic vein [7].

8.2.5 *Medial Antebrachial Cutaneous Nerve*

The medial antebrachial cutaneous nerve originates from the medial cord of the brachial plexus and houses sensory cell bodies from the C8 and T1 nerve roots [6]. It progresses distally along the upper arm, traversing the brachial fascia with the basilic vein, approximately 10 cm proximal to the medial epicondyle. Upon emerging from the brachial fascia, the medial antebrachial cutaneous nerve bifurcates into two principal branches—anterior and posterior—both continuing their course toward the wrist (Fig. 8.4). The anterior branch penetrates the brachial fascia at the anterior aspect of the elbow and courses subcutaneously in the forearm, while the posterior branch crosses the elbow in a more posterior position on the ulnar side.

8.3 Sonoanatomy

8.3.1 *Distal Biceps Brachii Tendon-Anterior View*

The transducer is positioned over the distal volar humerus to visualize two layers of muscles: the biceps brachii above and the brachialis below (Fig. 8.5a, b). The lateral aspect of the biceps brachii originates from its long head, while the medial portion arises from its short head. As the transducer is moved distally, these two components converge to form the distal biceps brachii tendon (Fig. 8.5c).

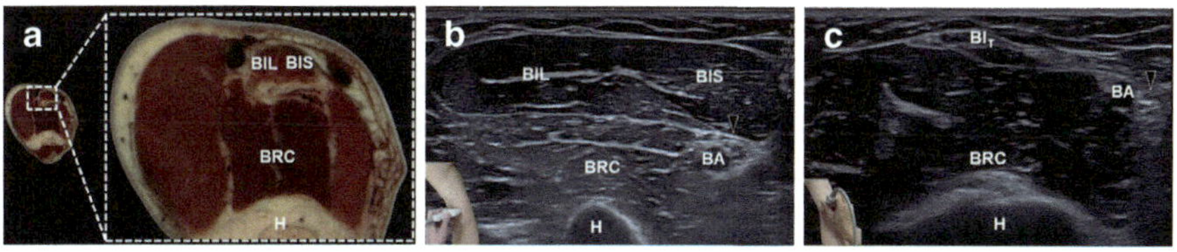

Fig. 8.5 The cadaveric image (**a**) and the corresponding sonoanatomy of the biceps brachii (**b**) are shown. As the transducer is moved distally, both heads of the biceps brachii converge to become the distal biceps brachii tendon (**c**). BA brachial artery; BIL long head of the biceps brachii; BIS short head of the biceps brachii; BI_T tendon of the biceps brachii; BRC brachialis; black arrowhead: median nerve; H humerus

Before reaching the elbow joint, the bony plane consisting of the coronoid fossa and radial fossa is identified first (Fig. 8.6a, b). Subsequently, another bony plane, characterized by the trochlea and capitellum covered with a cartilage layer, becomes apparent. At this point, a thin layer of fascia, known as the lacertus fibrosus, extends from the distal biceps brachii tendon, covering the superficial portion of the brachial artery and median nerve (Fig. 8.7a–c).

Moving further distally, the distal biceps brachii tendon starts to descend, casting a hypoechoic shadow due to anisotropy. The lateral part of the distal biceps brachii

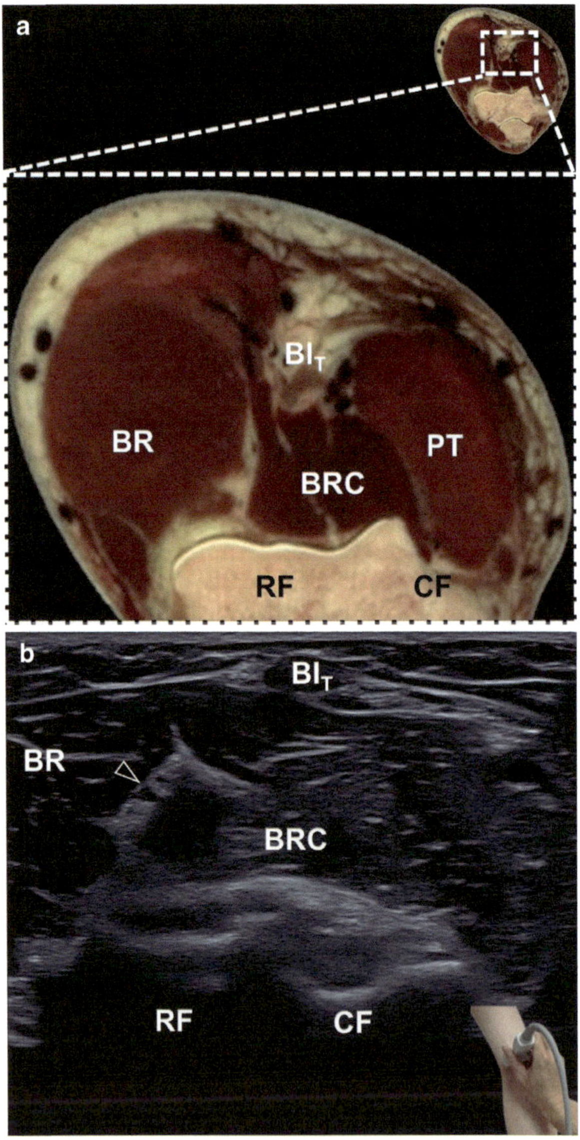

Fig. 8.6 The cadaveric image (**a**) and the corresponding sonoanatomy (**b**) of the radial and coronoid fossa of the humerus in the axial plane are shown. Black arrowhead: radial nerve; BI_T tendon of the biceps brachii; BRC brachialis; BR brachioradialis; CF coronoid fossa of the humerus; RF radial fossa of the humerus; PT pronator teres

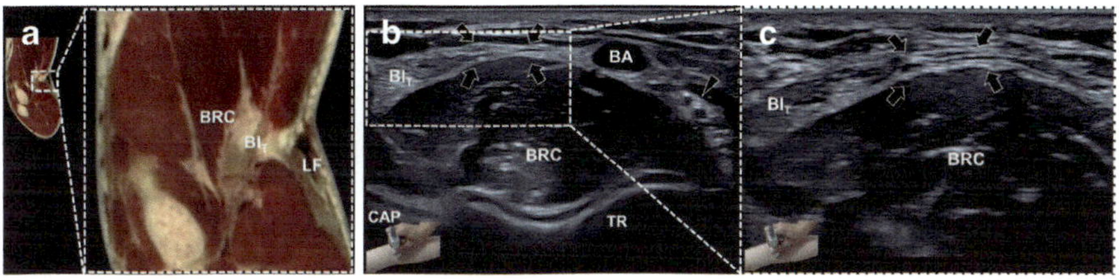

Fig. 8.7 The cadaveric image of the lacertus fibrosus in the sagittal oblique cross-sectional view (**a**), the corresponding sonoanatomy (**b**), and the image examined using a higher frequency transducer (**c**). LF and black arrows: lacertus fibrosus; black arrowhead: median nerve; BA brachial artery; BI_T biceps brachii tendon; BRC brachialis; TR trochlea; CAP capitellum

tendon, associated with the long head, descends first, followed by the medial part related to the short head (Fig. 8.8a, b). To visualize the distal attachment of the biceps brachii tendon, maximal supination of the elbow is necessary. Subsequently, the transducer is rotated 90 degrees to align with the long axis of the forearm, allowing visualization of the distal biceps brachii tendon inserting on the radial tuberosity (Fig. 8.9a, b).

8.3.2 *Distal Biceps Brachii Tendon-Medial View*

During the examination, it is recommended to flex and supinate the elbow. The transducer should be positioned along the long axis of the forearm, similar to the view used for examining the common flexor of the wrist. This perspective, also known as the pronator window [8], is chosen because the pronator teres originates most cranially on the medial epicondyle among the common flexors of the wrist and has the most cranial myotendinous junction (Fig. 8.10a, b).

While moving the transducer from medial to lateral, the brachialis muscle becomes evident, attaching to the coronoid process of the proximal ulna. The brachialis muscle is divided into a superficial and a deep head. The superficial head is larger and more medially positioned compared to the deep head. A prominent intramuscular tendon within the superficial head attaches to the ulnar tuberosity (Fig. 8.11a, b), while the less prominent intramuscular tendon of the deep head inserts into the coronoid process of the ulna (Fig. 8.11c) [9]. Furthermore, the distal attachment of the superficial head of the brachialis would be located more distal than the deep head of the brachialis, also shown by the cadaveric study done by Leonello et al. [10].

The long axis of the median nerve (Fig. 8.12a, b) and brachial artery (Fig. 8.12c) can be sequentially visualized from medial to lateral. Once the brachial artery is identified, a slight adjustment of the transducer allows for the visualization of the distal attachment of the biceps brachii tendons. In this view, the attachment of the long head (Fig. 8.13a, b) can be clearly observed more cranially than the attachment of the short head (Fig. 8.14a, b) on the radial tuberosity. Importantly, the examinee

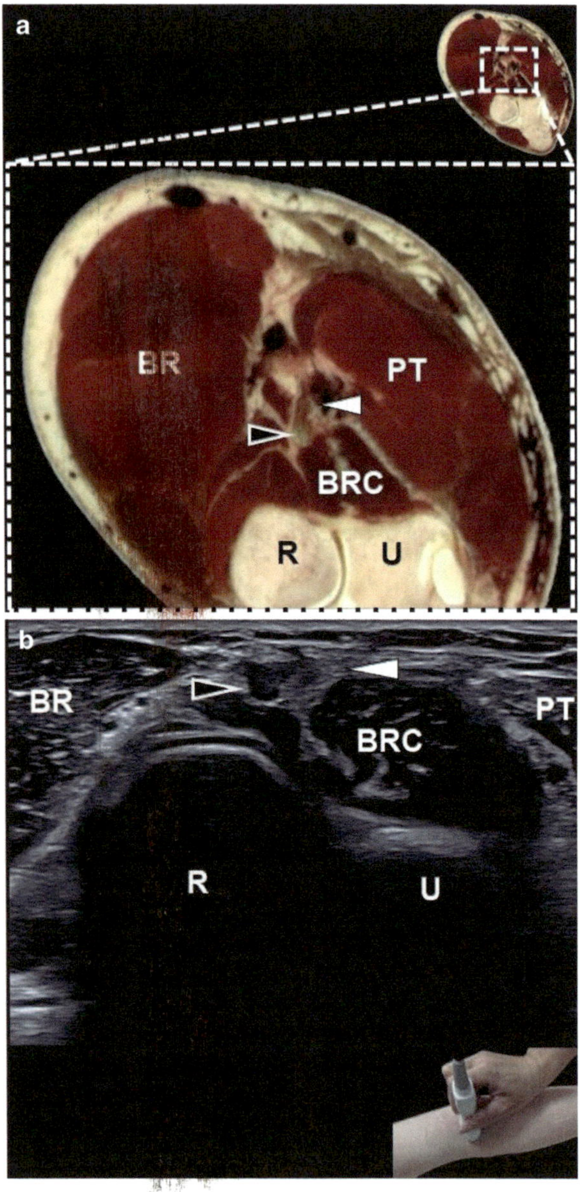

Fig. 8.8 The cadaveric image (**a**) and the corresponding sonoanatomy (**b**) of the tendon of the biceps brachii in the short-axis view. White arrowheads: short head of the biceps brachii tendon; black arrowheads: long head of the biceps brachii tendon; BRC brachialis; BR brachioradialis; PT pronator teres; R radius; U ulna

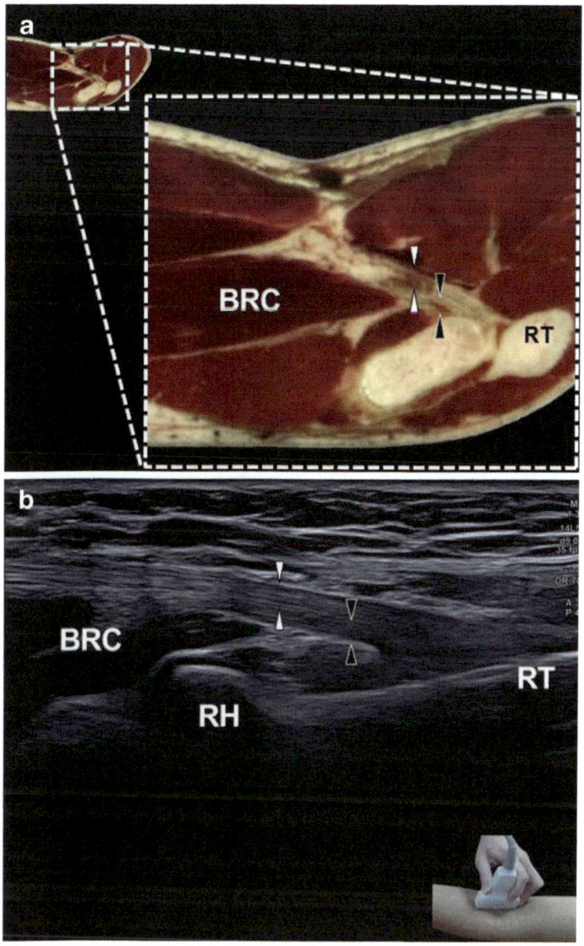

Fig. 8.9 The cadaveric image (**a**) and the corresponding sonoanatomy (**b**) show the distal tendon of the biceps brachii and its insertion in the long axis. White arrowheads: short head of the biceps brachii; black arrowheads: long head of the biceps brachii; BRC brachialis; RH radial head; RT radial tuberosity

can be instructed to supinate and pronate the forearm, facilitating the observation of the biceps brachii tendon rotating with the radial head. This dynamic maneuver serves as an effective way to differentiate between the biceps brachii and brachialis tendons.

8.3.3 Distal Biceps Brachii Tendon-Posterior View

The examinee's elbow is flexed and positioned on the examination table, followed by flexing the wrist and pronating the forearm. This particular view is commonly referred to as the cobra view (Fig. 8.15a) [11], named after the gesture resembling a cobra's stance. The transducer is then placed over the proximal aspect of the dorsal forearm, allowing clear identification of the supinator connecting the radius and

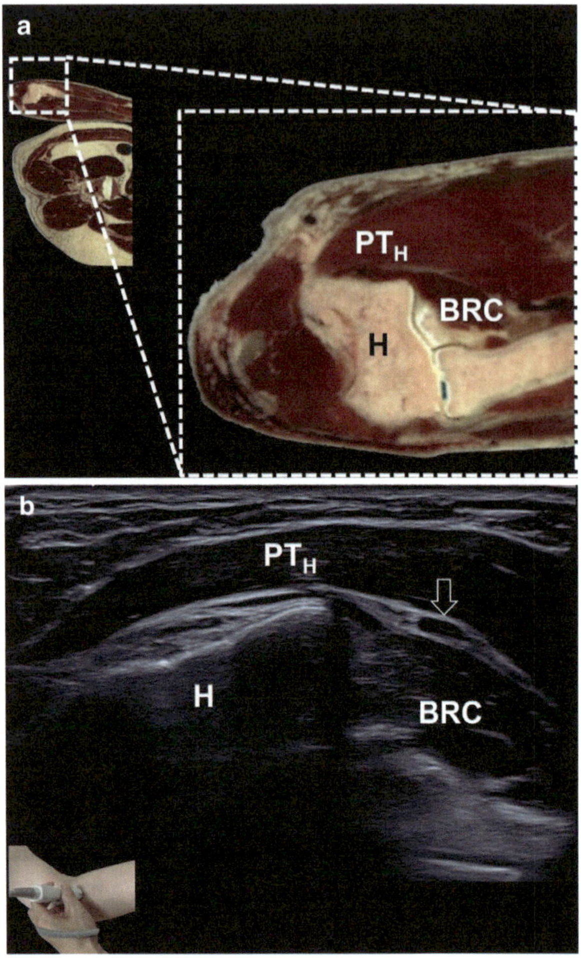

Fig. 8.10 The cross-sectional cadaveric image (**a**) and the corresponding sonoanatomy (**b**) of the humeral head of the pronator teres in its long axis. PT_H humeral head of the pronator teres; BRC brachialis; black arrow: median nerve; H humerus

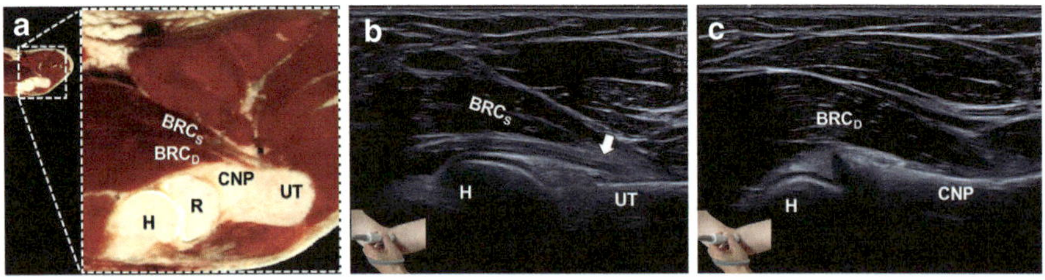

Fig. 8.11 The cadaveric image (**a**), corresponding sonoanatomy of the superficial head of the brachialis (**b**), and the deep head of the brachialis (**c**) in long axis. BRC_S superficial head of the brachialis; white arrow: tendon of the superficial head of the brachialis; BRC_D deep head of the brachialis; UT ulnar tuberosity; CNP coronoid process of the ulna; R radius; H humerus

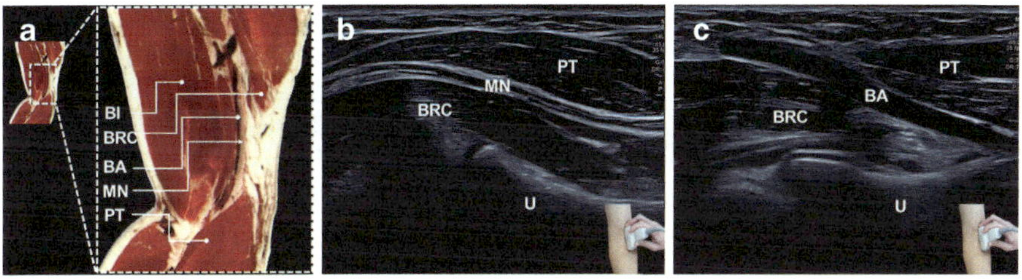

Fig. 8.12 The cadaveric image (**a**), the corresponding sonoanatomy of the median nerve (**b**), and the brachial artery (**c**) in the long axis. BI: biceps brachii; BA brachial artery; BRC brachialis; MN median nerve; PT pronator teres; U ulna

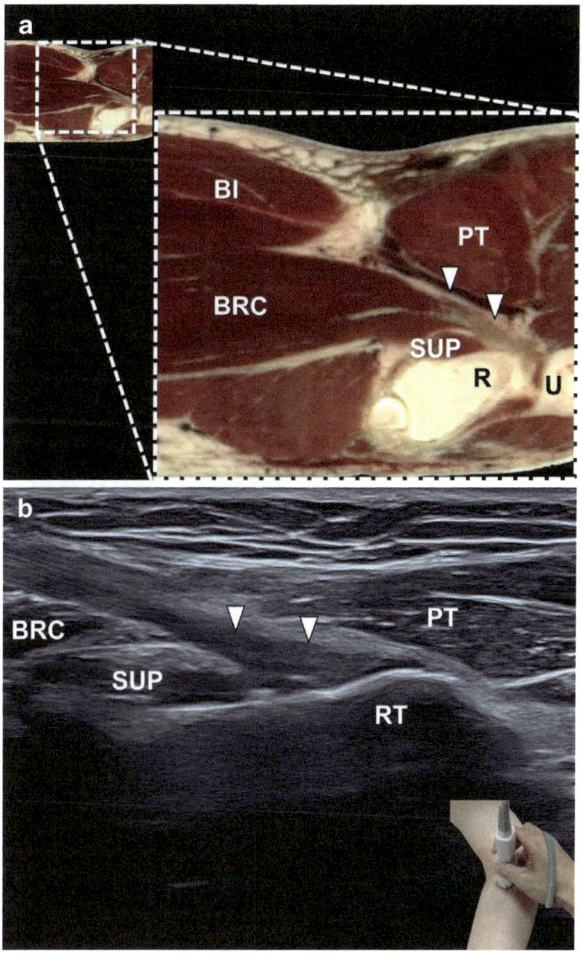

Fig. 8.13 The cadaveric image in the coronal cross-section (**a**) and the corresponding sonoanatomy (**b**) of the long head tendon of the biceps brachii (white arrowheads) in the long axis. BRC brachialis; BI biceps brachii; SUP supinator; RT radius tuberosity; PT pronator teres; R radius; U ulna

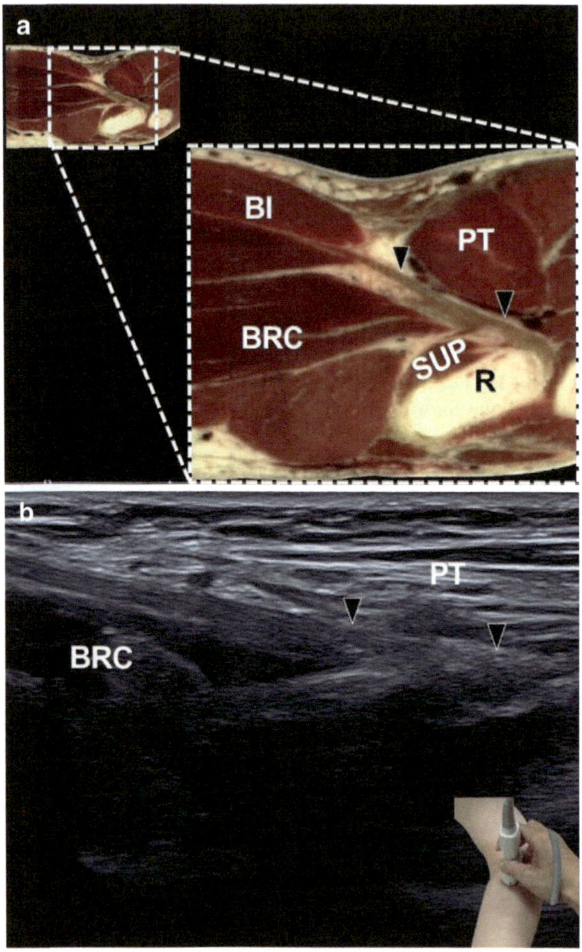

Fig. 8.14 The cadaveric image in the coronal cross-section (**a**) and the corresponding sonoanatomy (**b**) of the short head tendon of the biceps brachii (black arrowheads) in the long axis. BI biceps brachii; BRC brachialis; SUP supinator; PT pronator teres; R radius

supinator crest (Fig. 8.15b). Moving the transducer more cranially with pronating the foearm, a hyperechoic structure resembling a bird beak comes into view, indicating the distal biceps brachii tendon (Fig. 8.15c). Aligning the transducer with the long axis of the distal biceps brachii tendon and shifting it to the ventral aspect of the elbow enhances the visualization of the proximal portion of the distal bicep's tendon and its myotendinous junction (Fig. 8.16a). The visibility is further facilitated by repeated pronation (Fig. 8.16b) and supination (Fig. 8.16c) of the forearm. The method can be specifically referred to as the ventral radial approach.

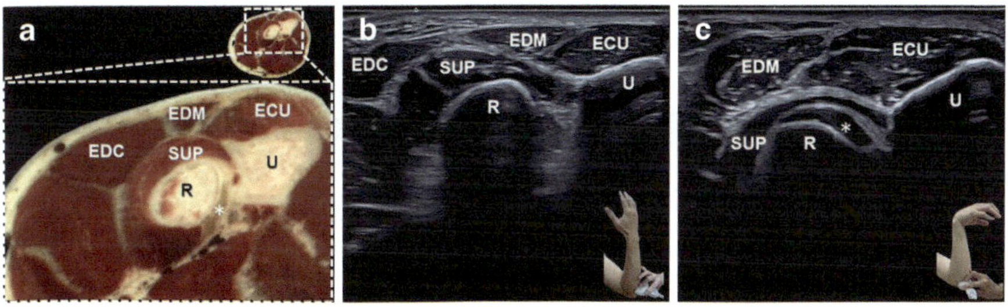

Fig. 8.15 The cadaveric image (**a**) and the corresponding sonoanatomy of the biceps brachii tendon (asterisks) during the posterior view. During forearm supination (**b**), the distal tendon of the biceps brachii is not visible, and during pronation (also known as the cobra's view), the distal tendon of the biceps brachii can be visualized (**c**). ECU extensor carpi ulnaris; EDC extensor digitorum communis; EDM extensor digiti minimi; SUP supinator; R radius; U ulna

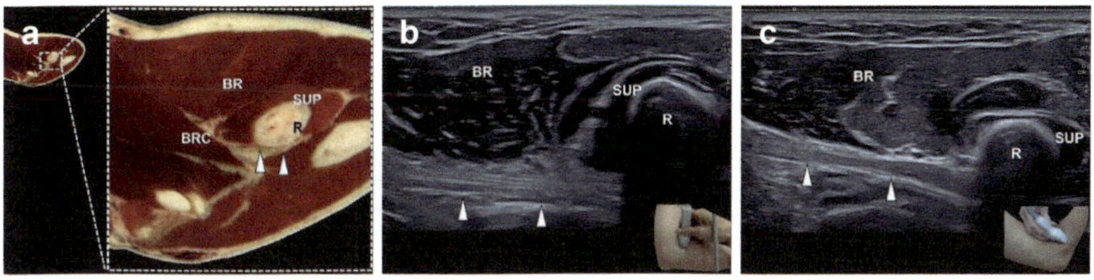

Fig. 8.16 The cadaveric image in the transverse cross-section (**a**) and the corresponding sonoanatomy of the tendon of the biceps brachii (white arrowheads) during forearm pronation (**b**) and supination (**c**). BR brachioradialis; BRC brachialis; SUP supinator; R radius

8.3.4 Relevant Nerves

The transducer is positioned in the axial plane on the distal humerus, revealing the radial nerve. This nerve displays a lateral fascicle representing its deep motor branch and a medial fascicle representing its superficial radial branch, situated between the brachioradialis and brachialis muscles. Conversely, the median nerve is observed between the brachialis and pronator teres muscles (Fig. 8.17a, b). As the transducer is moved distally, the median nerve traverses a passage formed between the humeral and ulnar heads of the pronator teres muscle. The median nerve gives off the anterior interosseous nerve, coursing through the interosseous membrane between the flexor pollicis longus and flexor digitorum profundus muscles (Fig. 8.18a, b).

Returning to the axial plane of the distal humerus, the lateral antebrachial cutaneous nerve is identified lateral to the distal biceps brachii tendon and alongside the cephalic vein (Fig. 8.19a, b). This nerve can be traced back to its main trunk, the musculocutaneous nerve, which is interposed between the biceps brachii and brachialis muscles (Fig. 8.20a, b). Additionally, the medial antebrachial cutaneous

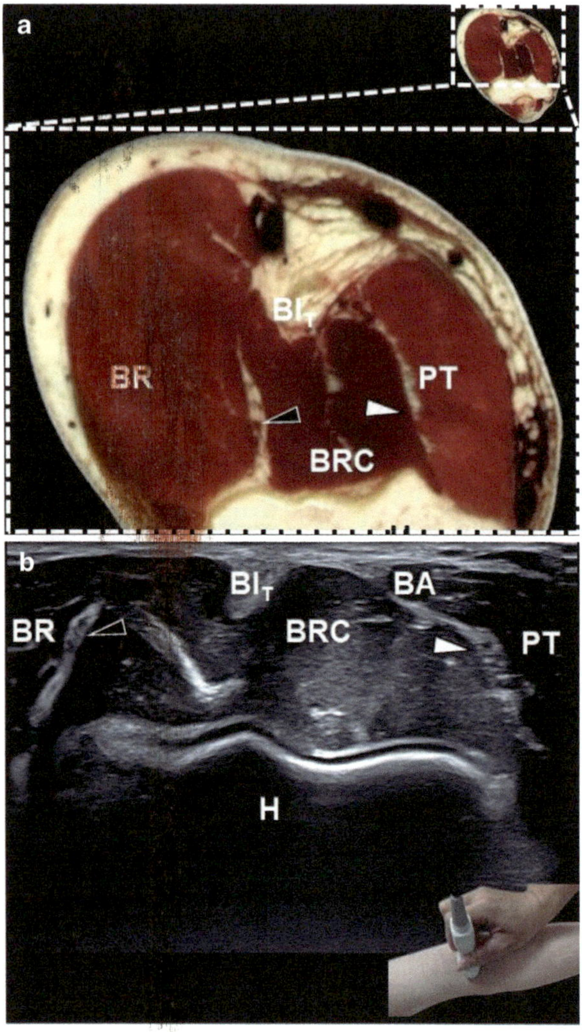

Fig. 8.17 The cadaveric image (**a**) and the corresponding sonoanatomy (**b**) of the radial nerve (black arrowheads) and median nerve (white arrowheads) in short axis are shown. BA brachial artery; BI_T tendon of the biceps brachii; BRC brachialis; BR brachioradialis; PT pronator teres; H humerus

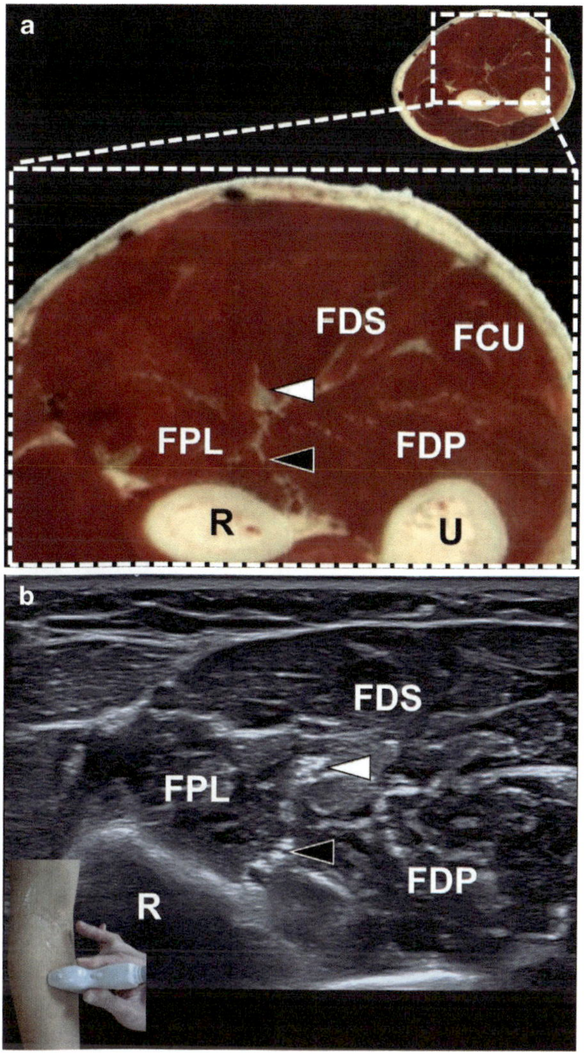

Fig. 8.18 The cadaveric image (**a**) and the corresponding sonoanatomy (**b**) of the anterior interosseous nerve (black arrowheads) in short axis. White arrowheads: median nerve; FDP flexor digirotum profundus; FDS flexor digitorum superficialis; FPL flexor pollicis longus; FCU flexor carpi ulnaris; R radius; U ulna

nerve is visualized medial to the median nerve and beside the basilic vein (Fig. 8.21a, b). Gentle pressure with the transducer is recommended to avoid the collapse of adjacent veins, facilitating the visualization of the cutaneous nerves.

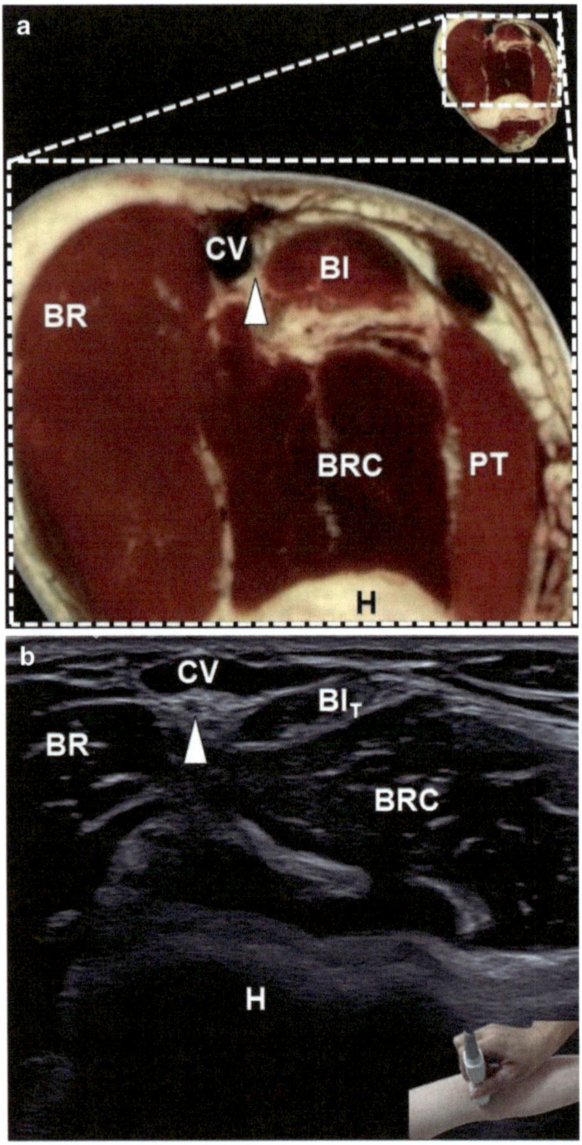

Fig. 8.19 The cadaveric image (**a**) and the corresponding sonoanatomy (**b**) of the lateral antebrachial cutaneous nerve (white arrowheads) in short axis at the distal humerus. BI biceps brachii; BI_T tendon of the biceps brachii; BRC brachialis; BR brachioradialis; CV cephalic vein; PT pronator teres; H humerus

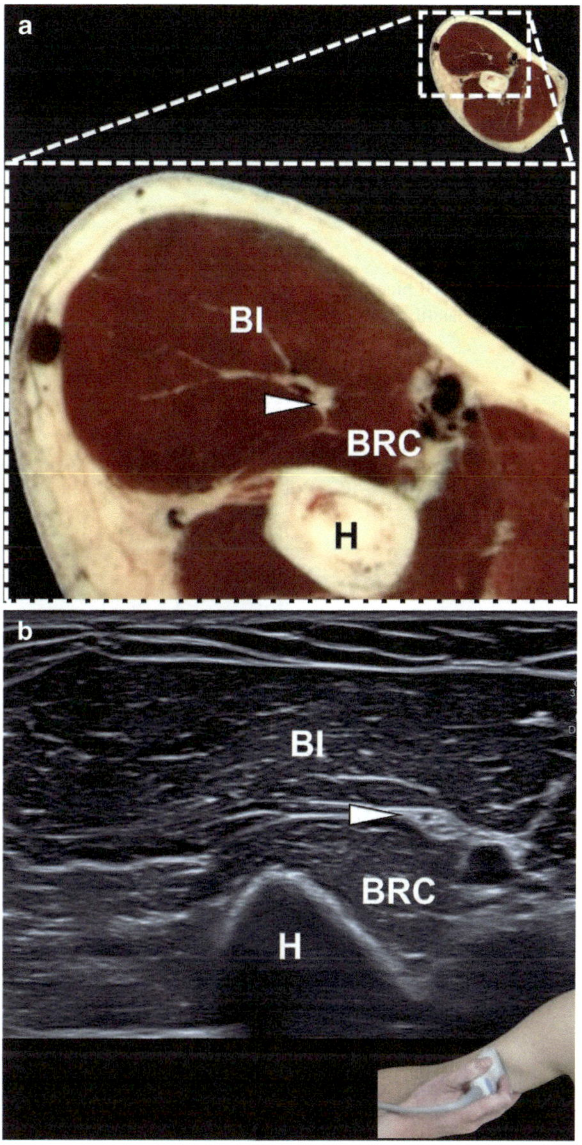

Fig. 8.20 The cadaveric image (**a**) and the corresponding sonographic anatomy (**b**) of the musculocutaneous nerve (white arrowheads) in short axis. BI: biceps brachii; BRC brachialis; H humerus

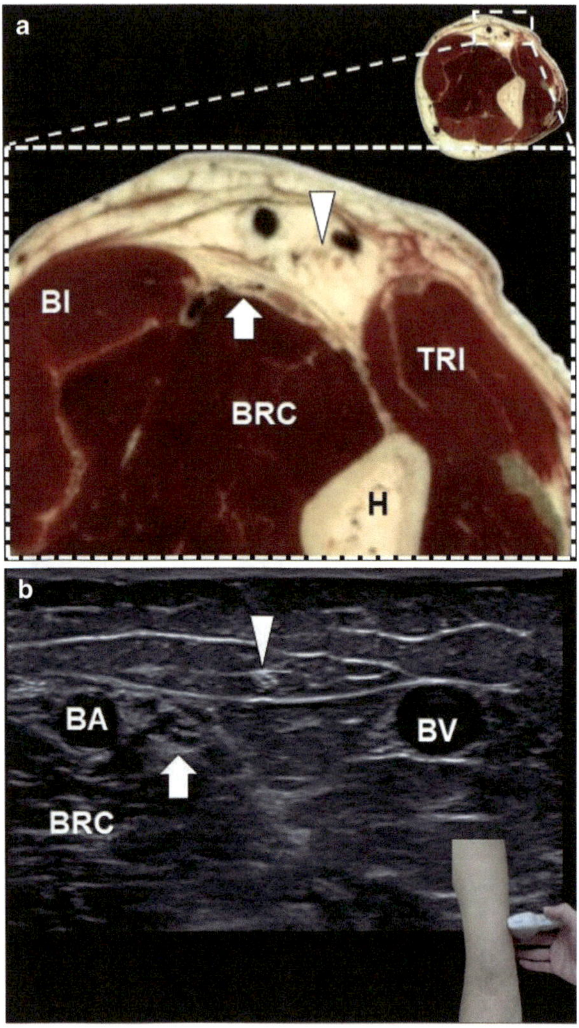

Fig. 8.21 The cadaveric image (**a**) and corresponding sonoanatomy (**b**) of the medial antebrachial cutaneous nerve (white arrowheads) in short axis. White arrows: median nerve; BA brachial artery; BRC brachialis; TRI triceps brachii; BI biceps brachii; BV basilic vein; H humerus

8.4 Pathologies

For individuals facing elongation or traumatic injury without evident tendon tearing, the long-axis ultrasound view may depict a consistently thickened and hypoechogenic distal biceps brachii tendon. The loss of fibrillary pattern affects the entire thickness and length, yet no discernible gaps are noted within the tendon (medial approach, Fig. 8.22a; posterior approach, Fig. 8.22b).

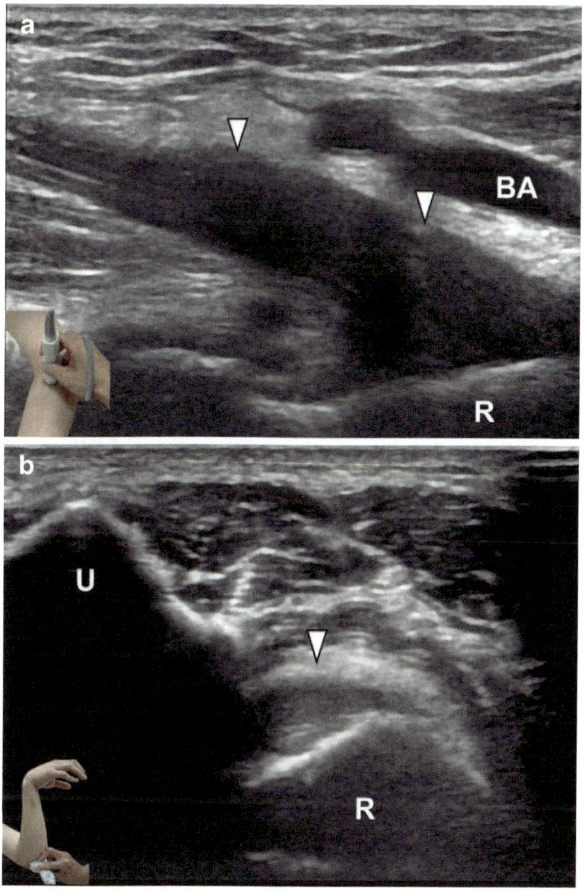

Fig. 8.22 Ultrasonography using the medial approach (**a**) and posterior approach (**b**) reveals a thickened and hypoechoic distal tendon of the biceps brachii (white arrowheads). BA brachial artery; R radius; U ulna

In cases of a low-grade partial tear at the attachment, the long-axis ultrasound view might reveal a minor partial detachment (involving less than 50% of the biceps brachii tendon) near the radial tuberosity (gray scale imaging, Fig. 8.23a; power Doppler imaging, Fig. 8.23b). The tendon defect may be filled with anechoic fluid, and the short-axis view could suggest a mild peritendinous effusion, potentially interpreted as bicipitoradial bursitis due to synovial irritation (medial approach, Fig. 8.24a; ventral radial approach, Fig. 8.24b; posterior approach, Fig. 8.24c).

For patients experiencing a high-grade partial tear, where the detachment affects more than 50% of the distal biceps brachii tendon, it is observed adjacent to the radial tuberosity. A hyperechogenic line corresponding to the torn tendon interface with peritendinous effusion may be visible (long axis, Fig. 8.25a; short axis, Fig. 8.25b), and a substantial anechoic defect is evident as most tendon fibers are torn.

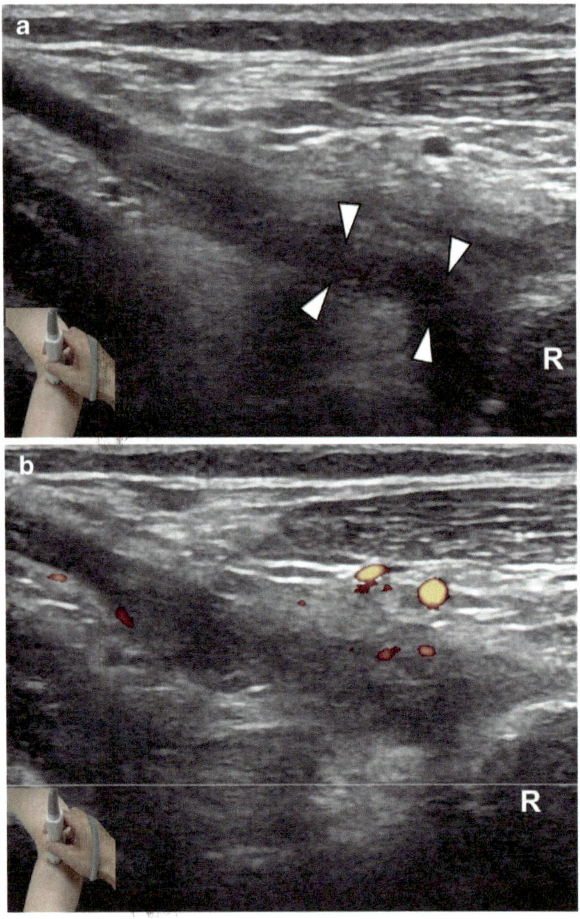

Fig. 8.23 Ultrasonography reveals swelling and loss of the fibrillary pattern in the distal tendon of the biceps brachii (especially over the long head), consistent with a partial-thickness tear (**a**), and hypervascularity is evident in power Doppler mode (**b**). White arrowheads: portion of the partial-thickness tear; R radius

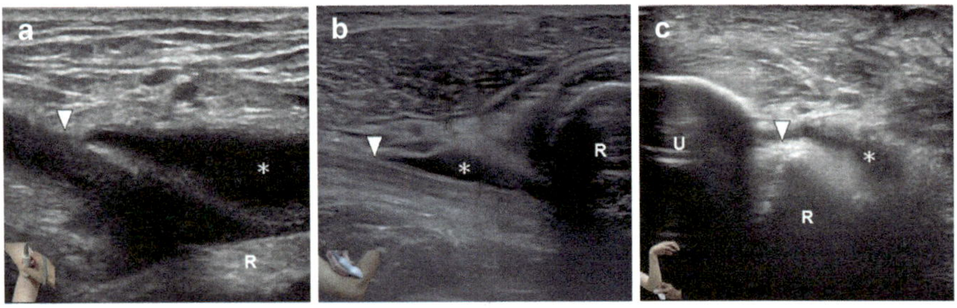

Fig. 8.24 Ultrasonography reveals anechoic fluid, which may indicate bicipitoradial bursitis, using the medial (**a**), ventral radial (**b**), and posterior (**c**) approaches. White arrowheads: distal tendon of the biceps brachii; asterisks: distended bicipitoradial bursa; R radius; U ulna

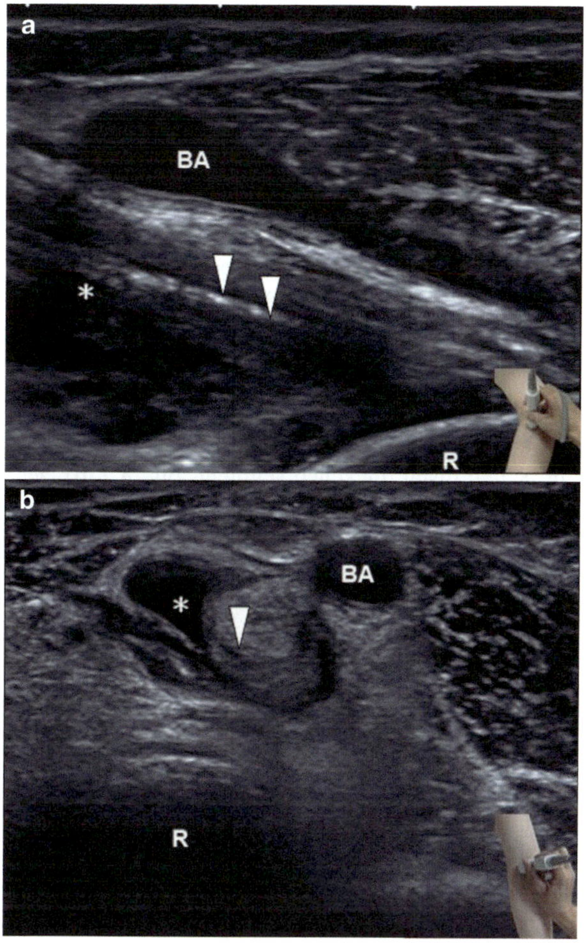

Fig. 8.25 Ultrasound imaging reveals a partial tear of the distal tendon of the biceps brachii, with peritendinous effusion visible at the interface in both the long-axis (**a**) and short-axis (**b**) views. White arrowheads: interface with peritendinous effusion; asterisks: effusion; BA brachial artery; R radius

In instances of a complete non-retracted tear of the distal biceps brachii tendon, there is mild observable tendon gapping. The short-axis view can unveil tendon hypertrophy and an altered echotexture in the disrupted tendon. In cases of a completely retracted tear, the distal biceps brachii tendon stump displays a wavy appearance, often accompanied by a hematoma near the stump (short axis at the tendon's attachment, Fig. 8.26a; short axis at the elbow crease, Fig. 8.26b; long axis, Fig. 8.26c). Selective involvement of the short head or long head tendon is also possible.

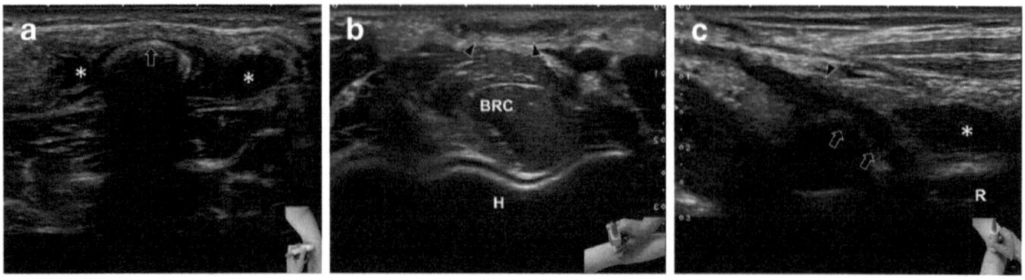

Fig. 8.26 Ultrasonography reveals a hematoma (asterisks) with intra-hematoma calcification (black arrows) at the attachment of the distal tendon of the biceps brachii (**a**), along with the absence of distal tendon fibers of the biceps brachii (black arrowheads) in both the short-axis (**b**) and long-axis views (**c**). BRC brachialis; R radius; H humerus

Patients with a partial distal biceps brachii tendon tear may display an enlarged and echogenic lateral antebrachial cutaneous nerve (proximal normal segment, Fig. 8.27a; distal thickened segment, Fig. 8.27b), accompanied by the absence of the normal fascicular echotexture in the short-axis view. In a study by Chiavaras et al. [12], 26 elbows in 13 patients underwent examination, leading to the identification of abnormalities in the lateral antebrachial cutaneous nerve using sonography. Symptomatic lateral antebrachial cutaneous nerves present fusiform enlargement, heightened echogenicity, and a loss of the normal fascicular echotexture. The average cross-sectional area of these symptomatic nerves measures 12.0 mm^2, with a maximum thickness of 3.5 mm, in contrast to 3.3 mm^2 with a maximum thickness of 1.3 mm observed in the contralateral normal elbows.

While distal biceps tendon pathologies rarely link to the medial antebrachial cutaneous nerve, the nerve remains susceptible to iatrogenic injury. Procedures such as venous punctures, injections for medial epicondylitis, or cubital tunnel releases carry the potential for nerve damage. Additionally, a subcutaneous lipoma could be a causative factor in the entrapment of the medial antebrachial cutaneous nerve [13]. In instances of medial antebrachial cutaneous neuropathy, ultrasound images may not reveal nerve swelling. However, employing sono-palpation to elicit a Tinel sign can be a valuable diagnostic aid.

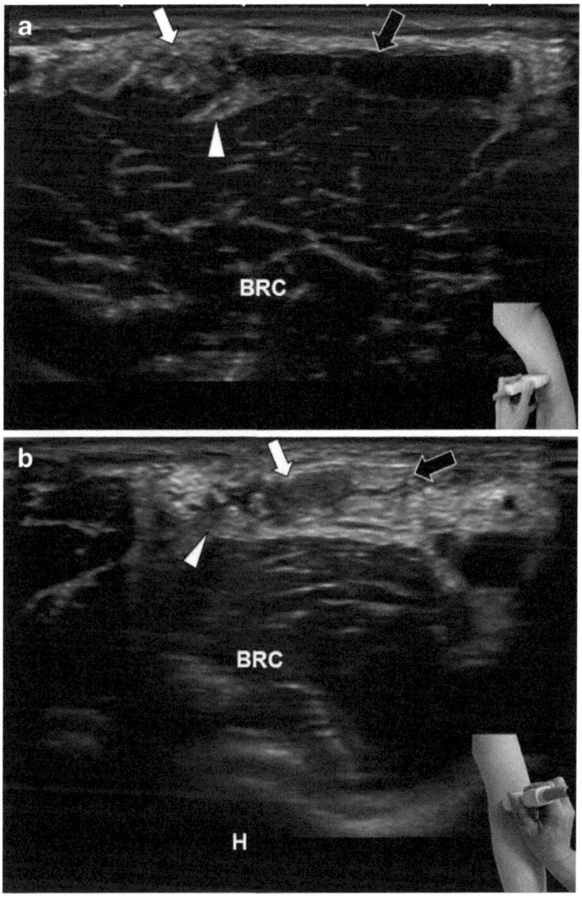

Fig. 8.27 Proximal normal segment (**a**) and distal thickened segment (**b**) of the lateral antebrachial cutaneous nerve (white arrowheads) in a case with partial tears of the distal tendon of the biceps brachii. White arrows: long head tendon of the distal biceps brachii; black arrows: short head tendon of the distal biceps brachii; BRC brachialis; H humerus

8.5 Ultrasound-Guided Injection

When administering an injection to the distal biceps brachii tendon, it is recommended to employ the posterior view, where the tendon is easily identifiable as it encircles the proximal radius. This approach presents the advantage of conducting the injection without the concern of collateral neurovascular damage, as all pertinent nerves and vessels are situated on the volar side of the proximal forearm. By positioning the transducer between the proximal posterior radius and ulna, the needle can be introduced using the in-plane approach, moving from the radial to ulnar aspect (Fig. 8.28a). In the case of injecting the bicipitoradial bursa, the transducer is positioned over the elbow crease to recognize the bursa encircling the distal biceps brachii tendon [14] (Fig. 8.28b). The needle is introduced using the in-plane

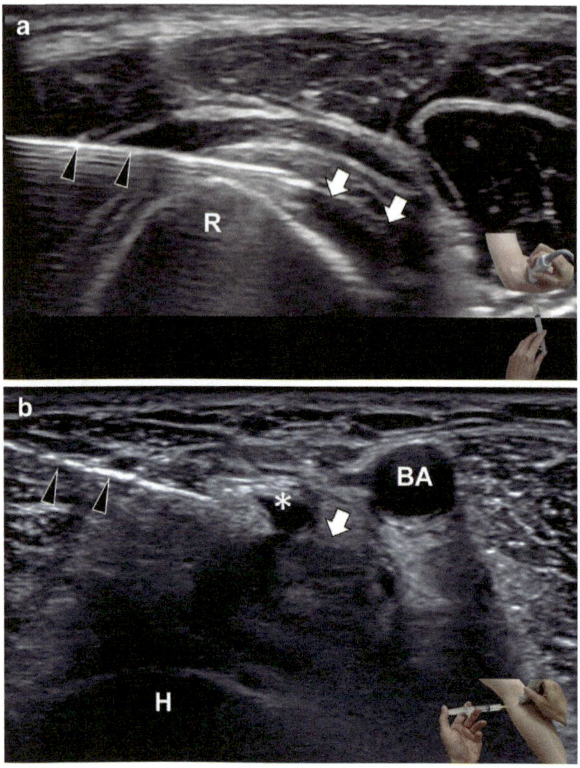

Fig. 8.28 Ultrasound-guided injection targeting the distal tendon of the biceps brachii (white arrows) (**a**) and the bicipitoradial bursa (asterisk) (**b**). Black arrowheads: needle trajectory; BA brachial artery; R radius; H humerus

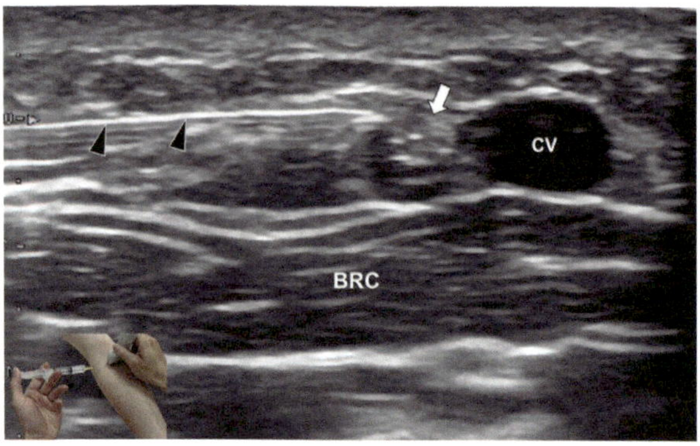

Fig. 8.29 Ultrasound-guided lateral antebrachial cutaneous nerve (white arrow) hydrodissection. Black arrowheads: needle trajectory; CV cephalic vein; BRC brachialis

approach from lateral to medial, navigating between the radial nerve and distal biceps brachii tendon. Additionally, the forearm is supinated to alleviate compression on the bicipitoradial bursa. If there is associated involvement of the adjacent lateral antebrachial cutaneous nerve (Fig. 8.29), consideration can be given to conducting ultrasound-guided perineural hydrodissection.

8.6 Conclusion

Among the three views for the distal biceps brachii tendon, the medial view (pronator window) is most effective for distinguishing its pathologies and determining which component (long head or short head) is affected. Conversely, the posterior view is optimal for injecting the distal biceps brachii tendon with minimal risk of neurovascular injury. In situations involving unresponsive patients, consideration should be given to the involvement of the adjacent lateral antebrachial cutaneous nerve, and ultrasound-guided perineural hydrodissection can be beneficial for alleviating symptoms.

Acknowledgments Images and illustrations adapted from cadaveric images provided by the Visible Human Project® of the National Library of Medicine. Excerpts featured in the VH Dissector are used with permission from Touch of Life Technologies Inc.

References

1. Safran MR, Graham SM. Distal biceps tendon ruptures: incidence, demographics, and the effect of smoking. Clin Orthop Relat Res. 2002:404.
2. Kulshreshtha R, Singh R, Sinha J, Hall S. Anatomy of the distal biceps Brachii tendon and its clinical relevance. Clin Orthop Relat Res. 2007:456.
3. Athwal GS, Steinmann SP, Rispoli DM. The distal biceps tendon: footprint and relevant clinical anatomy. J Hand Surg Am. 2007;32(8):1225–9.
4. Mazzocca AD, Cohen M, Berkson E, et al. The anatomy of the bicipital tuberosity and distal biceps tendon. J Shoulder Elb Surg. 2007;16(1):122–7.
5. Skaf AY, Boutin RD, Dantas RW, et al. Bicipitoradial bursitis: MR imaging findings in eight patients and anatomic data from contrast material opacification of bursae followed by routine radiography and MR imaging in cadavers. Radiology. 1999;212(1):111–6.
6. Chang KV, Mezian K, Nanka O, et al. Ultrasound imaging for the cutaneous nerves of the extremities and relevant entrapment syndromes: from anatomy to clinical implications. J Clin Med. 2018;7(11)
7. Beldner S, Zlotolow DA, Melone CP Jr, Agnes AM, Jones MH. Anatomy of the lateral antebrachial cutaneous and superficial radial nerves in the forearm: a cadaveric and clinical study. J Hand Surg Am. 2005;30(6):1226–30.
8. Smith J, Finnoff JT, O'Driscoll SW, Lai JK. Sonographic evaluation of the distal biceps tendon using a medial approach: the pronator window. J Ultrasound Med. 2010;29(5):861–5.
9. Ilayperuma I, Uluwitiya SM, Nanayakkara BG, Palahepitiya KN. Re-visiting the brachialis muscle: morphology, morphometry, gender diversity, and innervation. Surg Radiol Anat. 2019;41(4):393–400.
10. Leonello DT, Galley IJ, Bain GI, Carter CD. Brachialis muscle anatomy. A study in cadavers. J Bone Joint Surg Am. 2007;89(6):1293–7.
11. Pierce JL, Nacey NC. Elbow ultrasound. Current Radiology Reports. 2016;4(10):51.
12. Chiavaras MM, Jacobson JA, Billone L, Lawton JM, Lawton J. Sonography of the lateral antebrachial cutaneous nerve with magnetic resonance imaging and anatomic correlation. J Ultrasound Med. 2014;33(8):1475–83.
13. Chang MC, Chang KV, Wu WT, Özçakar L. Ultrasound imaging for painful lipomatosis: cutaneous nerves really matter! Am J Phys Med Rehabil. 2020;99(7):e88–e9.
14. Chang KV, Wu WT, Ozcakar L. An uncommon cause of anterior elbow pain: diagnosis and injection for bicipitoradial bursitis using ultrasonography. Kaohsiung J Med Sci. 2017;33(4):212–3.

Part III
Wrist and Hand

Chapter 9
De Quervain's Disease Reimagined

Ke-Vin Chang, Wei-Ting Wu, and Yuan-Yuan Tsai

9.1 Introduction

De Quervain tenosynovitis, coined by the Swiss surgeon Fritz de Quervain in 1895, gained initial recognition through his description. Adachi et al. [1] conducted a study highlighting De Quervain's disease as a significant contributor to wrist pain. The research involved 402 participants (804 hands), revealing a 3.7% prevalence of De Quervain's disease (15 out of 402 individuals). The prevalence across age groups showed 9.8% in their forties, 3.6% in their fifties, 1.8% in their sixties, 3.9% in their seventies, and 3.7% in their eighties. Females exhibited a notably higher prevalence compared to males. No significant differences were noted in mean age, hand dominance, height, weight, labor activity intensity, or the presence of medical complications.

Symptoms associated with De Quervain's disease include pain and swelling near the base of the thumb, along with challenges in moving the thumb and wrist during grasping or pinching activities. The study by Clarke and colleagues [2] found that histopathology did not suggest inflammation but indicated thickening of the tendon sheath and the accumulation of mucopolysaccharide, a marker for myxoid degeneration. Presently, ultrasound is widely acknowledged as a valuable diagnostic tool for De Quervain's disease. This chapter will delve into the sonoanatomy near the first dorsal compartment of the wrist and discuss the safe and effective application of ultrasound-guided injections.

K.-V. Chang (✉) · W.-T. Wu · Y.-Y. Tsai
Bei-Hu Branch, National Taiwan University Hospital, Taipei, Taiwan

K.-V. Chang (ed.), *Ultrasonography of Musculoskeletal Pain*,
https://doi.org/10.1007/978-981-96-6787-1_9

9.2 Regional Anatomy

The abductor pollicis longus tendon originates from the posterior surface of the proximal half of the radius, ulna, and interosseous membrane, ultimately inserting onto the base of the first metacarpal bone (Fig. 9.1). In a cadaveric study conducted by Marí-Gorreto et al. [3], which involved the examination of 30 upper limbs, it was observed that the abductor pollicis longus tendon's main structure could exist as either a single tendon (19 instances/63.3%) or be divided into two or three independent tendons, categorized as the double type (8 instances/26.7%) or triple type (3 instances/10%). Furthermore, variations were noted in the insertion of the abductor pollicis longus main tendon, with instances of insertion into the abductor pollicis brevis muscle (2 instances/6.66%) or the opponens pollicis muscle (2 instances/6.66%).

The extensor pollicis brevis has its origin on the posterior surface of the distal third of the radius and the interosseous membrane, inserting onto the posterior aspect of the base of the proximal phalanx of the thumb (Fig. 9.1). According to Jabir

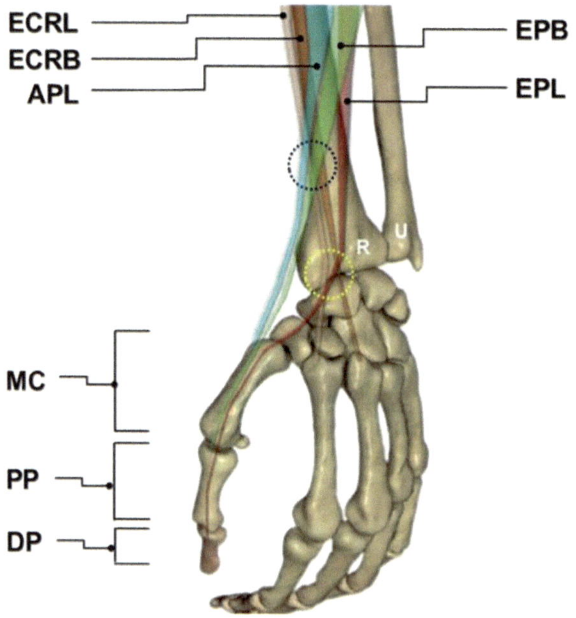

Fig. 9.1 The illustration depicts the abductor pollicis longus tendon, extensor pollicis brevis tendon, and their insertions. The black dashed circle indicates the proximal intersection, where the abductor pollicis longus and extensor pollicis brevis muscles cross over the second dorsal extensor compartment. The yellow dashed circle indicates the distal intersection, where the extensor pollicis longus muscle crosses over the second dorsal extensor compartment. APL abductor pollicis longus; EPB extensor pollicis brevis; ECRL extensor carpi radialis longus; ECRB extensor carpi radialis brevis; EPL extensor pollicis longus; MC metacarpal; PP proximal phalanx; DP distal phalanx; R radius; U ulna

et al.'s review, there is variability in the anatomical relationships of the extensor pollicis brevis with the abductor pollicis longus. The extensor pollicis brevis may either run in a distinct tendon compartment or share a common tendon sheath with the abductor pollicis longus. Within the first extensor compartment, which houses the abductor pollicis longus and extensor pollicis brevis, a separation is observed in 30–60% of cases, attributed to a complete or partial septum. Additionally, it is noted that the extensor pollicis brevis tendon might have an origin from the same muscle belly as the abductor pollicis longus tendon. In certain instances, the extensor pollicis brevis tendon may extend into the extensor hood of the thumb. These variations highlight the complex and diverse anatomical considerations associated with the extensor pollicis brevis and its relationship with neighboring structures.

The abductor pollicis longus and extensor pollicis brevis receive innervation from the posterior interosseous nerve (Fig. 9.2). According to findings from the cadaveric study conducted by Jariwala et al. [4], following its emergence from the lower border of the supinator, the posterior interosseous nerve undergoes division subsequent to supplying the extensor pollicis longus. The resulting branches exhibit distinct courses: the medial branch concludes its trajectory in the extensor indicis proprius, while the lateral branch continues distally, coursing along the interosseous membrane beneath the extensor pollicis longus. Upon issuing its final motor branch, the posterior interosseous nerve persists in its distal course as a unified sensory branch, ultimately terminating in the fourth extensor compartment across all specimens.

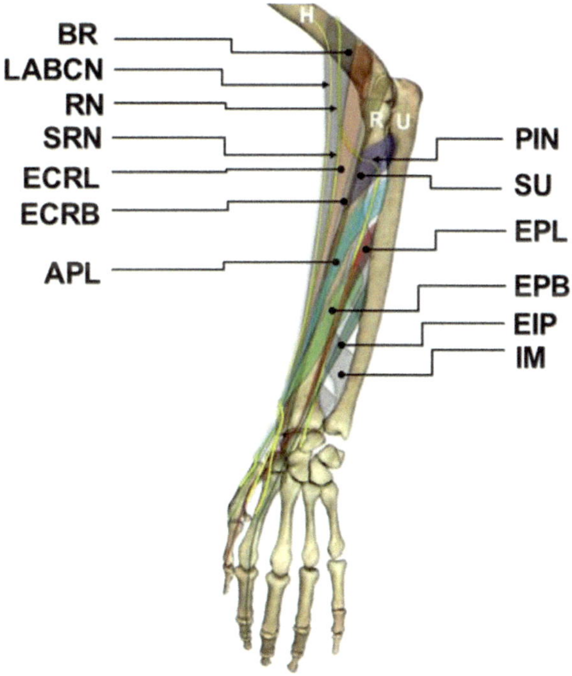

Fig. 9.2 The illustration shows the pathway of the posterior interosseous nerve (PIN) along with related nerves and the muscles they innervate. LABCN lateral antebrachial cutaneous nerve; RN radial nerve; SRN superficial radial nerve; APL abductor pollicis longus; EPB extensor pollicis brevis; ECRL extensor carpi radialis longus; ECRB extensor carpi radialis brevis; EPL extensor pollicis longus; EIP extensor indicis proprius; SU supinator; BR brachioradialis; IM interosseous membrane; R radius; U ulna; H humerus

Another pertinent nerve in this context is the superficial radial nerve (Fig. 9.3). Originating beneath the brachioradialis muscle, between the heads of the extensor carpi radialis longus and brachioradialis muscles, the superficial radial nerve demonstrates distinctive branching patterns. The initial branch, extending radially and progressing along the volar aspect of the forearm, is responsible for innervating the radial aspect of the thumb [5]. Continuing distally, the remaining segment of the main trunk of the superficial radial nerve travels radially to Lister's tubercle of the radius. Subsequently, two to five branches, such as the dorsal medial or dorsal lateral branches, emerge from the superficial radial nerve and traverse the tendon of the extensor pollicis longus. The point of divergence between the main trunk and its first branch creates a fork that overlays the extensor retinaculum on the radial aspect of the wrist. Notably, the superficial radial nerve closely associates with the cephalic vein in its course, emphasizing the intricate anatomical relationships within this region.

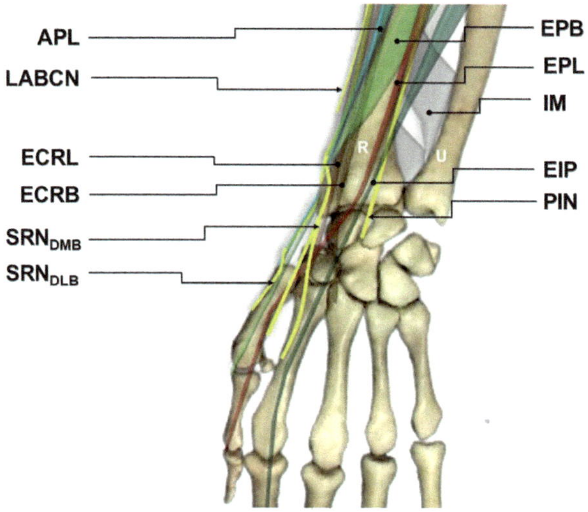

Fig. 9.3 The illustration depicts the course of the superficial radial nerve and its terminal branches. SRN_{DMB} dorsal medial branch of the superficial radial nerve; SRN_{DLB} dorsal lateral branch of the superficial radial nerve; APL abductor pollicis longus; EPB extensor pollicis brevis; ECRL extensor carpi radialis longus; ECRB extensor carpi radialis brevis; EPL extensor pollicis longus; EIP extensor indicis proprius; LABCN lateral antebrachial cutaneous nerve; PIN posterior interosseous nerve; IM interosseous membrane; R radius; U ulna

9.3 Sonoanatomy

9.3.1 Dorsal Wrist Extensor Compartments

The transducer is positioned over the radial styloid to visualize the abductor pollicis longus on the radial side and the extensor pollicis brevis on the ulnar side within the first dorsal extensor compartment (Fig. 9.4a, b). To explore other compartments of the dorsal wrist, the transducer can be smoothly moved from the radial to ulnar aspect.

As it moves towards the ulnar side, two notches on the distal radius accommodate the extensor carpi radialis longus on the radial side and the extensor carpi radialis brevis on the ulnar side (Fig. 9.4b). After identifying the short axis of the extensor carpi radialis longus and extensor pollicis brevis at the radial styloid, the transducer can be traced along their paths to their insertions on the bases of the second (short axis, Fig. 9.5a, b; long axis, Fig. 9.5c, d) and third (short axis, Fig. 9.6a, b; long axis, Fig. 9.6c, d) metacarpals, first in the short axis and then in the long axis view. Progressing toward the more ulnar aspect, the recognition of Lister's tubercle, a

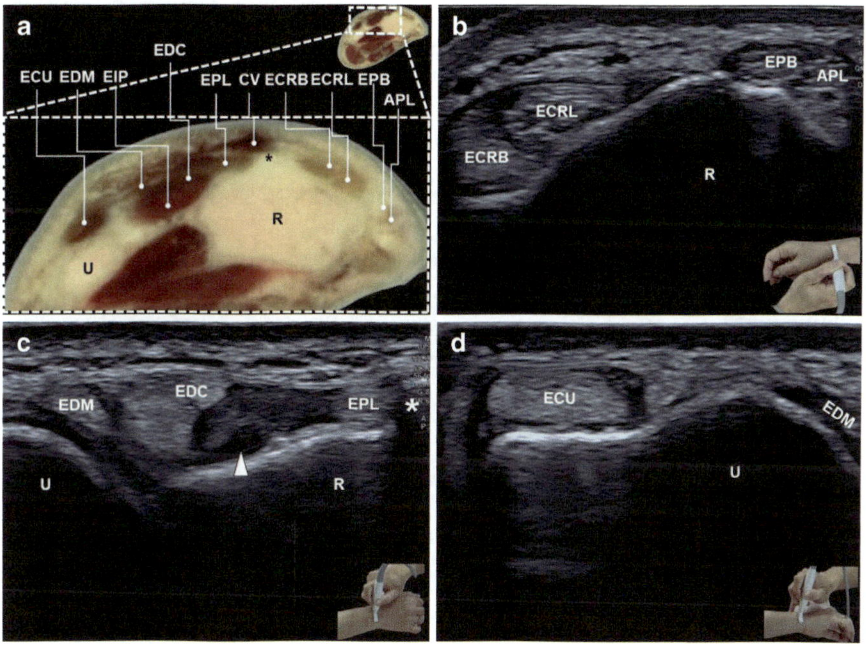

Fig. 9.4 The cadaveric image in the axial plane (**a**) and the corresponding sonoanatomy in the axial view illustrate the first to second (**b**), third to fifth (**c**), and sixth (**d**) dorsal wrist extensor compartments from the radial to ulnar aspect. White arrowhead: extensor indicis proprius tendon; asterisks: Lister's tubercle; CV cephalic vein; APL abductor pollicis longus; EPB extensor pollicis brevis; ECRL extensor carpi radialis longus; ECRB extensor carpi radialis brevis; EPL extensor pollicis longus; EDC extensor digitorum communis; EIP extensor indicis proprius; EDM extensor digiti minimi; ECU extensor carpi ulnaris; R radius; U ulna

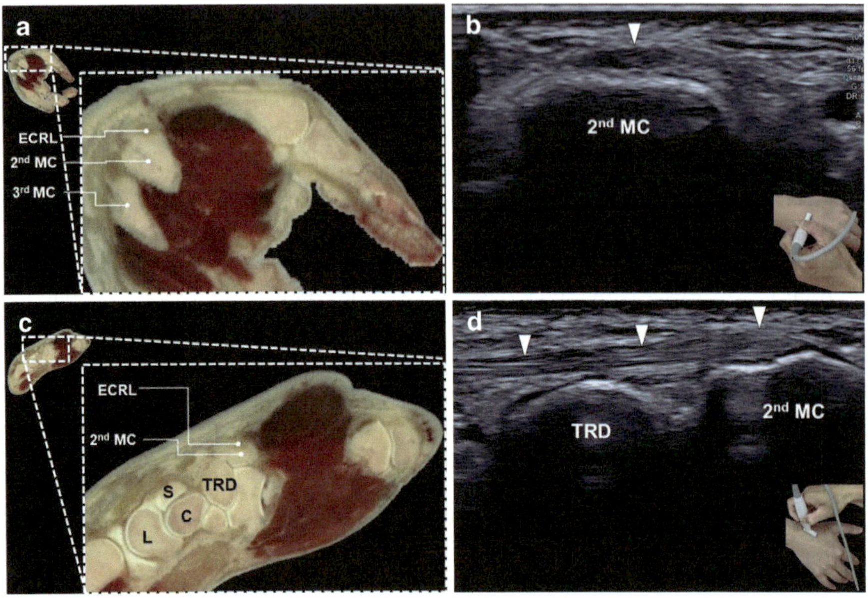

Fig. 9.5 The cadaveric image and corresponding sonoanatomy illustrate the distal insertion of the extensor carpi radialis longus tendon in the short-axis (**a**, **b**) and long-axis (**c**, **d**) views, respectively. White arrowheads and ECRL: extensor carpi radialis longus tendon; MC metacarpal; L lunate; S scaphoid; C capitate; TRD trapezoid

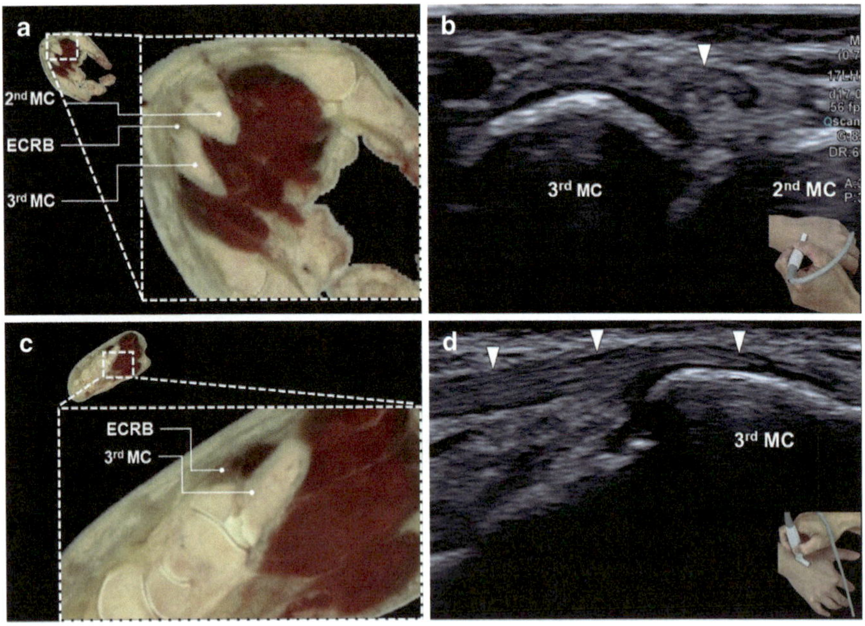

Fig. 9.6 The cadaveric image and corresponding sonoanatomy illustrate the extensor carpi radialis brevis tendon at its distal insertion in the short-axis (**a**, **b**) and long-axis (**c**, **d**) views, respectively. MC metacarpal; ECRB and white arrowheads: extensor carpi radialis brevis

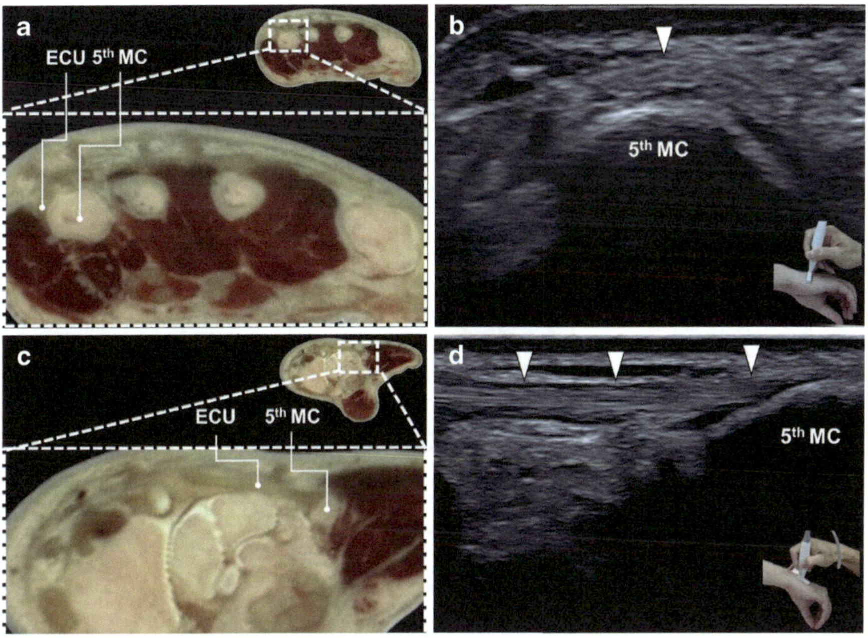

Fig. 9.7 The cadaveric images and corresponding sonoanatomy illustrate the distal insertion of the extensor carpi ulnaris tendon in the short-axis (**a**, **b**) and long-axis (**c**, **d**) views, respectively. ECU and white arrowheads: extensor carpi ulnaris; MC metacarpal

bony prominence on the distal radius, indicates the presence of the third compartment on the ulnar side of the tubercle, which is traversed by the extensor pollicis longus (Fig. 9.4c).

Further laterally, the fourth compartment becomes evident, accommodating the extensor digitorum communis and extensor indicis proprius (Fig. 9.4c). Even more laterally, the fifth compartment appears at the distal radio-ulnar joint, where the extensor digiti minimi is located (Fig. 9.4d). On the distal ulnar styloid, the sixth compartment is identified, housing the extensor carpi ulnaris. After identifying the extensor carpi ulnaris at the ulnar styloid, the transducer can be moved distally to visualize the tendon's distal insertion in both the short-axis (Fig. 9.7a, b) and long-axis views (Fig. 9.7c, d).

9.3.2 Thumb Extensor Tendon Origin

The transducer is repositioned to the axial plane on the radial styloid, following the course of the abductor pollicis longus and extensor pollicis brevis towards the dorsal forearm. The distal myotendinous junctions of the abductor pollicis longus and extensor pollicis brevis converge over the second dorsal extensor compartment

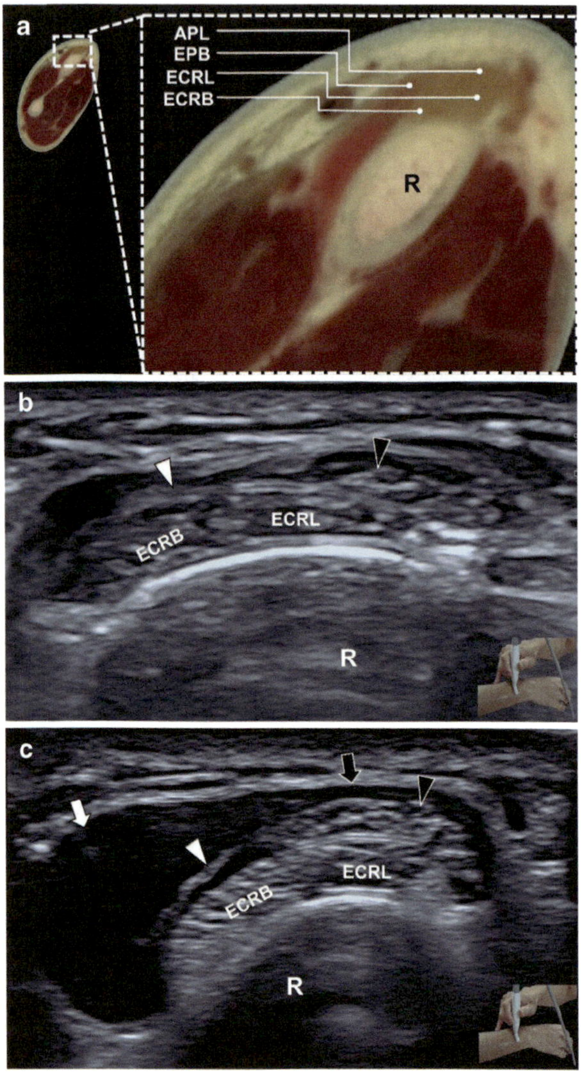

Fig. 9.8 The cadaveric image (**a**) and the corresponding sonoanatomy illustrate the proximal intersection from the distal aspect (**b**) to the proximal aspect (**c**). White arrowheads: extensor pollicis brevis tendon; white arrow: extensor pollicis brevis muscle; black arrowheads: abductor pollicis longus tendon; black arrow: abductor pollicis longus muscle; APL abductor pollicis longus; EPB extensor pollicis brevis; ECRL extensor carpi radialis longus; ECRB extensor carpi radialis brevis; R radius

(Fig. 9.8a, b), whereas the muscular portions of the abductor pollicis longus and extensor pollicis brevis become more prominent at a cranial level (Fig. 9.8c). Shifting the transducer more cranially reveals a sequential view of the abductor pollicis longus, extensor pollicis brevis, extensor pollicis longus, and extensor indicis proprius from the radial to ulnar aspects (Fig. 9.9a, b).

Tracking their origin on the dorsal forearm, the abductor pollicis longus, extensor pollicis longus, and extensor indicis proprius can be identified, while the extensor pollicis brevis terminates on the interosseous membrane (short axis, Fig. 9.10a, c; long axis, Fig. 9.10b, d).

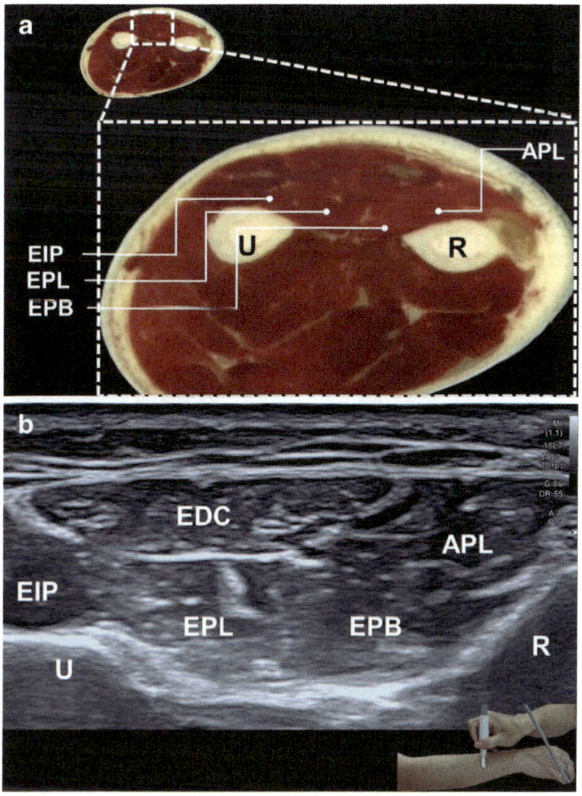

Fig. 9.9 The cadaveric image in the axial plane (**a**) and the corresponding sonoanatomy (**b**) illustrate the muscle belly of the dorsal wrist extensors. APL abductor pollicis longus; EPB extensor pollicis brevis; EPL extensor pollicis longus; EIP extensor indicis proprius; EDC extensor digitorum communis; R radius; U ulna

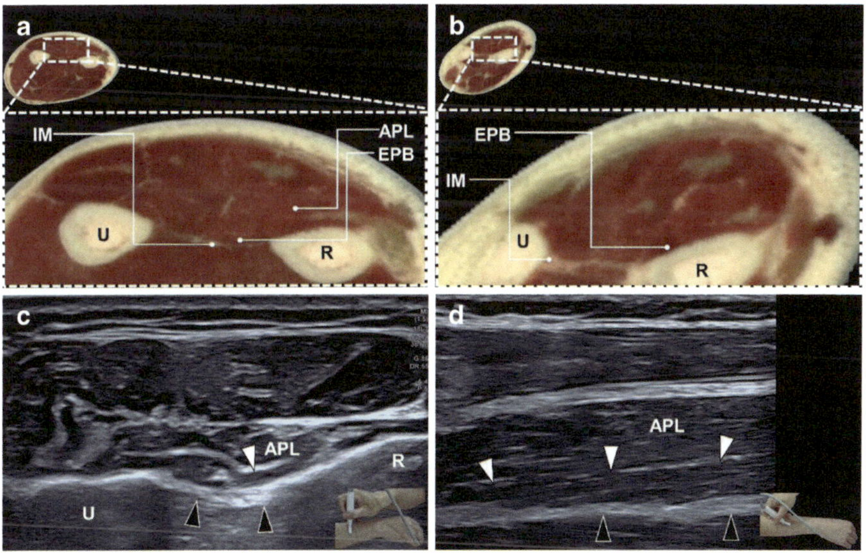

Fig. 9.10 The cadaveric images and the corresponding sonoanatomy illustrate the extensor pollicis brevis in short-axis (**a**, **c**) and long-axis (**b**, **d**) views, respectively. EPB and white arrowheads: extensor pollicis brevis; IM and black arrowheads: interosseous membrane; APL abductor pollicis longus; R radius; U ulna

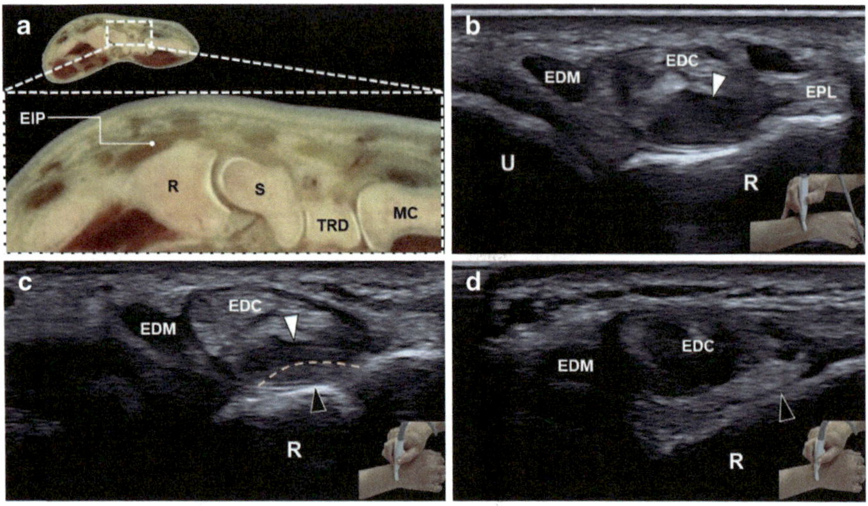

Fig. 9.11 The cadaveric image (**a**) displays the extensor indicis proprius muscle in the long axis. The sonoanatomy images show the extensor indicis proprius in short axis at the distal muscle belly (**b**), myotendinous junction (**c**), and distal tendon (**d**) levels. The pink dashed line in (**c**) marks the myotendinous junction. White arrowheads: extensor indicis proprius muscle; black arrowheads: extensor indicis propius tendon; EPL extensor pollicis longus; EDC extensor digitorum communis; EIP extensor indicis propius; EDM extensor digiti minimi; R radius; S scaphoid; TRD trapezoid; MC metacarpal

The extensor indicis proprius is a muscle located adjacent to the extensor pollicis brevis in the dorsal forearm. To confirm the extensor indicis proprius (Fig. 9.11a), positioning the transducer over the radial styloid level allows visualization of the fourth dorsal extensor compartment, with further cranial movement for verification. In contrast to the extensor digitorum communis, the extensor indicis proprius exhibits a more distal myotendinous junction. Consequently, when the transducer is moved in the cranial to caudal direction, identification of a tendon emerging from a relatively more distal muscle belly confirms it as the extensor indicis proprius (distal muscle belly, Fig. 9.11b; myotendinous junction, Fig. 9.11c; tendinous portion, Fig. 9.11d).

9.3.3 Thumb Distal Tendon Insertion

Repositioning the transducer to the distal radius in the axial plane reveals the presence of the abductor pollicis longus and extensor pollicis brevis within the first dorsal extensor compartment. As the transducer is moved distally, spanning the articular gap between the scaphoid and radius, these two tendons move beyond the confines of the extensor retinaculum, exposing the underlying radial artery (Fig. 9.12a–c). Continuing past the trapezium, the abductor pollicis longus

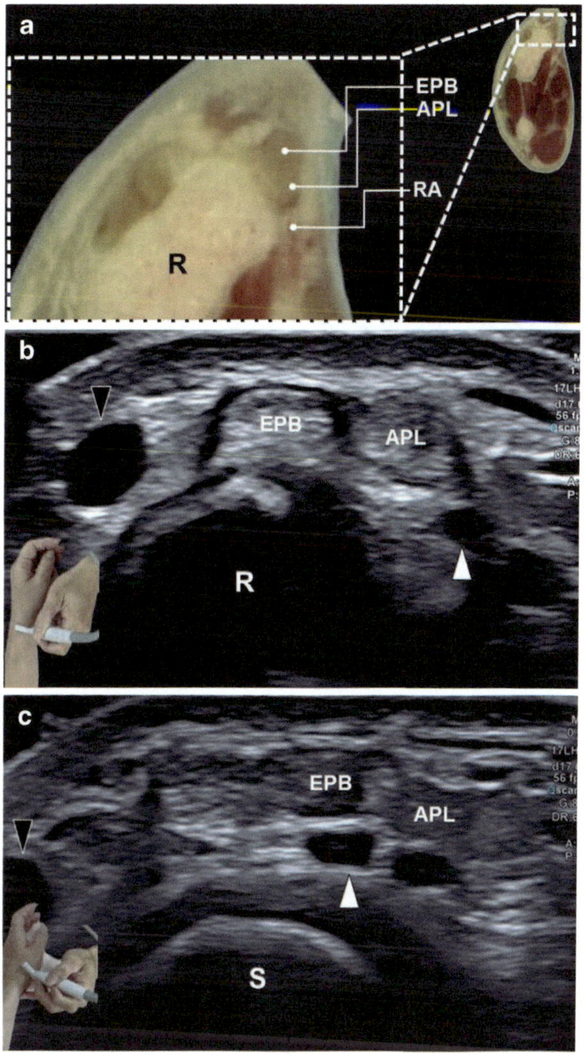

Fig. 9.12 The cadaveric image (**a**) and the sonoanatomy demonstrate the relationship between the abductor pollicis longus, extensor pollicis brevis, and the radial artery at the levels of the radius (**b**) and scaphoid (**c**), respectively. Black arrowheads: cephalic vein; RA and white arrowheads: radial artery; APL abductor pollicis longus; EPB extensor pollicis brevis; R radius; S scaphoid

becomes visible, attaching to the base of the first metacarpal bone (short axis, Fig. 9.13a, c; long axis, Fig. 9.13b, d). In contrast, the extensor pollicis brevis, running parallel and ulnar to the abductor pollicis longus, progresses forward until it connects to the base of the proximal phalanx (short axis, Fig. 9.14a, c; long axis, Fig. 9.14b, d).

Concerning the extensor pollicis longus, readjusting the transducer to the distal radius is necessary to visualize it within the third compartment (Fig. 9.4c), positioned ulnar to Lister's tubercle. Moving the transducer distally toward the dorsal aspect of the thumb, the extensor pollicis longus courses over the second dorsal extensor compartment, which houses the extensor carpi radialis longus and extensor

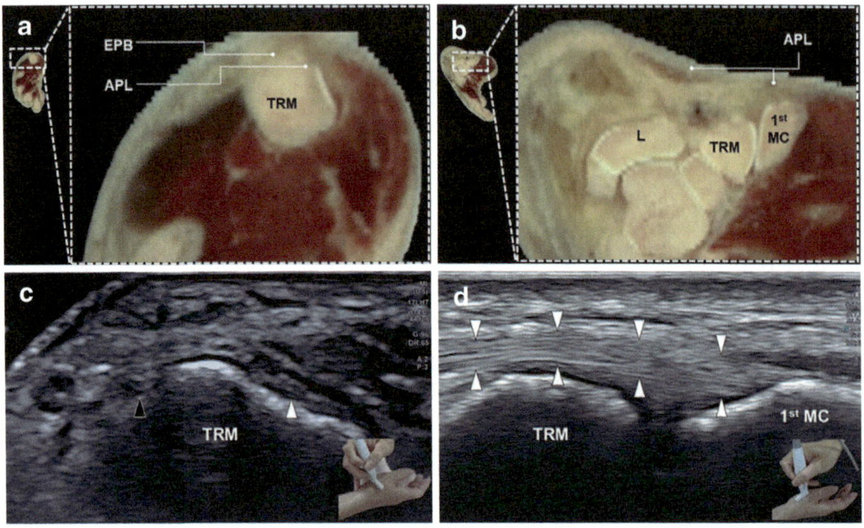

Fig. 9.13 The cadaveric images and the corresponding sonoanatomy illustrate the abductor pollicis longus tendon in the short-axis (**a**, **c**) and long-axis (**b**, **d**) views, respectively. APL and white arrowheads: abductor pollicis longus tendon; EPB and black arrowhead: extensor pollicis brevis tendon; TRM trapezium; L lunate; 1st MC first metacarpal

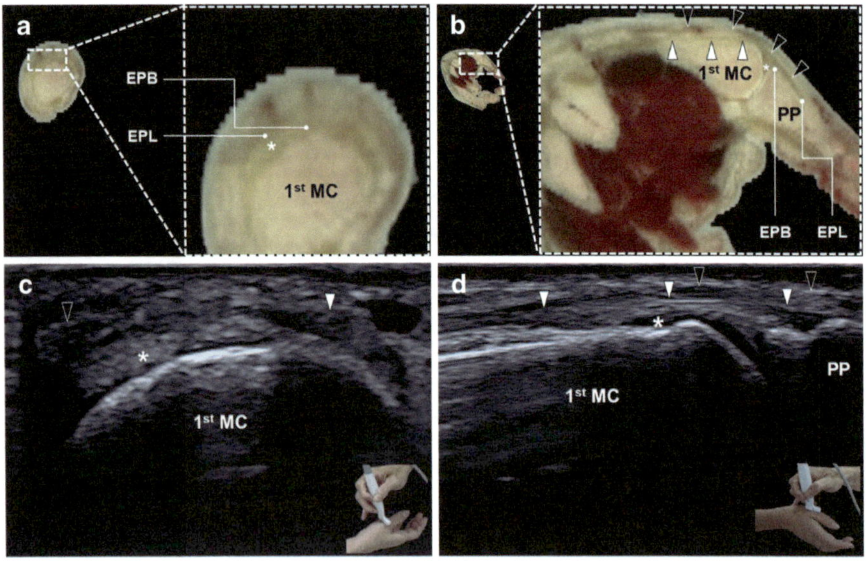

Fig. 9.14 The cadaveric image and the corresponding sonoanatomy illustrate the insertion of the extensor pollicis brevis tendon in the short-axis (**a**, **c**) and long-axis (**b**, **d**) views, respectively. EPB and white arrowheads: extensor pollicis brevis; EPL and black arrowheads: extensor pollicis longus; white asterisk: dorsal plate; MC metacarpal; PP proximal phalanx

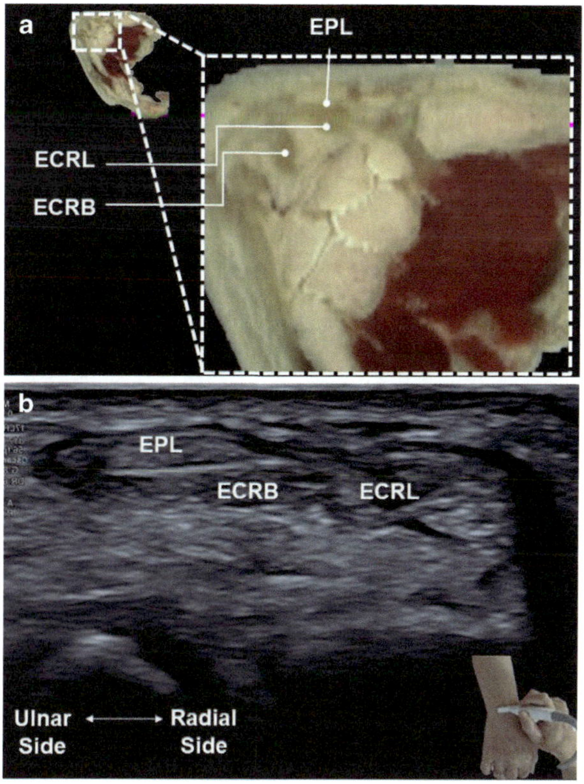

Fig. 9.15 The cadaveric image (**a**) and the corresponding sonoanatomy (**b**) illustrate the distal intersection junction that extensor pollicis longus tendon courses above the second compartment. EPL extensor pollicis longus; ECRB extensor carpi radialis brevis; ECRL extensor carpi radialis longus

carpi radialis brevis (Fig. 9.15a, b). Subsequently, the extensor pollicis longus tendon continues its distal trajectory until it attaches to the base of the distal phalanx. Once the short axis of these tendons is successfully depicted (Fig. 9.16a, c), redirecting the transducer to the tendon's long axis allows for the observation of their attachment either to the metacarpal bone or phalanx (Fig. 9.16b, d).

9.3.4 Relevant Nerves

To locate the terminal segment of the posterior interosseous nerve, position the transducer over the distal radius, specifically on the fourth dorsal extensor compartment. Within this compartment, the posterior interosseous nerve appears as an ovoid hypoechoic structure, situated at the base (Fig. 9.17a, b). It typically resides between the tendons of the extensor digitorum communis and extensor indicis proprius. Upon tracking more proximally, the posterior interosseous nerve becomes identifiable as it ascends from the interosseous membrane, traversing the gap between the extensor pollicis brevis and extensor pollicis longus (Fig. 9.18a, b). Subsequently, it

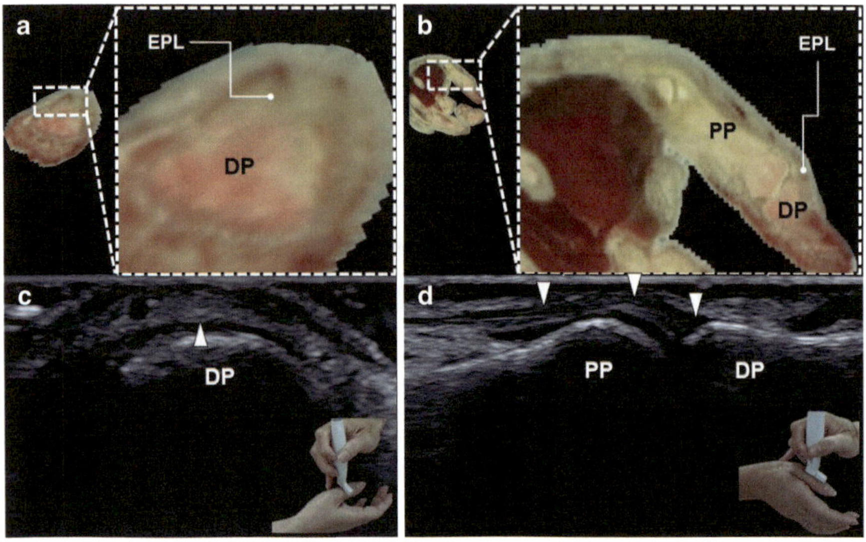

Fig. 9.16 The cadaveric image and the corresponding sonoanatomy (**c**, **d**) illustrate the insertion of the extensor pollicis longus tendon in the short-axis (**a**, **c**) and long-axis (**b**, **d**) views, respectively. EPL and white arrowheads: extensor pollicis longus; PP proximal phalanx; DP distal phalanx

Fig. 9.17 The cadaveric image (**a**) and corresponding sonoanatomy (**b**) illustrate the posterior interosseous nerve situated at the base of the fourth compartment. PIN and white arrowhead: posterior interosseous nerve; PIA and black arrowhead: posterior interosseous artery; white asterisk: Lister's tubercle; EPL extensor pollicis longus; EDC extensor digitorum communis; EIP extensor indicis propius; EDM extensor digiti minimi; R radius; U ulna

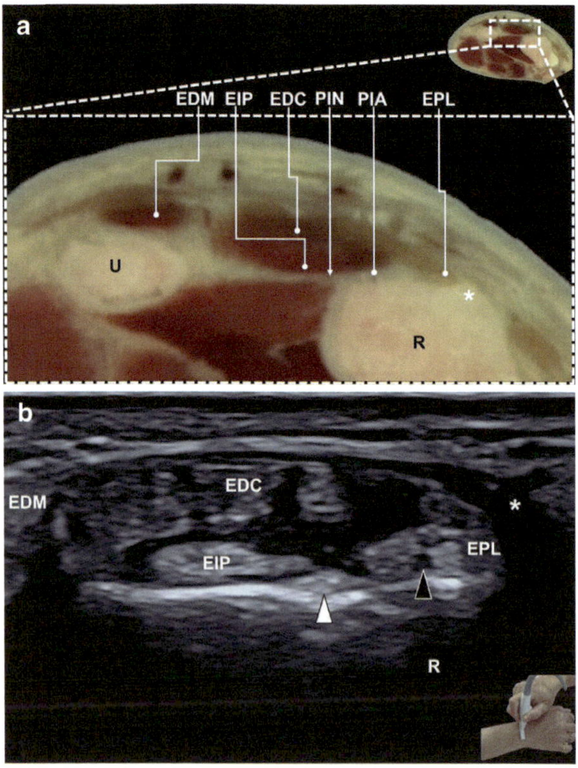

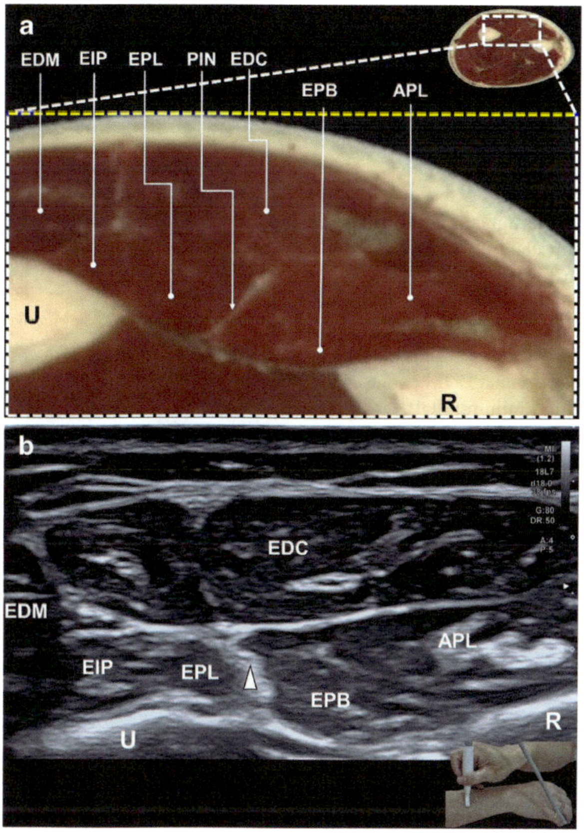

Fig. 9.18 The cadaveric image (**a**) and corresponding sonoanatomy in the axial view (**b**) illustrate the posterior interosseous nerve between the extensor pollicis brevis and extensor pollicis longus muscle. PIN and white arrowhead: posterior interosseous nerve; APL abductor pollicis longus; EPB extensor pollicis brevis; EPL extensor pollicis longus; EDC extensor digitorum communis; EIP extensor indicis propius; EDM extensor digiti minimi; R radius; U ulna

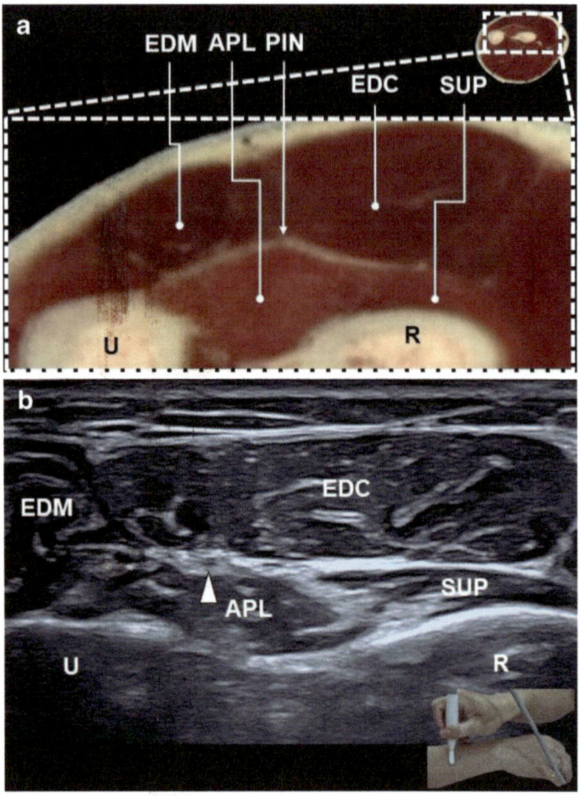

Fig. 9.19 The cadaveric image (**a**) and corresponding sonoanatomy in axial view (**b**) illustrate the posterior interosseous nerve between the abductor pollicis longus and extensor digitorum communis muscle. PIN and white arrowhead: posterior interosseous nerve; APL abductor pollicis longus; EDC extensor digitorum communis; EDM extensor digiti minimi; SUP supinator; R radius; U ulna

courses through the fascial plane between the extensor digitorum communis and the muscles responsible for thumb abduction and extension (Fig. 9.19a, b).

To locate the superficial radial nerve, the transducer is positioned over the volar distal forearm, allowing for visualization of the nerve's course alongside the radial artery beneath the brachioradialis muscle (Fig. 9.20a, c). As the nerve progresses distally, it separates from the radial artery, pierces the antebrachial fascia, and emerges into the subcutaneous layer between the brachioradialis and extensor carpi radialis longus (Fig. 9.20b, d). It then divides into the dorsal medial and dorsal lateral branches at the level where the brachioradialis tendon inserts onto the distal

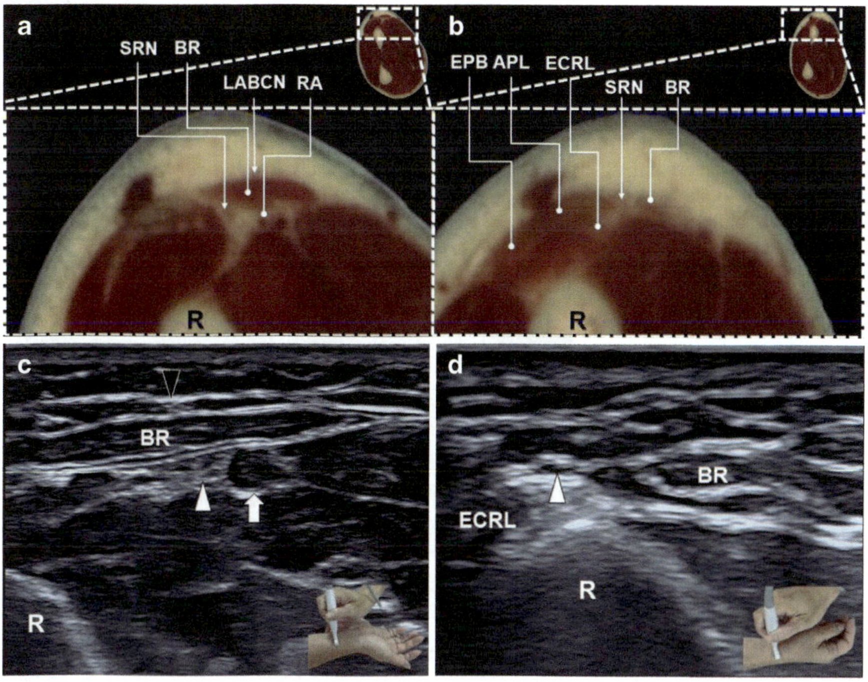

Fig. 9.20 The cadaveric images in the axial plane and the corresponding sonoanatomy in the axial view demonstrate the superficial radial nerve beneath the brachioradialis muscle (**a**, **c**) and depict the nerve emerging through the antebrachial fascia, lateral to the brachioradialis (**b**, **d**). SRN and white arrowheads: superficial radial nerve; RA and white arrow: radial artery; LABCN and black arrowhead: lateral antebrachial cutaneous nerve; APL abductor pollicis longus; EPB extensor pollicis brevis; ECRL extensor carpi radialis longus; BR brachioradialis; R radius

radius (Fig. 9.21a, b). The dorsal medial branch of the superficial radial nerve traverses over the first dorsal extensor compartment, ultimately supplying the dorsal radial aspect of the hand and dorsal ulnar aspect of the thumb (Fig. 9.22a, b). The dorsal lateral branch of the superficial radial nerve follows a radial trajectory adjacent to the first dorsal extensor compartment, providing innervation to the dorsal lateral aspect of the thumb (Fig. 9.23a, b).

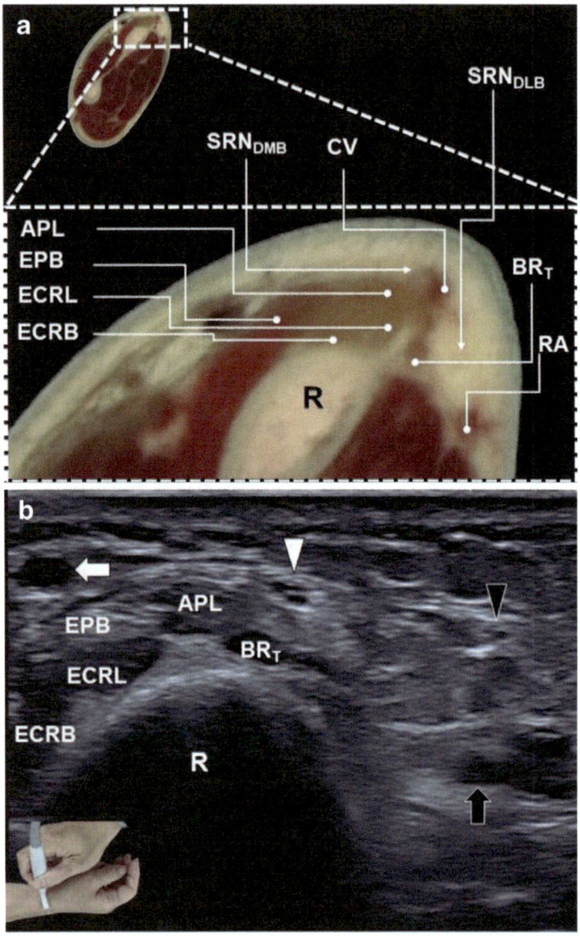

Fig. 9.21 The cadaveric image (**a**) and the corresponding sonoanatomy in the axial view (**b**) illustrate the dorsal medial and lateral branches of the superficial radial nerve at the level where the brachioradialis attaches to the distal radius. SRN_{DMB} and white arrowhead: dorsal medial branch of the superficial radial nerve; SRN_{DLB} and black arrowhead: dorsal lateral branch of the superficial radial nerve; CV and white arrow: cephalic vein; RA and black arrow: radial artery; APL abductor pollicis longus; EPB extensor pollicis brevis; ECRL extensor carpi radialis longus; ECRB extensor carpi radialis brevis; BR_T brachioradialis tendon; R radius

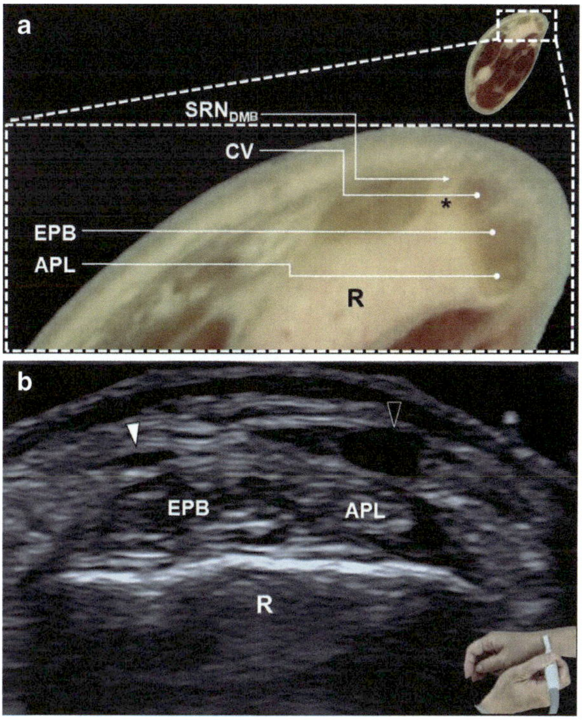

Fig. 9.22 The cadaveric image (**a**) and the corresponding sonoanatomy (**b**) demonstrate the dorsal medial branch of the superficial radial nerve as it is positioned to cross the first dorsal extensor compartment. SRN$_{DMB}$ and white arrowhead: dorsal medial branch of the superficial radial nerve; CV and black arrowhead: cephalic vein; black asterisk: radial styloid; APL abductor pollicis longus; EPB extensor pollicis brevis; R radius

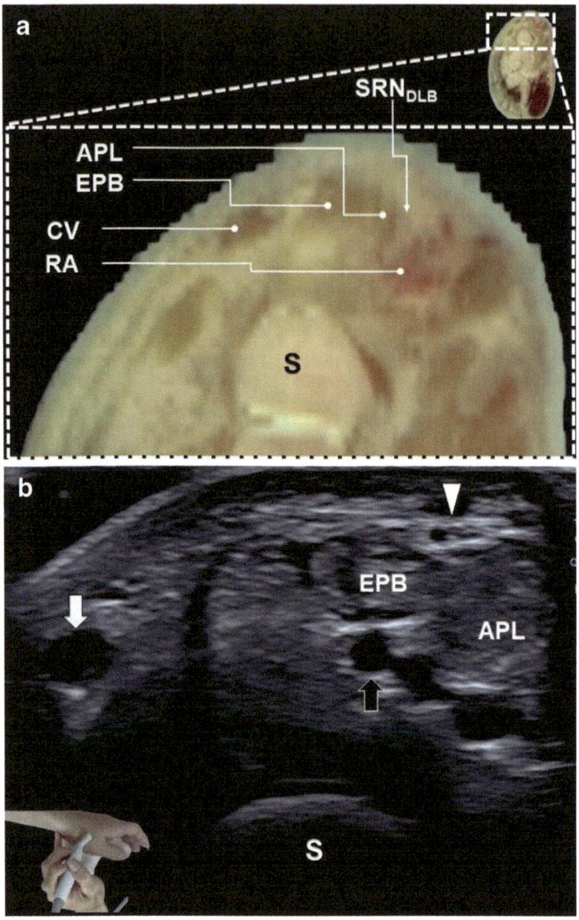

Fig. 9.23 The cadaveric image (**a**) and the corresponding sonoanatomy (**b**) illustrate the dorsal lateral branch of the superficial radial nerve in a short-axis view at the level of the scaphoid. SRN_{DLB} and white arrowhead: dorsal lateral branch of the superficial radial nerve; CV and white arrow: cephalic vein; RA and black arrow: radial artery; APL abductor pollicis longus; EPB extensor pollicis brevis; S scaphoid

9.4 Pathologies

In individuals diagnosed with De Quervain's disease, it is typical to observe localized swelling of the abductor pollicis longus and extensor pollicis brevis tendons near the radial styloid. The overlying retinaculum of the first dorsal extensor compartment often appears thickened with hypervascularity (Fig. 9.24a, b). Within this compartment, there may be either complete or partial separation, and the presence of a septum increases the likelihood of exclusive involvement of either the abductor pollicis longus or extensor pollicis brevis tendons for developing tenosynovitis (Fig. 9.24c).

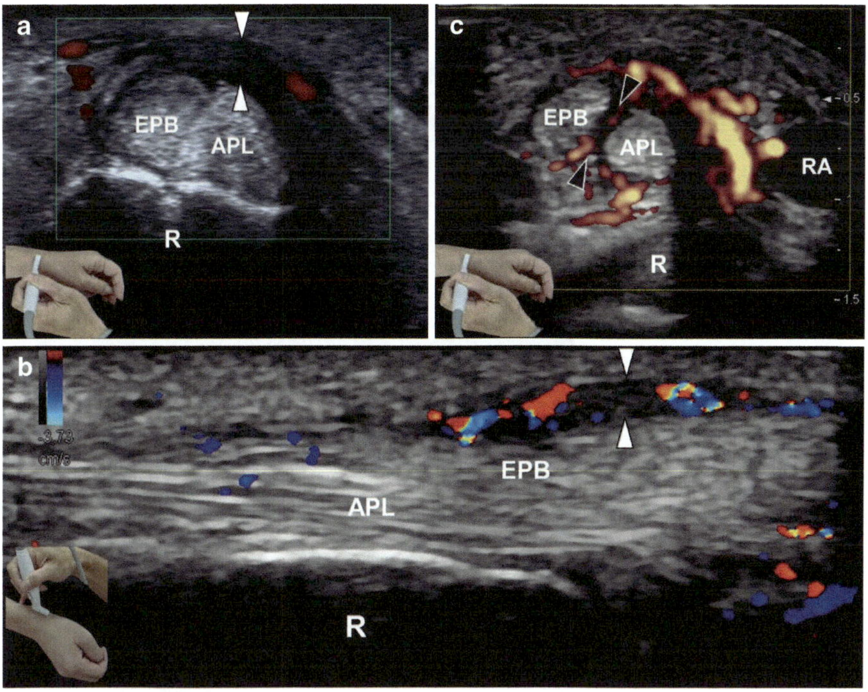

Fig. 9.24 The short-axis (**a**) and long-axis (**b**) ultrasound images reveal hypervascularity on power Doppler and a thickened retinaculum (white arrowheads) of the first dorsal extensor compartment. In another case of De Quervain's disease, a septum (black arrowheads) is visible within the first dorsal extensor compartment (**c**). RA radial artery; APL abductor pollicis longus; EPB extensor pollicis brevis; R radius

In patients with proximal (Fig. 9.25a) or distal intersection syndrome (Fig. 9.25b), hypervascularity can be observed in the tendon sheath and encircling retinaculum of the underlying extensor carpi radialis brevis and longus tendons. Additionally, multiple tendon slits within the first dorsal extensor compartment are commonly visualized in patients with De Quervain's disease (Fig. 9.25c). The primary trunk of the superficial radial nerve may become irritated, leading to greater swelling compared to the asymptomatic contralateral side. In cases where nerve swelling is not evident, the sonotinel sign, involving the use of a transducer to compress the superficial radial nerve, can be a helpful diagnostic technique.

Another concern involves the inability to extend the thumb. If the extensor pollicis brevis is fully torn, the patient can still extend the first interphalangeal joint because the extensor pollicis longus remains intact. However, the inability to extend the first carpometacarpal joint leads to dorsal subluxation of the first

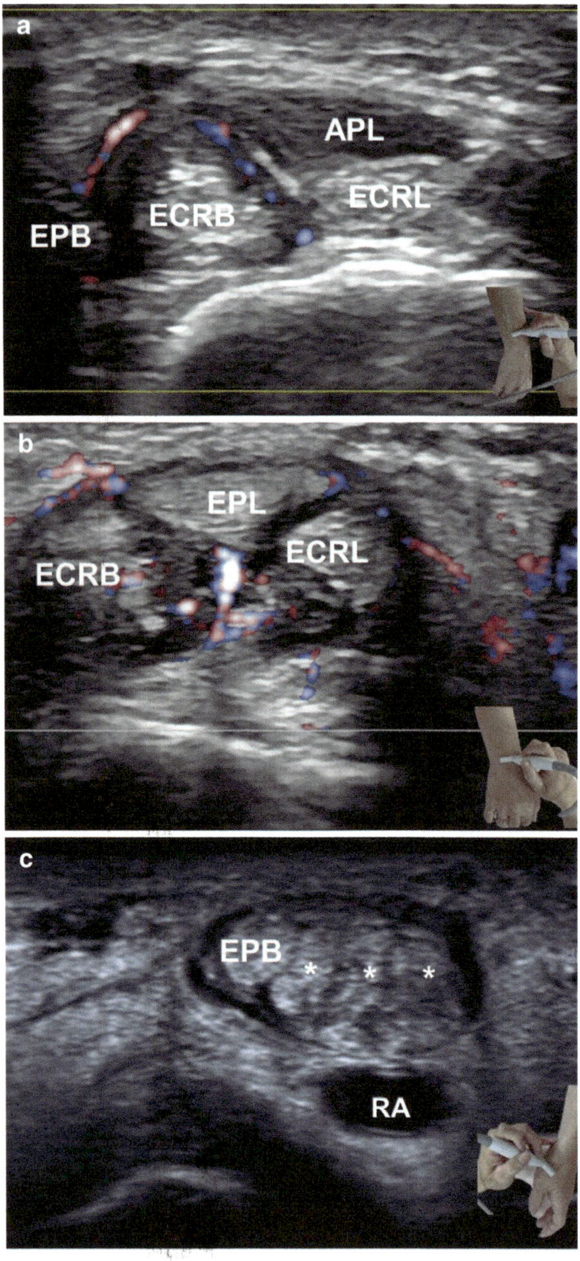

Fig. 9.25 The ultrasound image reveals hypervascularity over the tendon sheath and retinaculum on Power Doppler at the proximal intersection (**a**) in one case and at the distal intersection (**b**) in another case. In a third case (**c**), multiple tendon splits (asterisks) within the first dorsal extensor compartment are observed. RA radial artery; APL abductor pollicis longus; EPB extensor pollicis brevis; ECRL extensor carpi radialis longus; ECRB extensor carpi radialis brevis; EPL extensor pollicis longus

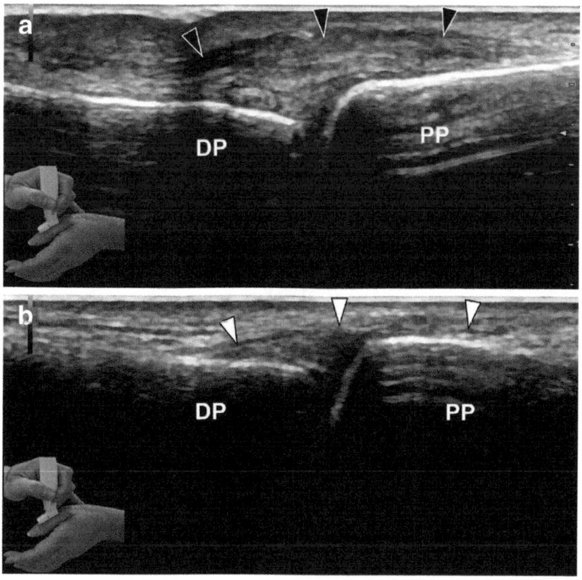

Fig. 9.26 The ultrasonography of partial tear of the extensor pollicis longus tendon (black arrowheads) (**a**), in comparison with a normal image (white arrowhead) (**b**). PP proximal phalanx; DP distal phalanx

carpometacarpal joint during attempts to extend the thumb. Ultrasound imaging might reveal an avulsion of the extensor pollicis brevis tendon along with swelling of the capsule of the first carpometacarpal joint [6]. When facing challenges in extending the first distal phalanx, suspicion should rise regarding the rupture/injury of the extensor pollicis longus. The tear could manifest at its insertion point over the distal phalanx (affected side, Fig. 9.26a; non-affected side, Fig. 9.26b), while ultrasound imaging may depict discontinuity in the extensor pollicis longus tendon, accompanied by a detached bony chip away from the distal phalanx. It is crucial to scrutinize the proximal portion of the extensor pollicis longus tendon as well, as it might exhibit rupture due to iatrogenic injury (such as corticosteroid intra-tendinous injection or attrition by a metal plate) (illustration of the extensor pollicis longus tendon, Fig. 9.27a; non-affected side, Fig. 9.27b; affected side, Fig. 9.27c; plain radiograph, Fig. 9.27d), with observable atrophy in the proximal muscle portion [7].

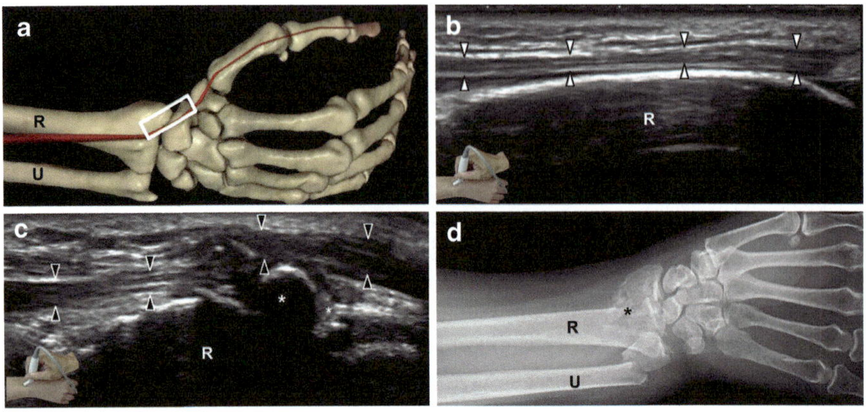

Fig. 9.27 The illustration depicts the extensor pollicis longus tendon and the placement of the ultrasound transducer for assessment (**a**). When compared to the healthy side (white arrowheads) (**b**), long-axis ultrasonography reveals a discontinuity in the tendon, indicating a partial tear of the extensor pollicis longus (black arrowheads) (**c**). A plain radiograph of the affected forearm shows displaced fractures of the radius and ulna (**d**). Asterisks: bony fragment that impinges the extensor pollicis longus; R radius; U ulna

9.5 Ultrasound-Guided Injection

For administering corticosteroid injections, such as triamcinolone acetonide (20 mg), in the treatment of De Quervain's disease, it is recommended to position the transducer in the short axis of the first dorsal extensor compartment. The focus should be placed on the area where the internal tendons exhibit the greatest swelling or where the surrounding retinaculum is significantly thickened. Confirming the location of the branches, typically the dorsal medial branch of the superficial radial nerve, in relation to the retinaculum is essential. If the nerve is located on the volar side of the retinaculum at the injection level, the needle is inserted from the dorsal to volar aspect, and vice versa if the nerve is on the dorsal side. The in-plane approach is recommended for advancing the needle until it pierces the retinaculum and enters the first compartment (Fig. 9.28a, b). In cases associated with superficial radial nerve entrapment, ultrasound-guided hydro-dissection can be performed using a 5% dextrose solution (Fig. 9.28c) [8]. A comprehensive systematic review examined studies on ultrasound-guided steroid injections for De Quervain's disease [9]. Among the 10 studies involving 379 wrists, 73.9% documented complete alleviation of symptoms. Compared to the landmark-guided technique, ultrasound-guided injections demonstrated significantly higher rates of symptom resolution and lower pain scores. The researchers concluded that ultrasound-guided steroid injections provide notable symptomatic relief due to accurate needle insertion, particularly in patients with anatomical variability involving sub-compartments [10]. However, in cases resistant to ultrasound-guided corticosteroid injection, ultrasound-guided retinaculum release using a specific blade can be considered as an alternative choice [11].

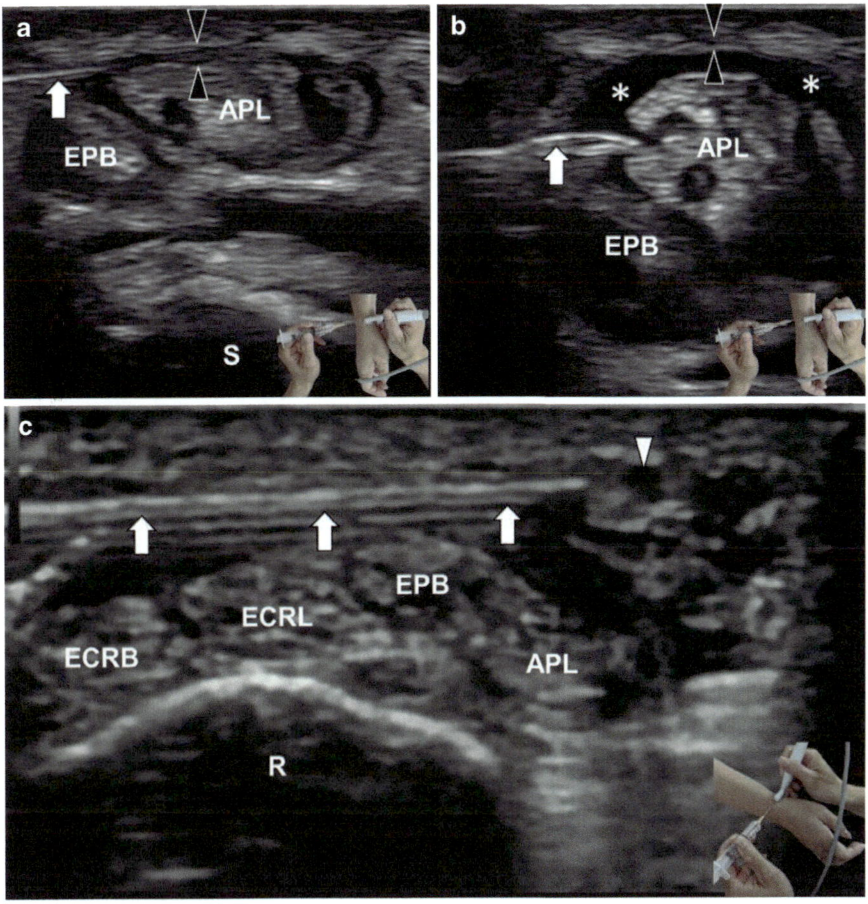

Fig. 9.28 The ultrasound-guided injection using the in-plane approach is administered inside the extensor retinaculum (black arrowheads) (**a**), with the anechoic injectate (asterisks) surrounding the abductor pollicis longus and extensor pollicis brevis (**b**). In another case, the ultrasound-guided injection using the in-plane approach is administered to the dorsal medial branch of the superficial radial nerve (white arrowhead) (**c**). White arrows: needle; APL abductor pollicis longus; EPB extensor pollicis brevis; ECRL extensor carpi radialis longus; ECRB extensor carpi radialis brevis; R radius; S scaphoid

9.6 Conclusion

The ultrasound diagnosis of De Quervain's disease is enhanced by visualizing the texture of the tendons within the first dorsal extensor compartment, along with the surrounding retinaculum and adjacent nerves. Recognizing the anatomical variations in the first extensor compartment is crucial for understanding the patient's elevated risk of developing De Quervain's disease and their resistance to conventional conservative treatments. Ultrasound-guided corticosteroid injection has proven to be both safe and effective in managing this condition, emphasizing the importance of precise needle placement to avoid complications related to the superficial radial nerve.

Acknowledgments Images and illustrations adapted from cadaveric images provided by the Visible Human Project® of the National Library of Medicine. Excerpts featured in the VH Dissector are used with permission from Touch of Life Technologies Inc.

References

1. Adachi S, Yamamoto A, Kobayashi T, et al. Prevalence of de Quervain's disease in the general population and risk factors. Kitakanto Med J. 2011;61(4):479–82.
2. Clarke MT, Lyall HA, Grant JW, Matthewson MH. The histopathology of de Quervain's disease. J Hand Surg Br. 1998;23(6):732–4.
3. Marí-Gorreto J, San-Millán M, Carrera A, et al. The anatomy of the tendon of abductor pollicis longus and its morphological variations: an anatomical approach emphasizing the clinical relevance. Ann Anat—Anat Anz. 2023;247:152068.
4. Jariwala A, Krishnan B, Soames R, Wigderowitz CA. Important anatomical relationships of the posterior interosseous nerve in the distal forearm for surgical planning: a cadaveric study. J Wrist Surg. 2014;3(1):60–3.
5. Robson AJ, See MS, Ellis H. Applied anatomy of the superficial branch of the radial nerve. Clin Anat. 2008;21(1):38–45.
6. Chang KV, Hung CY, Ozcakar L. Ultrasound imaging for the extensor pollicis brevis tendon: when martial arts caused partial rupture. Am J Phys Med Rehabil. 2015;94(2):e22.
7. Chen YC, Wu WT, Mezian K, Ricci V, Ozcakar L, Chang KV. Dynamic ultrasound examination for extensor Pollicis longus tendon rupture after palpation-guided corticosteroid injection. Diagnostics (Basel). 2023;13(5)
8. Chang KV, Hung CY, Ozcakar L. Snapping thumb and superficial radial nerve entrapment in De Quervain disease: ultrasound imaging/guidance revisited. Pain Med. 2015;16(11):2214–5.
9. He KS, He KS, Cheah A, Al-Halabi B, Danino MA, Efanov JI. Unblinding de Quervain: a systematic review of ultrasound-guided injection of corticosteroids for treatment of stenosing tenosynovitis of the 1st extensor compartment. J Med Radiat Sci. 2023;70(3):319–26.
10. Chang KV, Hung CY, Ozcakar L. Ultrasound imaging for precise diagnosis and injection of isolated extensor pollicis brevis tenosynovitis: it is not always a simple de Quervain disease. Am J Phys Med Rehabil. 2015;94(3):255.
11. Croutzet P, Guinand R, Mares O, Apard T, Candelier G, David I. Ultrasound-guided de Quervain's tendon release, feasibility, and first outcomes. J Wrist Surg. 2019;8(6):513–9.

Chapter 10
Exploring the Painful Thenar Region

Ke-Vin Chang, Wei-Ting Wu, and Shao-Yu Chi

10.1 Introduction

In 2004, a Finnish study [1] investigated the prevalence of osteoarthritis in the carpometacarpal joint of the thumb among adults aged 30 and older. The research, spanning from 1978 to 1980, followed 3595 subjects over time, evaluating work disability and mortality. Findings revealed a higher prevalence of thumb carpometacarpal osteoarthritis in women, correlated with an elevated body mass index. No significant link was found with physical workload history. While advanced osteoarthritis predicted increased mortality rates in men, it did not predict work disability. In 2021, a meta-analysis [2] examined radiographic thumb base osteoarthritis in the general population, involving 16 articles. The study highlighted a greater prevalence in females, with rates of 5.8% for males and 7.3% for females at 50 years, escalating to 33.1% for males and 39.0% for females at 80 years. The odds of having radiographic osteoarthritis increased by 1.06 per year of age, with higher odds in females. This research underscores a robust association between age, gender, and the prevalence of radiographic thumb base osteoarthritis. Considering the challenges of an aging society, the prevalence of thumb pain related to degenerative pathologies is expected to rise.

Presently, ultrasound has gained significance in assessing thumb pain, exploring pathologies beyond osteoarthritis. Superior to radiography, ultrasound allows for a detailed examination of tendons, muscles, ligaments, and nerves, in addition to the carpometacarpal joint. Ultrasound also facilitates safer periarticular injections, avoiding harm to the superficial palmar arch and recurrent motor branch of the median nerve. The subsequent chapter will delve into issues relevant to ultrasound diagnosis and guided injections.

K.-V. Chang (✉) · W.-T. Wu · S.-Y. Chi
Bei-Hu Branch, National Taiwan University Hospital, Taipei, Taiwan

K.-V. Chang (ed.), *Ultrasonography of Musculoskeletal Pain*,
https://doi.org/10.1007/978-981-96-6787-1_10

10.2 Regional Anatomy

10.2.1 Flexor Carpi Radialis

The origin of the flexor carpi radialis is at the medial epicondyle through a common tendon. In the proximal forearm, it is positioned between the pronator teres on the radial side, the palmaris longus on the ulnar side, and the flexor digitorum superficialis underneath. Initially featuring a slender and aponeurotic structure, the muscle undergoes an increase in size and culminates in a tendon that passes through a canal located in the radial part of the transverse carpal ligament (Fig. 10.1). Following this path, it courses above the scaphoid and through a groove in the sheath over the trapezium, also referred to as the trapezial ridge. A cadaveric study [3] has revealed that the flexor carpi radialis tendon has fibers attaching to the trapezial ridge. Ultimately, the tendon is inserted into the base of the second metacarpal bone, with a slip extending to the base of the third metacarpal bone.

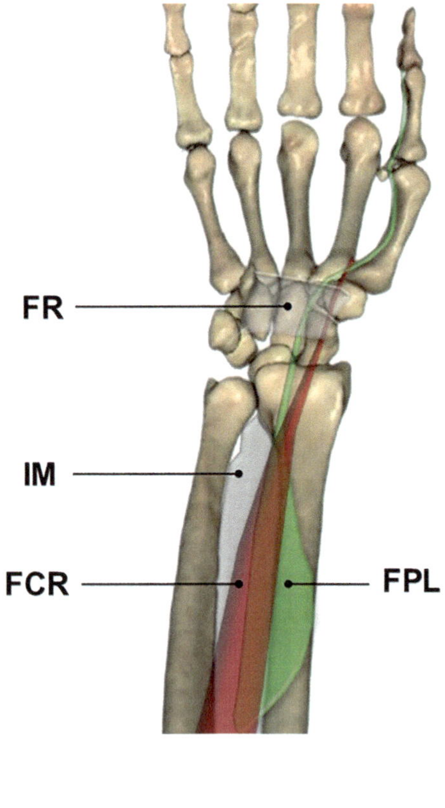

Fig. 10.1 The illustration depicts the anatomy of the flexor carpi radialis and flexor pollicis longus, highlighting their relationship with the flexor retinaculum. FCR flexor carpi radialis; FR flexor retinaculum; FPL flexor pollicis longus; IM interosseous membrane

10.2.2 Flexor Pollicis Longus

The flexor pollicis longus muscle arises on the volar aspect of the radius and the adjacent interosseous membrane, just distal to the radial tuberosity. It courses along the radial aspect of the volar forearm before transitioning into a long tendinous slip that traverses deep to the transverse carpal ligament within the carpal tunnel (Fig. 10.1). As the flexor pollicis longus tendon progresses, it becomes enveloped by the synovial sheath of the radial bursa. Continuing along the first metacarpal, it passes between the two sesamoid bones situated on the volar aspect of the thumb metacarpophalangeal joint. The flexor pollicis longus concludes its course by insert ing at the volar base of the distal phalanx of the thumb.

10.2.3 Ligament of the First Carpometacarpal Joint

The first carpometacarpal joint comprises seven ligaments, and a detailed examination emphasizes the crucial ones due to their intricate nature. An illustration of the dorsal thumb carpometacarpal ligaments reveals the dorsal deltoid ligament complex, including the dorsal radial ligament, dorsal central ligament, and posterior oblique ligament [4] (Fig. 10.2). Originating from the dorsal tubercle of the trapezium, these ligaments insert on the first metacarpal. Conversely, a scrutiny of the volar thumb carpometacarpal ligaments highlights the volar anterior oblique ligament and ulnar collateral ligament, coursing from the trapezial ridge onto the volar base of the first metacarpal. In contrast, the intermetacarpal ligament is an extracapsular ligament connecting the second metacarpal to the first metacarpal base (Fig. 10.3).

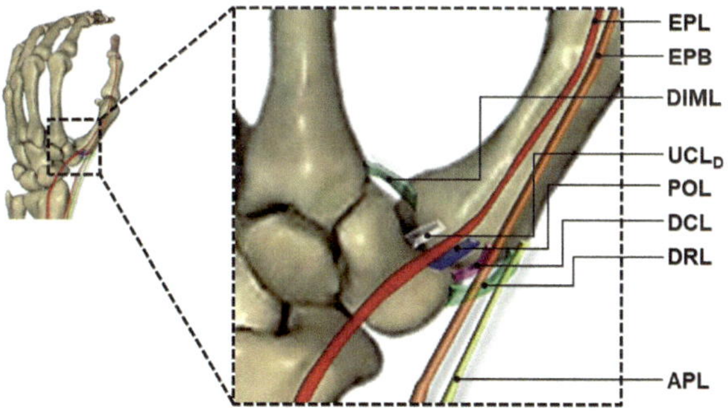

Fig. 10.2 The illustration depicts the dorsal aspect of the first carpometacarpal joint, along with the surrounding ligaments and tendinous structures. APL abductor pollicis longus; DRL dorsal radial ligament; EPB extensor pollicis brevis; DCL dorsal central ligament; POL posterior oblique ligament; EPL extensor pollicis longus; UCL_D dorsal portion of the ulnar collateral ligament; DIML dorsal intermetacarpal ligament

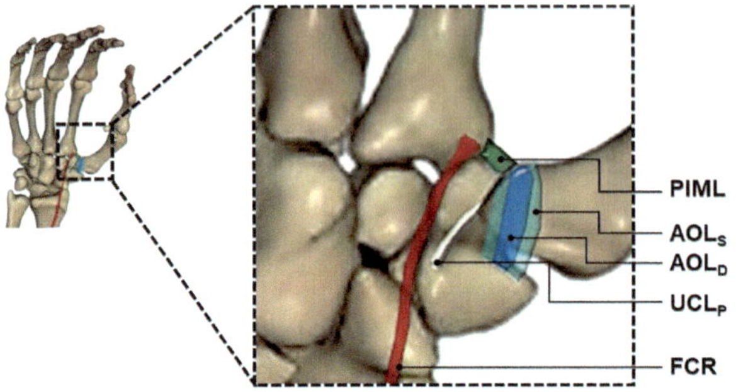

Fig. 10.3 The illustration depicts the volar aspect of the first carpometacarpal joint, along with the surrounding ligaments and tendinous structures. AOL_S superficial band of the anterior oblique ligament; AOL_D deep band of the anterior oblique ligament; UCL_P palmar portion of the ulnar collateral ligament; PIML palmar intermetacarpal ligament; FCR flexor carpi radialis

10.2.4 Thenar and Relevant Muscles

The thenar muscles constitute a group of three muscles: abductor pollicis brevis, flexor pollicis brevis (comprising superficial and deep heads), and opponens pollicis. Among these, the abductor pollicis brevis is the most lateral and superficial (Fig. 10.4). The abductor pollicis brevis originates from the tubercles of the scaphoid and trapezium bones, as well as the flexor retinaculum. It inserts on the lateral aspect of the base of the proximal phalanx of the thumb and the radial sesamoid bone. The flexor pollicis brevis consists of both superficial and deep heads. The superficial head originates from the flexor retinaculum and the tubercle of the trapezium bone, while the deep head is derived from the trapezoid and capitate bones. Its insertion point is on the lateral aspect of the base of the proximal phalanx of the thumb, extending to the radial sesamoid bone. In contrast, opponens pollicis extends from the trapezium bone and flexor retinaculum to the first metacarpal bone, positioning itself deeper than the aforementioned two muscles. All three muscles are innervated by the recurrent motor branch of the median nerve, except for the deep head of the flexor pollicis brevis muscle, which receives its innervation from the deep motor branch of the ulnar nerve.

Additional muscles responsible for thumb movement include the abductor pollicis longus, extensor pollicis brevis, extensor pollicis longus, and adductor pollicis. Since the preceding three muscles have already been covered in the discussion on “De Quervain’s Disease Reimagined,” our exclusive focus will now be on the adductor pollicis. The adductor pollicis muscle stands out for its unique triangular shape, comprising two heads. The oblique head originates from the capitate and the bases of the second and third metacarpals, while the transverse head originates from the volar aspect of the third metacarpal. These two heads converge as fibers course

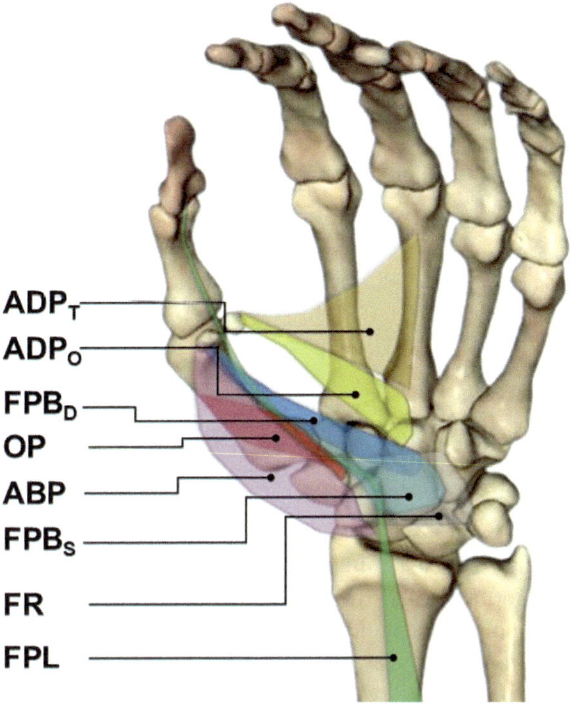

Fig. 10.4 The illustration depicts the anatomy of the thenar muscles. ABP abductor pollicis brevis; ADP$_O$ oblique head of the adductor pollicis; ADP$_T$ transverse head of the adductor pollicis; FPB$_D$ deep head of the flexor pollicis brevis; FPB$_S$ superficial head of the flexor pollicis brevis; OP opponens pollicis; FPL flexor pollicis longus; FR flexor retinaculum

laterally, forming the tendon of the adductor pollicis, which attaches to the medial aspect of the proximal phalanx of the thumb and the extensor hood. Innervation of the adductor pollicis is provided by the deep branch of the ulnar nerve.

10.2.5 Recurrent Motor Branch of the Median Nerve

In the study conducted by Kozin et al. [5], the recurrent motor branch of the median nerve was categorized into three types. Type I, though uncommon, passed through the transverse carpal ligament. Type II nerves traveled distally to the transverse carpal ligament through a distinct, obliquely oriented fascia that also originated from the transverse carpal ligament and inserted on the undersurface of the palmar aponeurosis. Type III nerves passed distally to the transverse carpal ligament without traversing the obliquely oriented fascia. The majority of recurrent motor branches originated from either the central portion of the median nerve or its radial aspect. Additionally, in 4% of the examined cadavers, more than one motor branch was identified (Fig. 10.5).

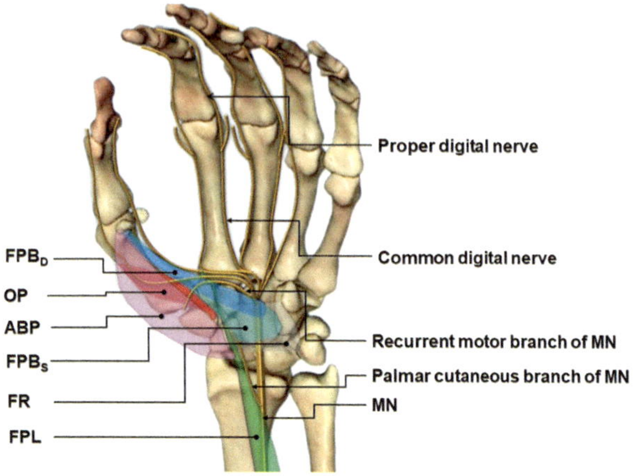

Fig. 10.5 The illustration of the recurrent motor branch and other terminal branches of the median nerve. ABP abductor pollicis brevis; FPB$_S$ superficial head of the flexor pollicis brevis; FPB$_D$ deep head of the flexor pollicis brevis; OP opponens pollicis; FPL flexor pollicis longus; FR flexor retinaculum; MN median nerve

10.3 Sonoanatomy

The transducer should be positioned between the scaphoid and pisiform to visualize the short axis of the flexor carpi radialis, located outside the flexor retinaculum and on top of the scaphoid (Fig. 10.6a, c). As the transducer is moved distally, the flexor carpi radialis comes into view, approximating a groove just medial to the trapezium (Fig. 10.6b, d). Beyond the carpal tunnel outlet, a cross-section of the flexor carpi radialis and the superficially running flexor pollicis longus is observed. Further distally, the flexor carpi radialis descends into the deeper region, ultimately inserting on the base of the second and third metacarpals. For optimal visualization of the terminal portion of the flexor carpi radialis in its long axis, it is advisable to compress the distal end of the transducer towards the metacarpal base (Fig. 10.7a, b). This helps counteract the impact of anisotropy and enhances the clarity of the imaging.

Returning to the carpal tunnel inlet in the axial plane, the flexor pollicis longus tendon is positioned beneath the transverse carpal ligament, in close proximity to the scaphoid and trapezium (Fig. 10.6a, b). After exiting the carpal tunnel and reaching the level of the first metacarpal base, the flexor pollicis longus tendon becomes enveloped by the superficial and deep heads of the flexor pollicis brevis muscle (Fig. 10.8a, c), and the long axis of the first metacarpal bone can be used to guide the transducer to visualize the tendon's long axis (Fig. 10.8b, d). Laterally adjacent to the superficial head of the flexor pollicis brevis, the abductor pollicis brevis shares the same layer with the flexor pollicis brevis. Below the abductor pollicis brevis lies the opponens pollicis, also positioned in the same layer as the flexor pollicis longus tendon. The distal trajectory of the flexor pollicis longus tendon reveals the radial

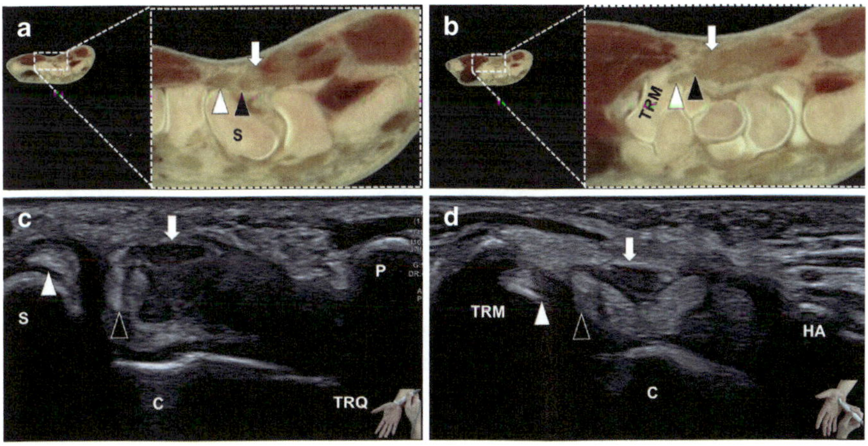

Fig. 10.6 The cadaveric images and the corresponding sonoanatomy show the flexor carpi radialis tendon in axial views at the inlet (**a**, **c**) and outlet (**b**, **d**) of the carpal tunnel. White arrowheads: tendon of the flexor carpi radialis; black arrowheads: tendon of the flexor pollicis longus; white arrows: median nerve; S scaphoid; P pisiform; TRM trapezium; TRQ triquetrum; C capitate; HA hamate

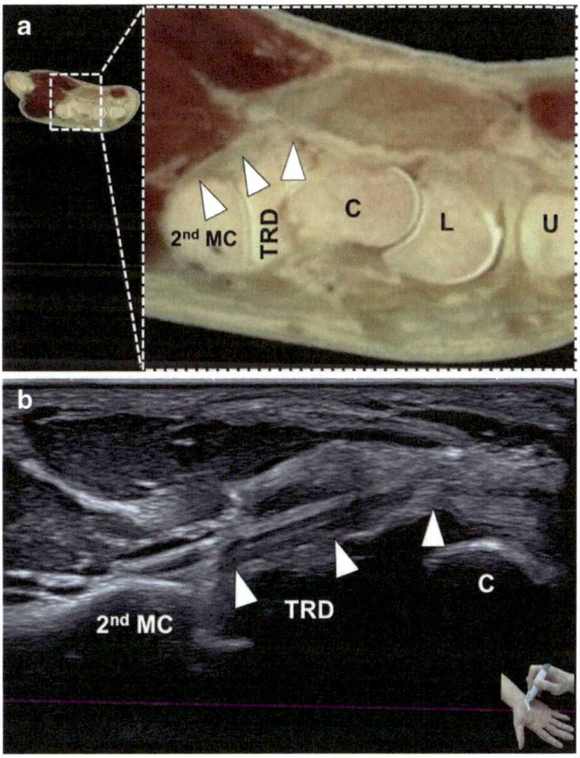

Fig. 10.7 The cadaveric image (**a**) and corresponding sonoanatomy (**b**) demonstrate the long-axis view of the flexor carpi radialis tendon insertion (white arrowheads). C capitate; L lunate; 2nd MC the second metacarpal bone; TRD trapezoid; U ulna

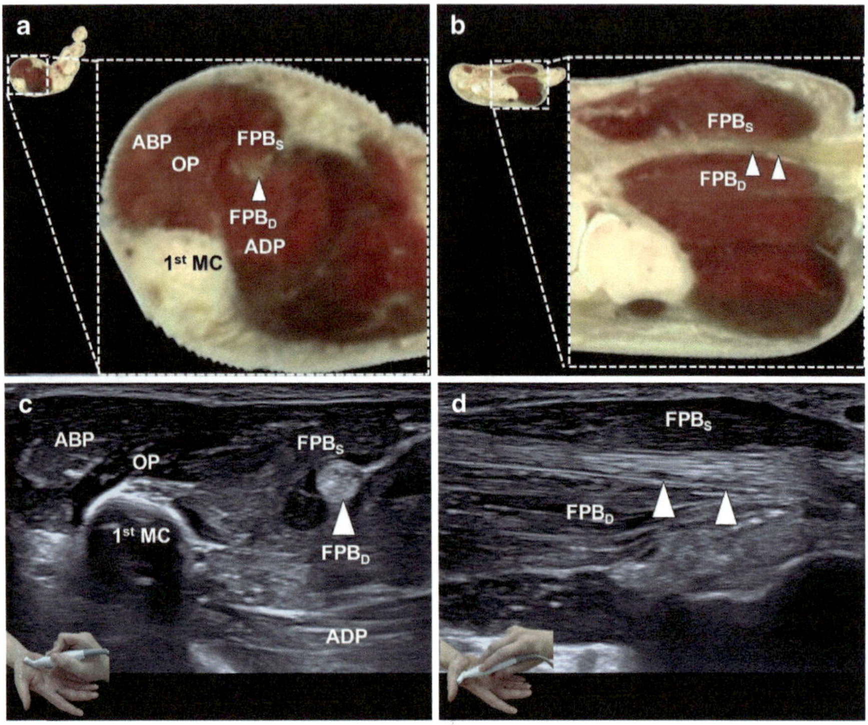

Fig. 10.8 The cadaveric images and corresponding sonoanatomy of the flexor pollicis longus tendon and surrounding thenar muscles at the level of the first metacarpal, shown in both short-axis (**a**, **c**) and long-axis (**b**, **d**) views. White arrowheads: flexor pollicis longus tendon; ABP abductor pollicis brevis; FPB$_S$ superficial head of the flexor pollicis brevis; FPB$_D$ deep head of the flexor pollicis brevis; OP opponens pollicis; ADP adductor pollicis; 1st MC the first metacarpal bone

sesamoid bone situated laterally at the metacarpal head, while the tendon is encircled by the A1 pulley. The volar plate can be seen between both sesamoid bones (Fig. 10.9a, b) [6].

The transducer is repositioned to visualize the long axis of the flexor carpi radialis tendon at its distal attachment on the second metacarpal bone (Fig. 10.7a, b). During thumb abduction, the transducer is shifted radially, revealing the short axis of the volar anterior oblique ligament and its proximal attachment on the trapezium (Fig. 10.10a, c). Rotating the transducer to align with the carpometacarpal joint exposes the long axis of the volar anterior oblique ligament (Fig. 10.10b, d). Positioning the transducer lateral to the insertion of the flexor carpal radialis and directing it laterally reveals the palmar portion of the ulnar collateral ligament at the first carpometacarpal joint (Fig. 10.11a, b). For the investigation of the palmar intermetacarpal ligament, the transducer can be placed on the base of the first and second metacarpal bones (Fig. 10.12a, c).

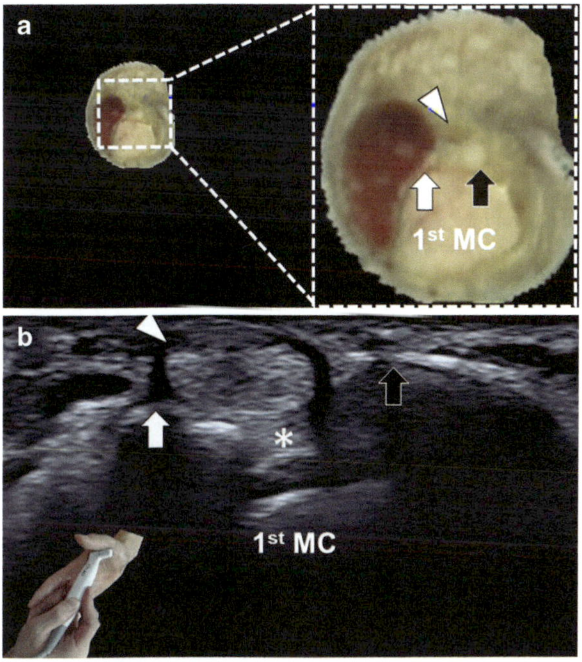

Fig. 10.9 The cadaveric image (**a**) and the corresponding sonoanatomy (**b**) of the flexor pollicis longus tendon at the level of the first metacarpal head in the short-axis view. Black arrows: radial sesamoid bone; white arrows: ulnar sesamoid bone; white arrowheads: tendon of the flexor pollicis longus; asterisk: volar plate; 1st MC the first metacarpal bone

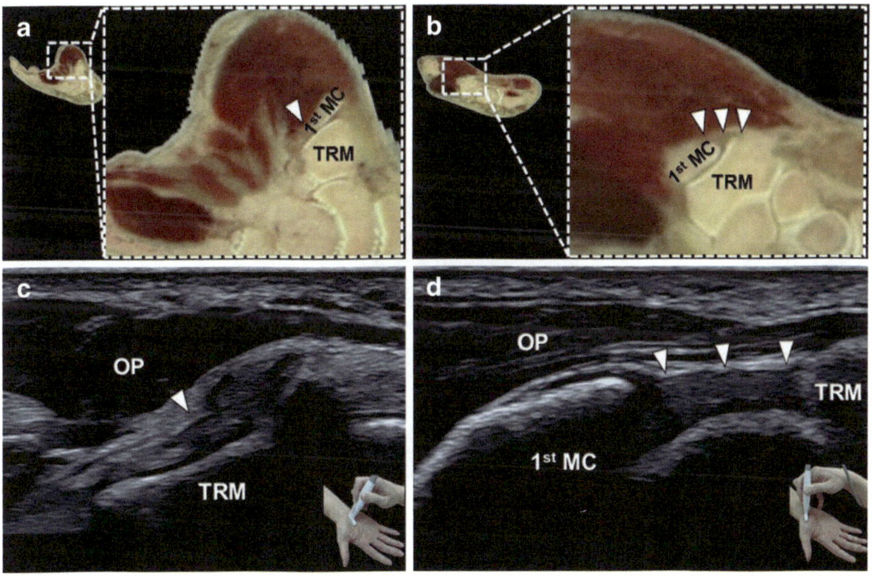

Fig. 10.10 The cadaveric images and the corresponding sonoanatomy of the anterior oblique ligament (white arrowheads) of the carpometacarpal joint in the short-axis (**a**, **c**) and long-axis (**b**, **d**) views. OP opponens pollicis; TRM trapezium; 1st MC the first metacarpal bone

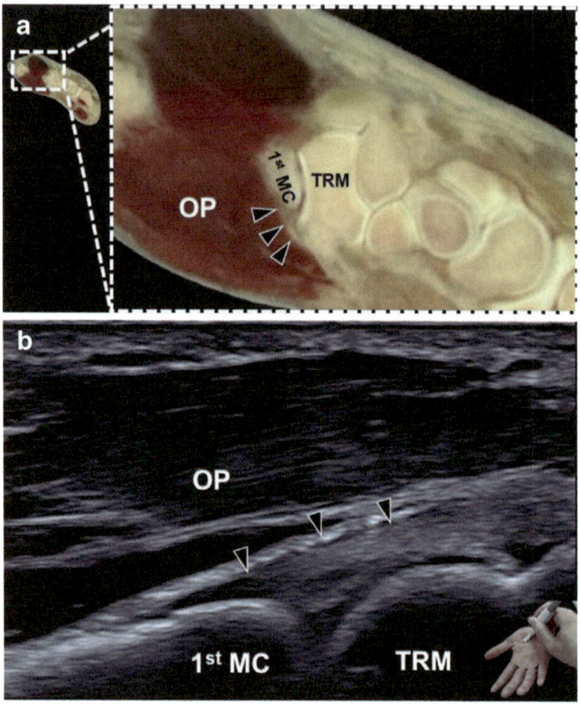

Fig. 10.11 The cadaveric image (**a**) and the corresponding sonoanatomy (**b**) of the palmar portion of the ulnar collateral ligament (black arrowheads) at the first carpometacarpal joint in the long-axis views. OP opponens pollicis; TRM trapezium; 1st MC the first metacarpal bone

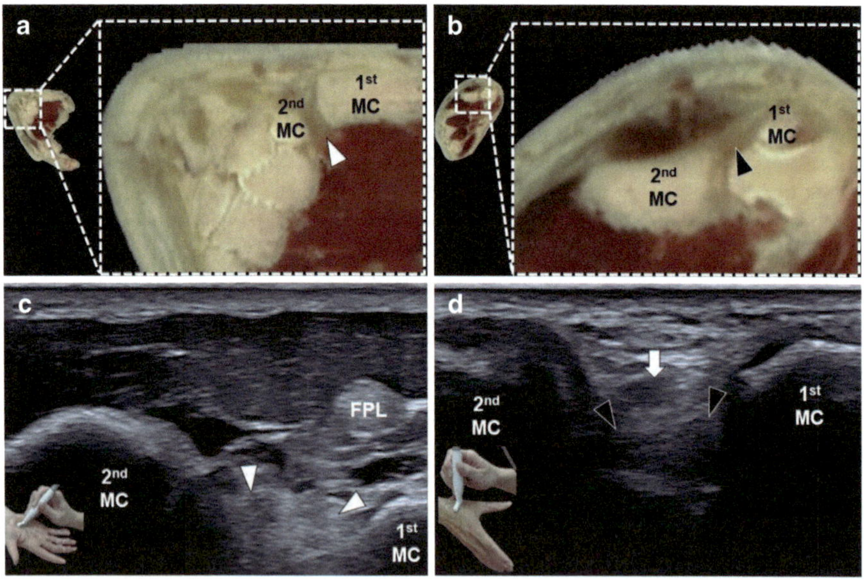

Fig. 10.12 The cadaveric images and the corresponding sonoanatomy of the palmar (**a**, **c**) and the dorsal (**b**, **d**) intermetacarpal ligament. White arrowheads: the palmar intermetacarpal ligament; black arrowheads: the dorsal intermetacarpal ligament; white arrow: the princeps pollicis artery; 1st MC the first metacarpal bone; 2nd MC the second metacarpal bone

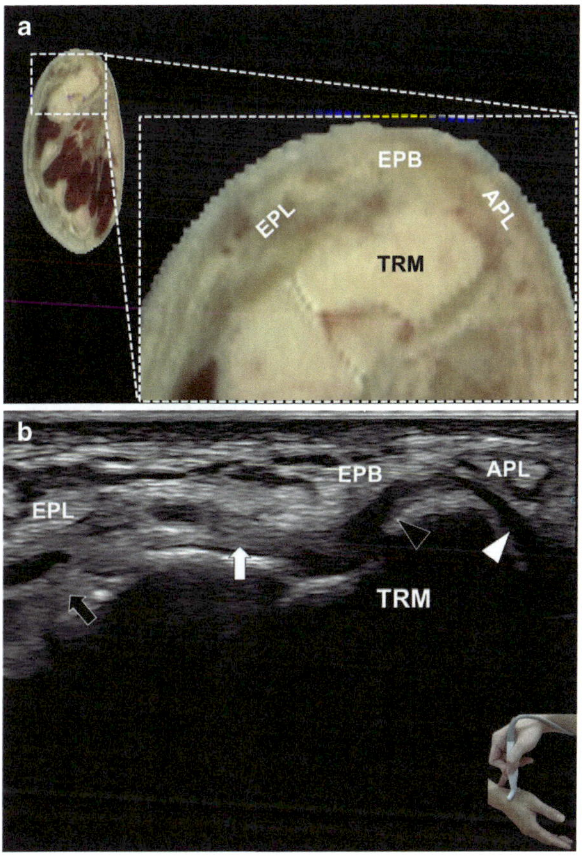

Fig. 10.13 The cadaveric image (**a**) and the corresponding sonoanatomy (**b**) of the dorsal ligaments complex of the first carpometacarpal joint in its short axis. White arrowhead: dorsal radial ligament; black arrowhead: dorsal central ligament; white arrow: posterior oblique ligament; black arrow: dorsal portion of the ulnar collateral ligament; APL abductor pollicis longus tendon; EPB extensor pollicis brevis tendon; EPL extensor pollicis longus tendon; TRM trapezium

As the transducer is aligned with the axial plane of the first carpometacarpal joint, the short axis of the dorsal ligament complex becomes visible beneath the extensor tendons of the thumb, allowing for an initial evaluation of its association with the joint (Fig. 10.13a, b). Next, by positioning the transducer along the long axis of the abductor pollicis longus, the dorsal radial ligament can be identified between the trapezium and the first metacarpal bone (Fig. 10.14a, b). When the transducer is placed medially along the extensor pollicis brevis tendon, the dorsal central ligament can be observed (Fig. 10.15a, b). The posterior oblique ligament is located medially to the dorsal central ligament, without the tendon crossing over it (Fig. 10.16a, b). Positioning the transducer over the first dorsal interosseous muscle and pivoting towards the ulnar side to connect with the base of the first and second metacarpals enhances the visualization of the dorsal intermetacarpal ligament (Fig. 10.12b, d).

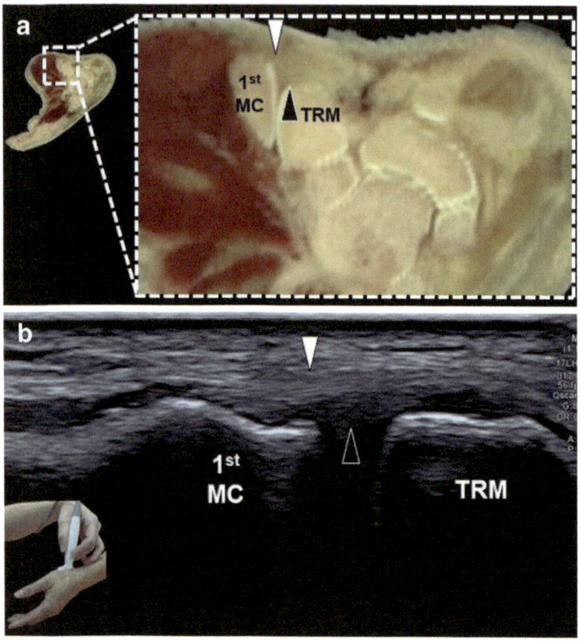

Fig. 10.14 The cadaveric image (**a**) and the corresponding sonoanatomy (**b**) of the dorsal radial ligament (black arrowheads) in its long axis. White arrowheads: the abductor pollicis longus tendon; TRM trapezium; 1st MC the first metacarpal bone

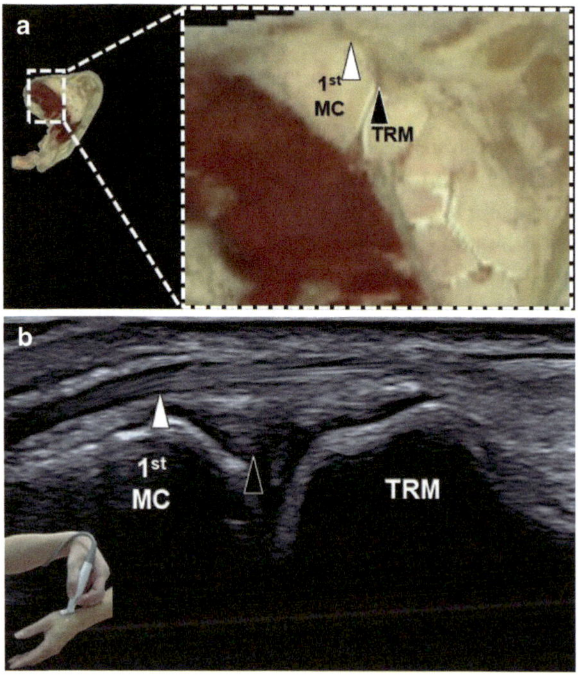

Fig. 10.15 The cadaveric image (**a**) and the corresponding sonoanatomy (**b**) of the dorsal central ligament (black arrowheads) in its long axis. White arrowheads: the extensor pollicis brevis tendon; TRM trapezium; 1st MC the first metacarpal bone

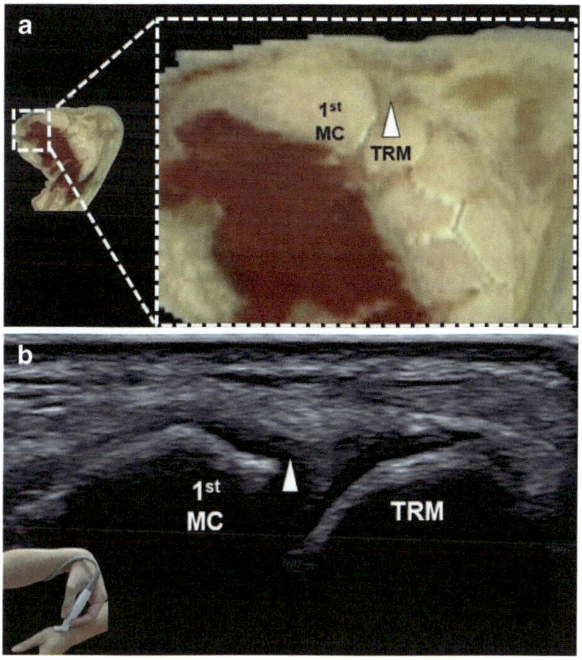

Fig. 10.16 The cadaveric image (**a**) and the corresponding sonoanatomy (**b**) of the posterior oblique ligament (white arrowheads) in the long-axis view. 1st MC the first metacarpal bone; TRM trapezium

Visualizing the recurrent motor branch of the median nerve involves initially placing the transducer along the long axis of the flexor pollicis longus, positioned atop the superficial head of the flexor pollicis brevis (Fig. 10.17a, c). On the superficial fascia of the thenar muscle, an arterial branch of the superficial palmar arch becomes apparent. Adjacent to this arterial branch, the recurrent motor branch of the median nerve is likely situated and can be observed in its short axis. Transitioning the distal end of the transducer from the radial to ulnar aspect allows for the observation of the recurrent motor branch of the median nerve as it courses through the ulnar edge of the thenar muscle, establishing connections with the main trunk or other branches of the median nerve (Fig. 10.17b, d).

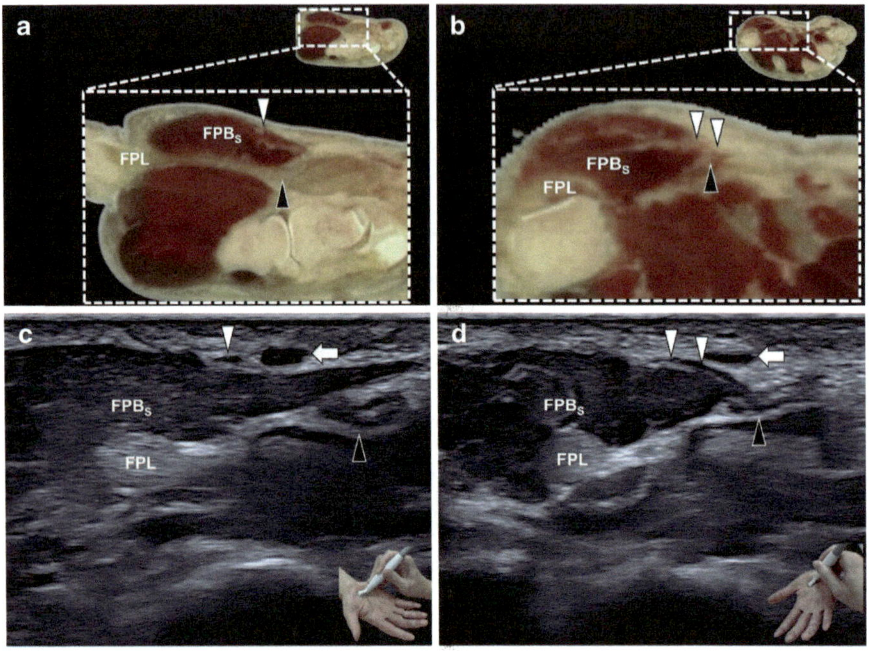

Fig. 10.17 The cadaveric images and the corresponding sonoanatomy of the recurrent motor branch of the median nerve (white arrowheads) in its short axis (**a**, **c**) and along its course branching from the median nerve in the long axis view (**b**, **d**). Black arrowheads: median nerve; white arrows: arterial branch of the superficial palmar arch; FPB_S superficial head of the flexor pollicis brevis; FPL flexor pollicis longus tendon

10.4 Pathologies

Tendinopathy of the flexor carpi radialis has been observed in connection with triscaphe or scapho–trapezium–trapezoid joint osteoarthritis [7]. Ultrasound images may reveal a swollen, irregular, and hypoechoic appearance of the flexor carpi radialis tendon at the level of and proximal to the scaphoid-trapezium-trapezoid complex, indicative of tendinopathy (long axis, Fig. 10.18a; short axis, Fig. 10.18b). Local loss of the fibrillar appearance and hyperemia at color Doppler may signify intratendinous neovascularization. In individuals with rheumatoid arthritis, Doppler ultrasound images may depict an active inflammatory pannus surrounding the flexor carpi radialis tendon. As the flexor carpi radialis is enclosed by a single tendon sheath, the tendon could be enveloped by an anechoic effusion, distending the synovial sheath in the presence of tenosynovitis. In cases of flexor carpi radialis tenosynovitis following trauma, consideration should be given to adjacent bony fractures, such as scaphoid fractures (long-axis ultrasound image, Fig. 10.19a; plain radiograph, Fig. 10.19b).

The anterior oblique ligament plays a crucial role in stabilizing the trapeziometacarpal joint, and its insufficiency is closely linked to degenerative joint disease. In

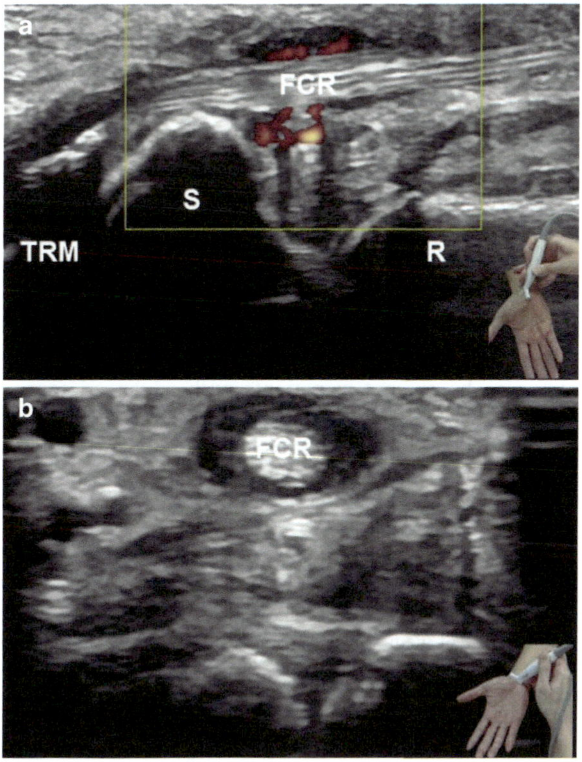

Fig. 10.18 The ultrasound images of flexor carpi radialis tendinopathy in its long-axis (**a**) and short-axis (**b**) views, with hypoechoic swelling of the tendon sheath and increased vascularity. FCR flexor carpi radialis tendon; R radius; S scaphoid; TRM trapezium

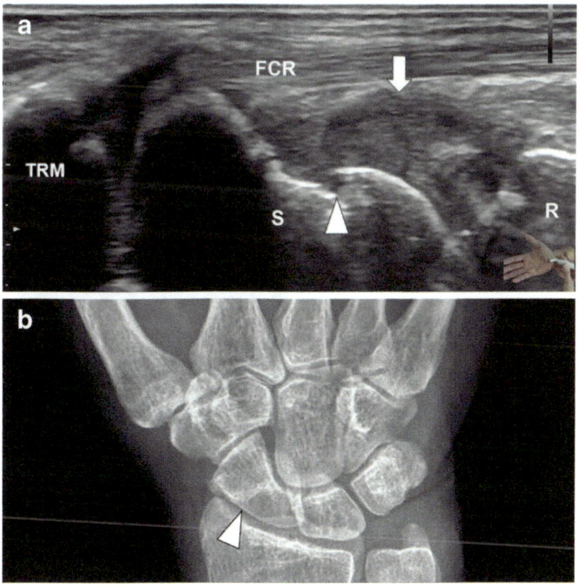

Fig. 10.19 The ultrasound image of a scaphoid fracture (white arrowheads) shows cortical irregularity, discontinuity in the scaphoid contour, and a surrounding hypoechoic hematoma (white arrow) (**a**), alongside the corresponding plain radiograph (**b**). FCR flexor carpi radialis tendon; S scaphoid; TRM trapezium; R radius

individuals with trapeziometacarpal joint arthritis, the presence of prominent osteophytes obstructs clear observation of both proximal and distal attachments (gray scale image, Fig. 10.20a; Power Doppler image, Fig. 10.20b). In cases displaying moderate osteoarthritic changes, the anterior oblique ligament can be observed extending over a metacarpal osteophyte, appearing to attach distally away from the joint line. An injured anterior oblique ligament is characterized by thickening and a hypoechoic appearance, along with disruption of the normal fibrillar band that extends between the trapezium and the base of the first metacarpal. The ligament may show discontinuity or avulsion, typically from its metacarpal insertion. Partial tears may be indicated by the separation of the periosteum from the base of the metacarpal. Furthermore, partial tears of the dorsal radial ligament (Fig. 10.21a), dorsal central ligament (Fig. 10.21b), and posterior oblique ligament (Fig. 10.21c) may also be present in patients with advanced carpometacarpal osteoarthritis. In cases of overstretching during thumb abduction in sports or traumatic injury, partial tears of the dorsal (Fig. 10.22a) and palmar (Fig. 10.22b) intermetacarpal ligaments may occur.

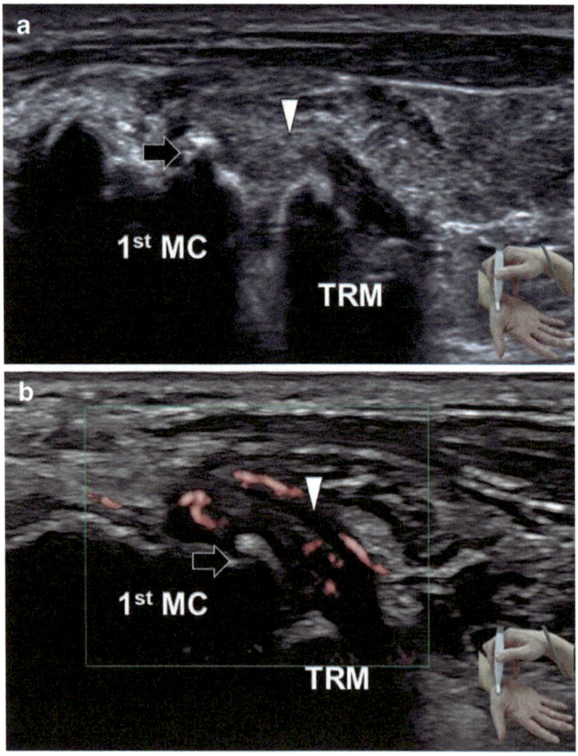

Fig. 10.20 The ultrasonography of osteoarthritis of the first carpometacarpal joint with the presence of osteophytes (black arrows) (**a**), swelling and increased vascularity of the anterior oblique ligament (white arrowheads) (**b**). TRM trapezium; 1st MC the first metacarpal bone

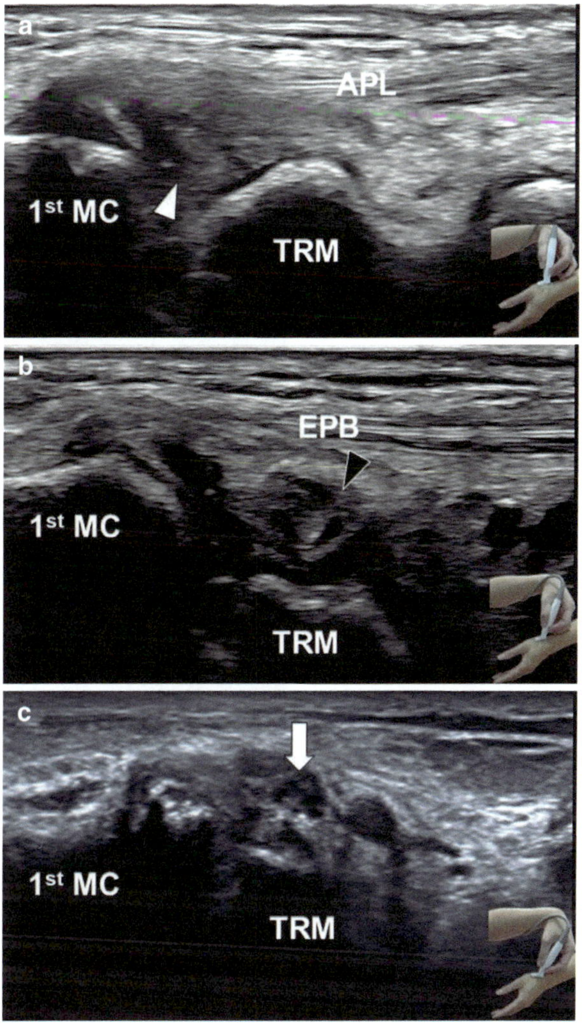

Fig. 10.21 Ultrasound images of osteoarthritis in the trapeziometacarpal joint show partial tears of the dorsal radial ligament (white arrowhead) (**a**), dorsal central ligament (black arrowhead) (**b**), and posterior oblique ligament (white arrow) (**c**). APL abductor pollicis longus tendon; EPB extensor pollicis brevis tendon; TRM trapezium; 1st MC the first metacarpal bone

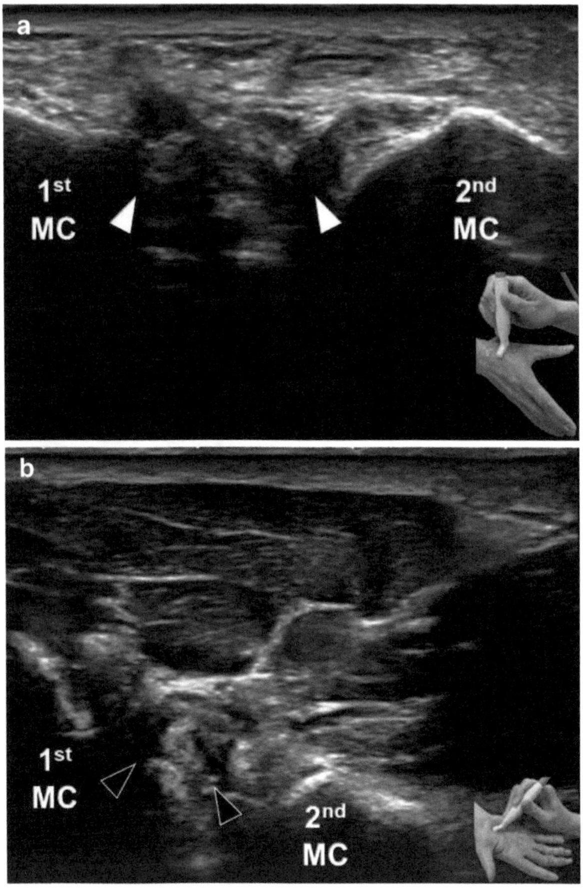

Fig. 10.22 Ultrasound images show partial tears of the dorsal (white arrowheads) (**a**) and palmar (black arrowheads) (**b**) intermetacarpal ligaments due to overstretching injuries during thumb abduction. 1st MC the first metacarpal bone; 2nd MC the second metacarpal bone

Trigger thumb may manifest as a momentary locking of the thumb during bending, followed by a painful snapping sensation during straightening. Ultrasound examinations can show varying degrees of thickening in the A1 pulley (short axis, Fig. 10.23a; long axis, Fig. 10.23b) and detect tendinosis or tenosynovitis, along with increased blood flow around the flexor pollicis longus tendon (short axis, Fig. 10.24a; long axis, Fig. 10.24b). Localized swelling of the flexor tendons below the pulley may result in the formation of a noticeable nodule. Dynamic scanning, performed during passive flexion and extension, typically illustrates challenging tendon gliding beneath the abnormal pulley. In severe instances, tears in the flexor pollicis longus tendons may be evident, presenting as discontinuity in ultrasound images of the tendon (short axis, Fig. 10.25a; long axis, Fig. 10.25b).

The pathologies affecting the recurrent motor branch of the median nerve are infrequent, often stemming from iatrogenic injuries during clinical procedures. Chang et al. [8] documented a case involving injury to the recurrent motor branch following a trigger point injection in the thenar muscle. Ultrasound imaging revealed

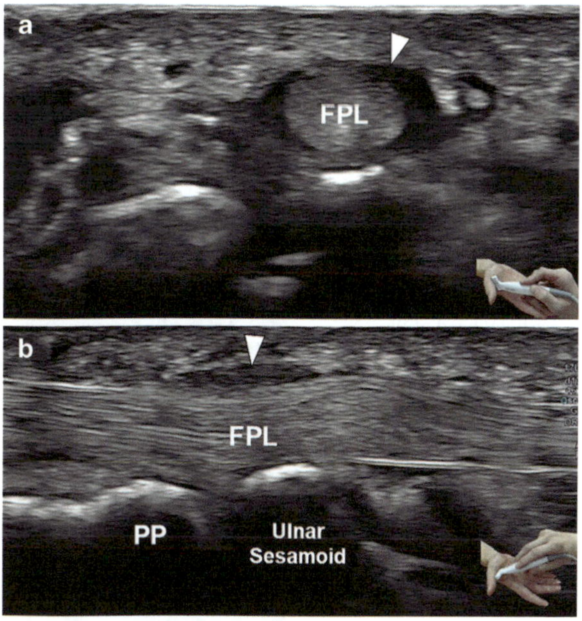

Fig. 10.23 Ultrasound images of a trigger thumb in both short-axis (**a**) and long-axis (**b**) views illustrate thickening of the A1 pulley (white arrowheads) and focal swelling of the flexor pollicis longus tendon proximal to the thickened A1 pulley. FPL flexor pollicis longus tendon; PP proximal phalanx of the thumb

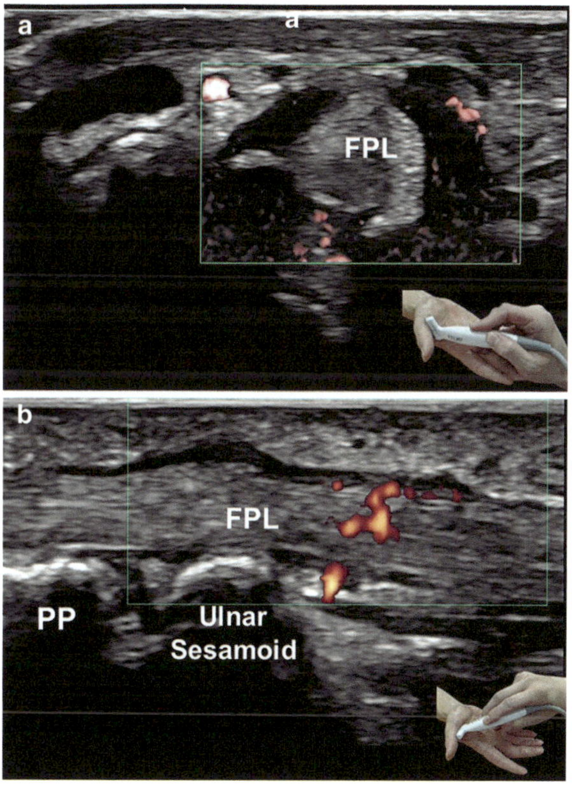

Fig. 10.24 Ultrasound images of flexor pollicis longus tenosynovitis in short-axis (**a**) and long-axis (**b**) views demonstrate increased vascularity in the tendon sheath. FPL flexor pollicis longus tendon; PP proximal phalanx of the thumb

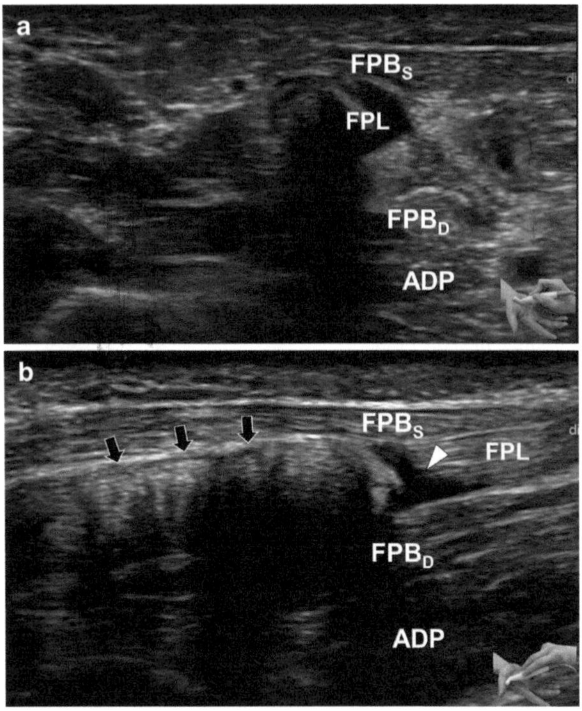

Fig. 10.25 Ultrasound images of flexor pollicis longus tendon rupture in short-axis (**a**) and long-axis (**b**) views. White arrowhead: the discontinued portion of the flexor pollicis longus tendon; black arrows: a retraction stump distal to the torn side; ADP adductor pollicis; FPB_S superficial head of the flexor pollicis brevis; FPB_D deep head of the flexor pollicis brevis; FPL flexor pollicis longus tendon

conspicuous swelling in the cross-section of the affected nerve (a normal distal segment, Fig. 10.26a; a proximal enlarged looping segment, Fig. 10.26b; a more proximal segment, Fig. 10.26c). Enlargement of the recurrent motor branch of the median nerve has been linked to carpal tunnel syndrome. Picasso et al. [9] conducted a study involving 32 patients and 50 controls, utilizing ultrasound imaging, and found that the nerve diameter was significantly larger in patients with carpal tunnel syndrome compared to the control group.

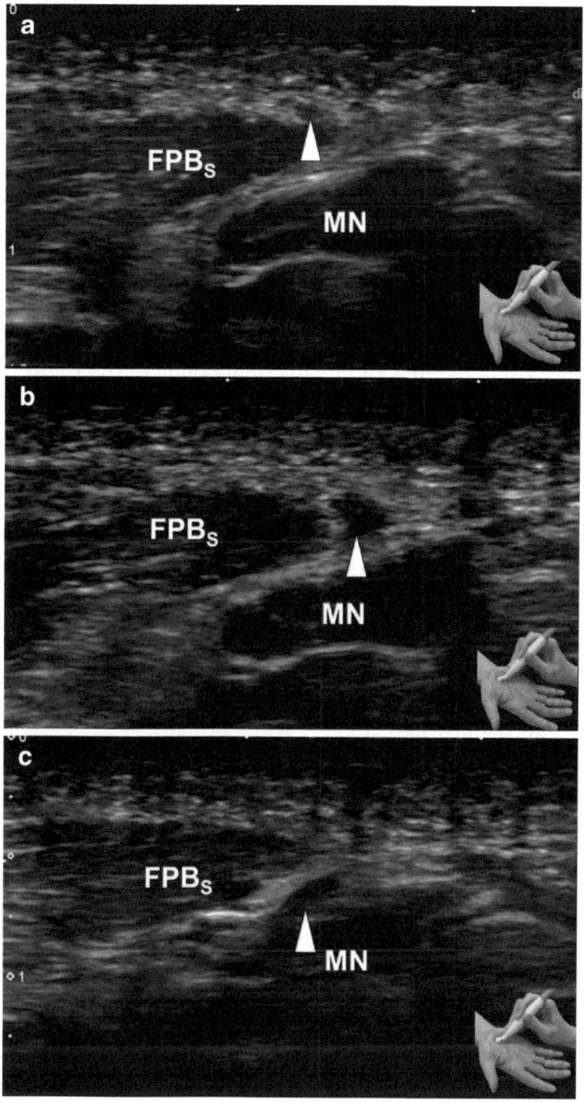

Fig. 10.26 The ultrasound images of the recurrent motor branch of the median nerve (white arrowheads) show a normal distal segment (**a**), a proximal enlarged looping segment (**b**), and a more proximal segment emerging from the main trunk (**c**). FPB$_S$ superficial head of the flexor pollicis brevis; MN main trunk of the median nerve

10.5 Ultrasound-Guided Injection

The most prevalent painful condition in the thumb region requiring intervention is flexor pollicis longus stenosing tenosynovitis. The injection is typically administered by positioning the transducer over the first metacarpal head along the tendon's short axis (Fig. 10.27). This in-plane approach targets the space between the tendon sheath and the tendon itself. To insert the needle from lateral to medial, the physician should guide the needle superficially over the radial sesamoid bone and direct it toward the flexor pollicis longus tendon at the level of the first metacarpal head.

When addressing the first carpometacarpal joint, particularly the volar joint aspect, the physician must carefully examine the recurrent motor branch of the median nerve to avoid inadvertent contact. The transducer can be positioned in the long axis of the joint to identify the joint gap and then guide the injection deep to the anterior oblique ligament (Fig. 10.28a). Alternatively, the transducer can be rotated to align with the joint's axial view for an in-plane ultrasound-guided injection deep to the anterior oblique ligament (Fig. 10.28b). Adhering to the same principle, injections on the dorsal aspect of the joint are feasible and comparatively easier than injections on the volar aspect, as there is no risk of injuring the recurrent motor branch of the median nerve (Fig. 10.29).

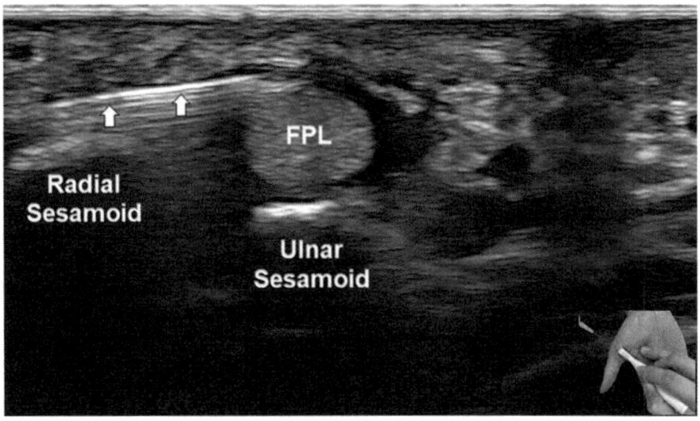

Fig. 10.27 Ultrasound-guided injection into the tendon sheath of the flexor pollicis longus using an in-plane approach. White arrows: needle trajectory; FPL flexor pollicis longus tendon

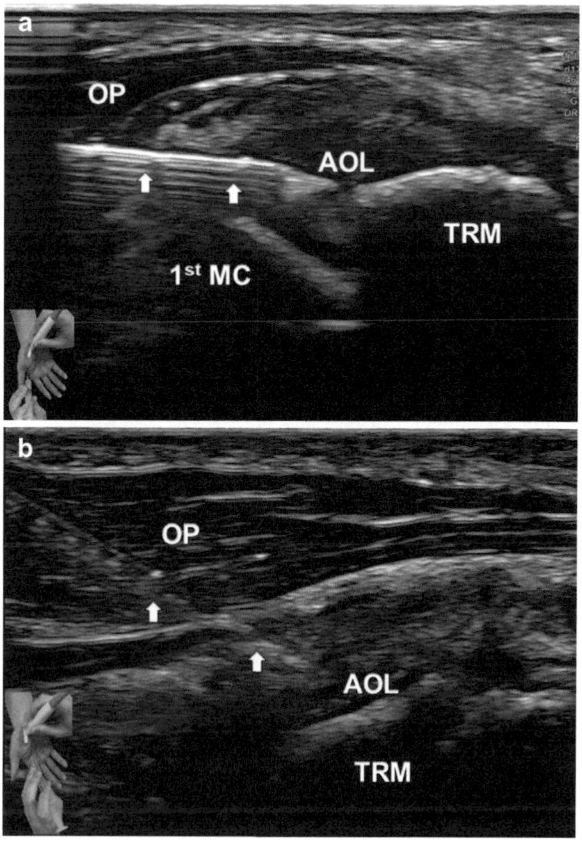

Fig. 10.28 Ultrasound-guided injection into the first carpometacarpal joint, aligned with the long axis (**a**) and short axis (**b**) of the anterior oblique ligament, using an in-plane approach. White arrows: needle trajectory; AOL anterior oblique ligament; OP opponens pollicis; TRM trapezium; 1st MC the first metacarpal bone

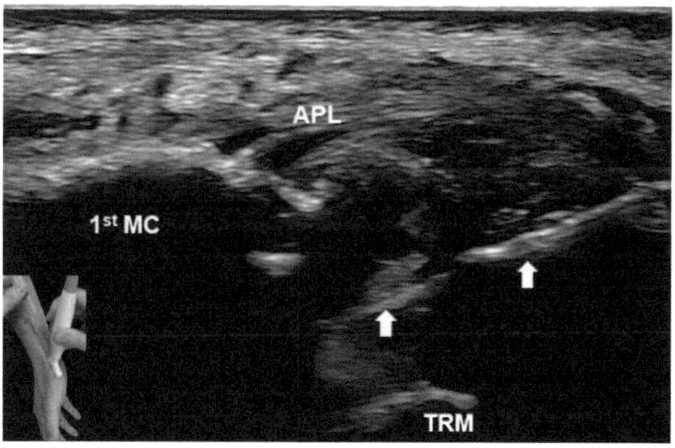

Fig. 10.29 Ultrasound-guided injection into the dorsal aspect of the first carpometacarpal joint using an in-plane approach. White arrows: needle trajectory; APL abductor pollicis longus tendon; 1st MC the first metacarpal bone; TRM trapezium

10.6 Conclusion

The study of thumb sonoanatomy, pathologies, and ultrasound-guided interventions yields a comprehensive grasp of structures and clinical factors. Essential components encompass the flexor carpi radialis, flexor pollicis longus, ligaments of the first carpometacarpal joint, the thenar muscles, and the recurrent branch of the median nerve. Examination of pathologies, including tendinopathy, ligament injuries, and trigger thumb, provides valuable insights for diagnostic interpretation. The section on ultrasound-guided injections emphasizes the importance of precision, particularly in proximity to critical structures such as the recurrent motor branch of the median nerve.

Acknowledgments Images and illustrations adapted from cadaveric images provided by the Visible Human Project® of the National Library of Medicine. Excerpts featured in the VH Dissector are used with permission from Touch of Life Technologies Inc.

References

1. Haara MM, Heliövaara M, Kröger H, et al. Osteoarthritis in the carpometacarpal joint of the thumb. Prevalence and associations with disability and mortality. J Bone Joint Surg Am. 2004;86(7):1452–7.
2. van der Oest MJW, Duraku LS, Andrinopoulou ER, et al. The prevalence of radiographic thumb base osteoarthritis: a meta-analysis. Osteoarthr Cartil. 2021;29(6):785–92.
3. Yeager K, Heifner J, Rubio F, Gray R, Orbay J, Mercer D. Flexor carpi Radialis tendon insertion onto the Trapezial ridge: an anatomic description. J Hand Surg Glob Online. 2023;5(1):55–7.
4. Ladd AL, Lee J, Hagert E. Macroscopic and microscopic analysis of the thumb carpometacarpal ligaments: a cadaveric study of ligament anatomy and histology. J Bone Joint Surg Am. 2012;94(16):1468–77.
5. Kozin SH. The anatomy of the recurrent branch of the median nerve. J Hand Surg Am. 1998;23(5):852–8.
6. Knisely B, Noland SS, Melville DM. Ultrasound versus MRI in the evaluation of the thumb metacarpophalangeal joint. J Ultrason. 2023;23(95):e214–e22.
7. Parellada AJ, Morrison WB, Reiter SB, et al. Flexor carpi radialis tendinopathy: spectrum of imaging findings and association with triscaphe arthritis. Skeletal Radiol. 2006;35(8):572–8.
8. Chang KV, Wu WT, Yang YC, Özçakar L. Ultrasound imaging and guided hydro-dissection for injury of the recurrent motor branch of the median nerve. Med Ultrason. 2021;23(2):239–40.
9. Picasso R, Zaottini F, Pistoia F, et al. Recurrent motor branch neuropathy in carpal tunnel syndrome: an ultrasound study. Muscle Nerve. 2023;68(2):184–90.

Chapter 11
Carpal Tunnel Syndrome Revisited

Ke-Vin Chang, Wei-Ting Wu, and Jia-Chi Wang

11.1 Introduction

The carpal tunnel functions as a narrow and rigid passage located at the base of the hand. Comprising the bottom and sides of the carpal tunnel are the carpal bones, while its upper boundary is formed by the transverse carpal ligament. Within this limited space, the median nerve and nine tendons, crucial for finger movement, travel from the forearm into the hand.

Carpal tunnel syndrome (CTS) typically arises due to heightened pressure on the median nerve within the carpal tunnel. According to a cross-sectional survey involving 969 respondents, the clinically confirmed prevalence of CTS was determined to be 9.6% [1]. This increased pressure can result from various factors, including activities involving repetitive hand and wrist movements, particularly those requiring forceful or prolonged flexing of the wrist. Certain medical conditions, such as diabetes, rheumatoid arthritis, and thyroid disorders, can further exacerbate this heightened pressure [2].

Common symptoms of CTS include numbness, tingling, or a "pins-and-needles" sensation in the thumb, index finger, middle finger, and part of the ring finger. In patients with moderate to severe CTS, grip strength diminishes, potentially causing difficulties in holding objects due to a loss of sensation and muscle control. Pain may radiate up the forearm and even into the shoulder, with discomfort often intensifying during the night.

The diagnosis of CTS generally encompasses a comprehensive assessment of medical history, a physical examination, and occasionally nerve conduction studies.

K.-V. Chang (✉) · W.-T. Wu
Bei-Hu Branch, National Taiwan University Hospital, Taipei, Taiwan

J.-C. Wang
Arkship Rehabilitation Clinic, New Taipei City, Taiwan

K.-V. Chang (ed.), *Ultrasonography of Musculoskeletal Pain*,
https://doi.org/10.1007/978-981-96-6787-1_11

Recent progress in the field has acknowledged ultrasound as a reliable diagnostic tool, a matter that will be extensively discussed in this chapter. Furthermore, in cases where patients do not exhibit improvement with non-invasive treatments, the application of ultrasound-guided hydrodissection, employing different regimens, has shown promise in providing relief from symptoms. This aspect will be thoroughly examined in the forthcoming sections of this chapter.

11.2 Regional Anatomy

The carpal tunnel, a composite structure of bone and fibrous tissue, is located on the volar aspect of the wrist. Its floor and lateral border are defined by the carpal bones, including the scaphoid, triquetrum, pisiform, trapezium, trapezoid, capitate, and hamate. The arrangement of proximal and distal carpal bones in two parallel arcs results in the lunate, situated in the middle of the proximal carpal row, falling proximal to the carpal tunnel inlet. Additionally, the scaphotriquetral ligament extends transversely between the finger flexor tendons and carpal bones.

The upper boundary of the carpal tunnel is marked by the transverse carpal ligament, inserting into the scaphoid tuberosity and pisiform, designating the level of the carpal tunnel inlet. This ligament further extends to the trapezium and the hook of the hamate, forming the distal portion of the carpal tunnel and serving as the carpal tunnel outlet. The flexor retinaculum can be segmented into three sections. The proximal portion courses deeply beneath the flexor carpi ulnaris and flexor carpi radialis. The middle portion is identified as the transverse carpal ligament. The distal portion consists of a thick aponeurosis connecting the thenar and hypothenar muscles [3].

Within the carpal tunnel, nine tendons and a nerve reside: the flexor pollicis longus, the four flexor digitorum superficialis, the four flexor digitorum profundus, and the median nerve. The flexor pollicis longus has its own synovial sheath enveloped by the radial bursa, while the flexor digitorum superficialis and profundus share a common synovial sheath encircled by the ulnar bursa. Both bursae originate proximal to the carpal tunnel, typically near the distal margin of the pronator quadratus muscle, and extend distally to the mid-palm level [4].

The larger ulnar bursa envelops the eight flexor digitorum tendons through three invaginations: a deep invagination between the carpal bones and the profundus tendons, a middle invagination between the profundus and superficialis tendons, and a superficial invagination between the superficialis tendons and the flexor retinaculum (Fig. 11.1). These invaginations stem from a common space at the most ulnar side of the flexor digitorum tendons. Notably, the ulnar bursa typically does not communicate with the flexor tendon sheaths of the index, middle, and ring fingers but terminates through short digital projections at the level of the metacarpal bones. Additionally, the tendons of the flexor carpi radialis, flexor carpi ulnaris, and palmaris longus travel outside the confines of the carpal tunnel.

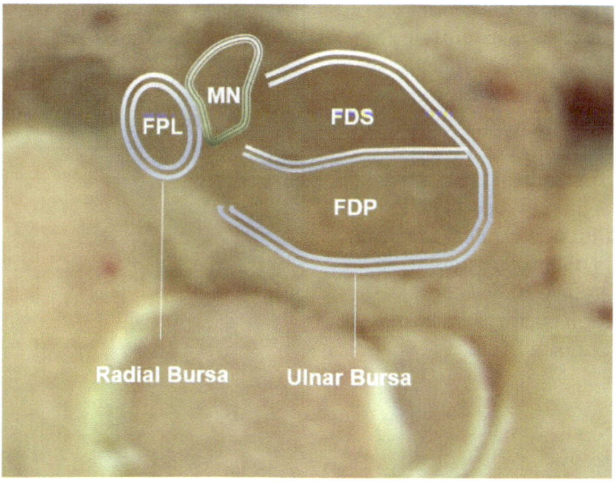

Fig. 11.1 Illustration of the radial and ulnar bursae. FPL flexor pollicis longus; FDS flexor digitorum superficialis; FDP flexor digitorum profundus; MN median nerve

11.3 Sonoanatomy

11.3.1 Axial View

11.3.1.1 Proximal to the Carpal Tunnel Inlet

Scanning of the carpal tunnel can commence from the distal one-third of the forearm in the axial plane, revealing the median nerve situated between the flexor digitorum superficialis and flexor digitorum profundus muscles. In this position, the median nerve is distinctly discernible from the ventral forearm muscles. However, placing the transducer more distally to reach the myotendinous junction of the ventral forearm muscles may pose challenges in distinguishing the median nerve from the tendinous part of the ventral forearm muscle.

Additionally, it is essential to note the topographic arrangement of the flexor digitorum superficialis muscle at the distal forearm. The muscular portion innervating the second digit is ulnar to that for the third digit. Consequently, the arrangement of the four digits for the flexor digitorum superficialis from the radial to ulnar aspect is as follows: third, second, fourth, and fifth finger (Fig. 11.2a, b) [5].

11.3.1.2 Carpal Tunnel Inlet

The transducer is then repositioned more distally to access the carpal tunnel inlet, with the scaphoid serving as the radial landmark and the pisiform as the ulnar landmark. The bony floor of the carpal tunnel consists of the capitate and triquetrum (or the hamate in certain cases). The scaphotriquetral ligament is observed lying on this bony floor, and the fibrillary connective tissue structure spanning the scaphoid and pisiform is identified as the transverse carpal ligament (Fig. 11.3a, b) [6].

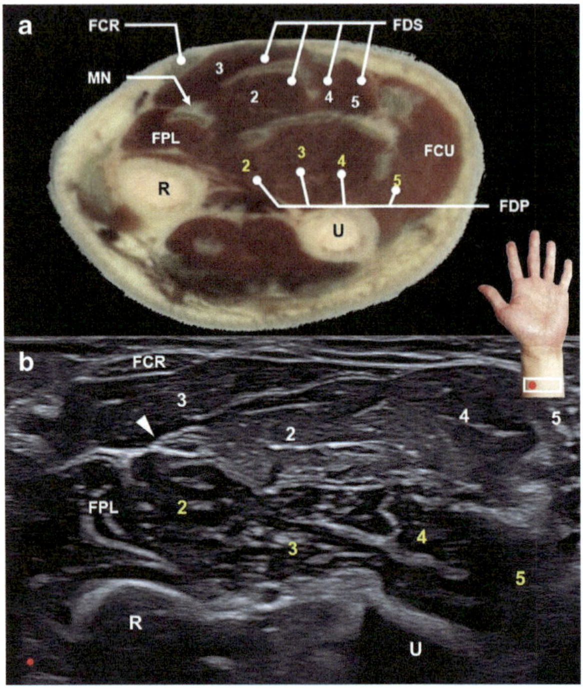

Fig. 11.2 Cadaveric cross-sectional imaging (**a**) and ultrasound imaging (**b**) of the distal volar forearm. MN and white arrowhead: median nerve; FCR flexor carpi radialis; FDS flexor digitorum superficialis; FPL flexor pollicis longus; FDP flexor digitorum profundus; FCU flexor carpi ulnaris; R radius; U ulna

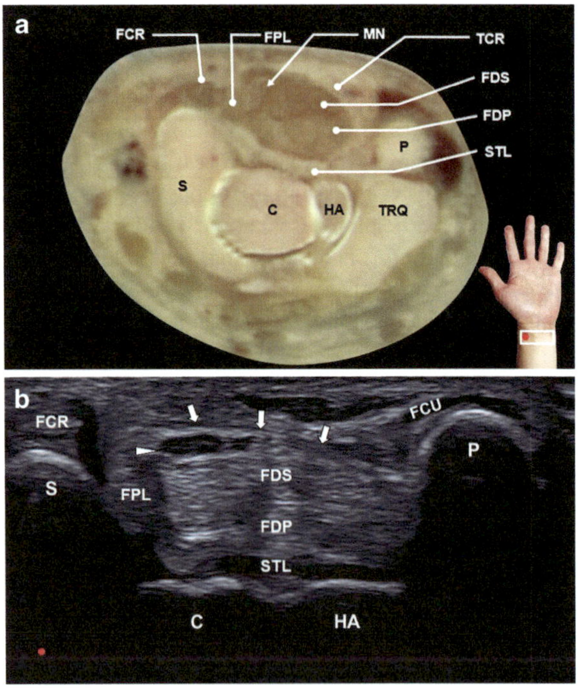

Fig. 11.3 Cadaveric cross-sectional imaging (**a**) and ultrasound imaging (**b**) of the carpal tunnel inlet. MN and white arrowhead: median nerve; TCR and white arrows: transverse carpal ligament; FCR flexor carpi radialis; FDS flexor digitorum superficialis; FPL flexor pollicis longus; FDP flexor digitorum profundus; FCU flexor carpi ulnaris; STL scaphotriquetral ligament; S scaphoid; C capitate; HA hamate; P pisiform; TRQ triquetrum

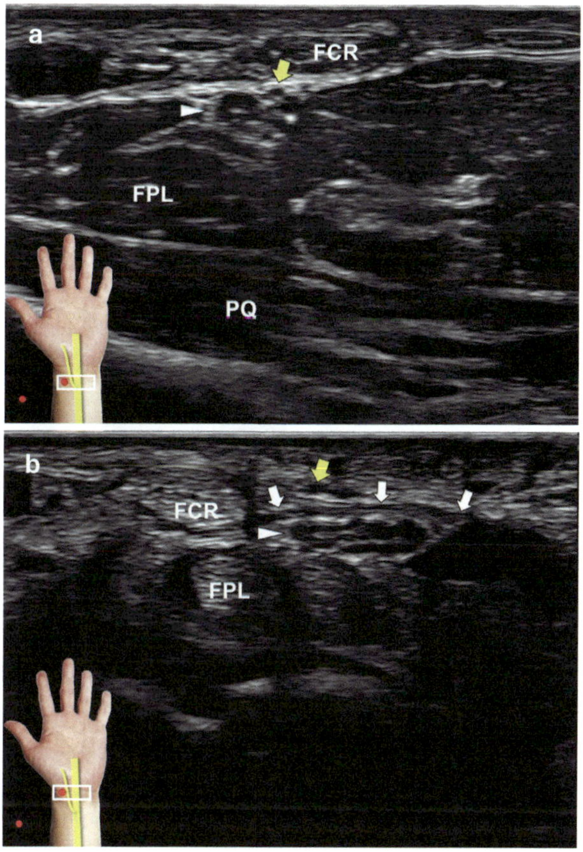

Fig. 11.4 Ultrasound imaging of the palmar cutaneous branch of the median nerve (yellow arrows) at the forearm (**a**) and the carpal tunnel (**b**) level. White arrows: transverse carpal ligament; white arrowheads: median nerve; FCR flexor carpi radialis; FPL flexor pollicis longus; PQ pronator quadratus

Beyond the transverse carpal ligament, the flexor carpi radialis tendon aligns itself over the scaphoid tubercle, while the palmaris longus tendon lies directly on the transverse carpal ligament. Simultaneously, the flexor carpi ulnaris tendon courses over the tip of the pisiform. Additionally, the palmar cutaneous branch of the median nerve emerges from the radial aspect of the median nerve, encircling the upper border of the median nerve before reaching the antebrachial fascia (Fig. 11.4a) [7]. This branch subsequently pierces the fascia and travels along the ulnar aspect of the flexor carpi radialis tendon (Fig. 11.4b). Within the carpal tunnel, the median nerve is positioned between the transverse carpal ligament and the finger flexor tendons, including the flexor pollicis longus, flexor digitorum superficialis (second finger), and flexor digitorum profundus (second finger).

It is essential to highlight that the median nerve exhibits a degree of mobility within the carpal tunnel. When participants are encouraged to flex and extend the second or third finger, the median nerve undergoes upward and downward movement within the space created by the flexor pollicis longus tendons (surrounded by the radial bursa) and the flexor digitorum tendons (enclosed by the ulnar bursa).

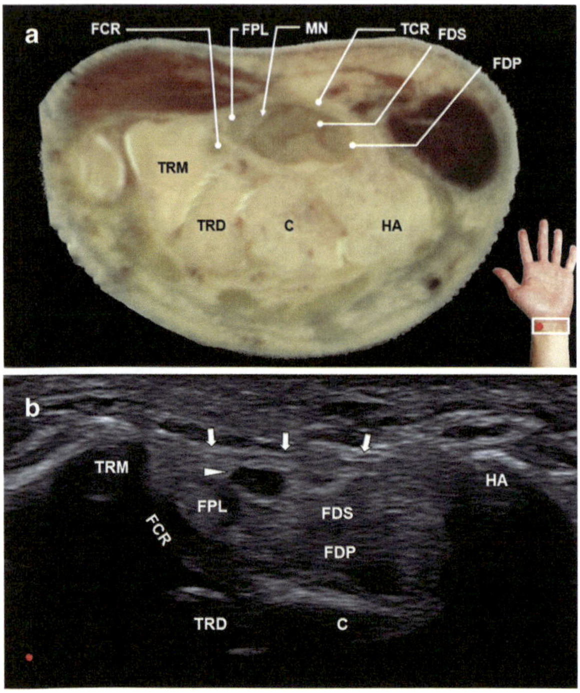

Fig. 11.5 Cadaveric cross-sectional imaging (**a**) and ultrasound imaging (**b**) of the carpal tunnel outlet. MN and white arrowhead: median nerve; TCR and white arrows: transverse carpal ligament; FCR flexor carpi radialis; FDS flexor digitorum superficialis; FPL flexor pollicis longus; FDP flexor digitorum profundus; TRM trapezium; TRD trapezoid; C capitate; HA hamate

11.3.1.3 Carpal Tunnel Outlet

Moving the transducer further distally, the carpal tunnel outlet is identified at the level linking the trapezium and hamate. The hamate is located more radially than the triquetrum, making the carpal tunnel outlet narrower than its inlet. Outside of the carpal tunnel, the flexor carpi radialis is visualized inside a groove over the trapezium. The bony floor is made by the trapezoid and capitate (Fig. 11.5a, b).

11.3.1.4 Distal to the Carpal Tunnel Outlet

Further distally, the median nerve undergoes division into common digital branches that provide innervation to the first, second, third, and the radial half of the fourth finger. It is noteworthy that the recurrent motor branch originates from the common digital branch, typically the one innervating the first finger [8]. This branch follows a course around the medial edge of the thenar muscle, surfacing before penetrating the thenar muscle for innervation. The transducer can be positioned in the short axis over the superficial head of the flexor pollicis brevis to visualize the recurrent motor branch on the surface of the muscle (Fig. 11.6a). Shifting the transducer proximally allows

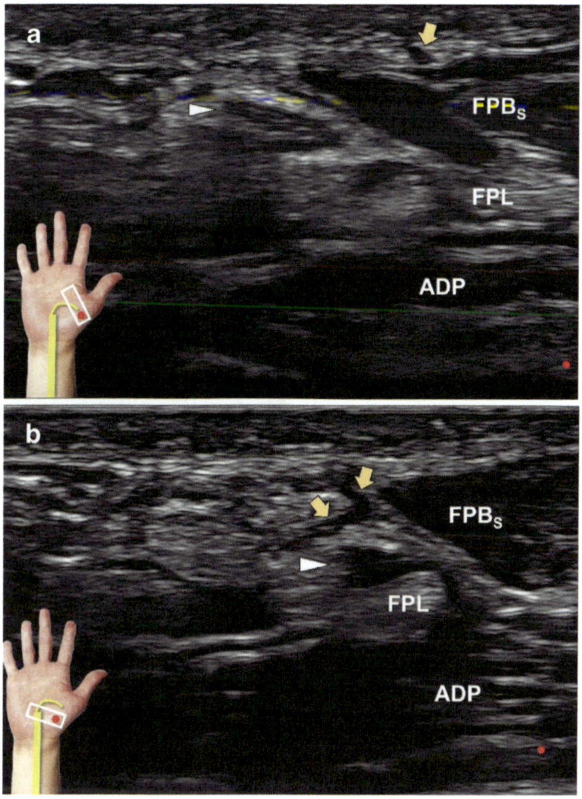

Fig. 11.6 Ultrasound imaging of the recurrent motor branch (yellow arrows) of the median nerve at the distal thenar region (**a**) and the proximal thenar region (**b**), where it joins the main trunk of the median nerve (white arrowheads). FPB$_S$ superficial head of the flexor pollicis brevis; FPL flexor pollicis longus; ADP adductor pollicis

visualization of the point where the nerve joins the main trunk of the median nerve (Fig. 11.6b). Additionally, distal to the carpal tunnel outlet, the transverse carpal ligament is replaced by an aponeurosis connecting the thenar and hypothenar muscles.

11.3.2 Long-Axis View

Following the examination of the carpal tunnel and adjacent structures in the axial view, the transducer can be rotated to align with the long axis of the distal forearm. This orientation proves most effective for identifying any entrapped segments of the median nerve before precisely measuring their cross-sectional area (Fig. 11.7a, b). Additionally, the examinee may be prompted to flex either the second or third finger, facilitating the recognition of reciprocal movement between the median nerve and the underlying tendons of the flexor digitorum superficialis and flexor digitorum profundus.

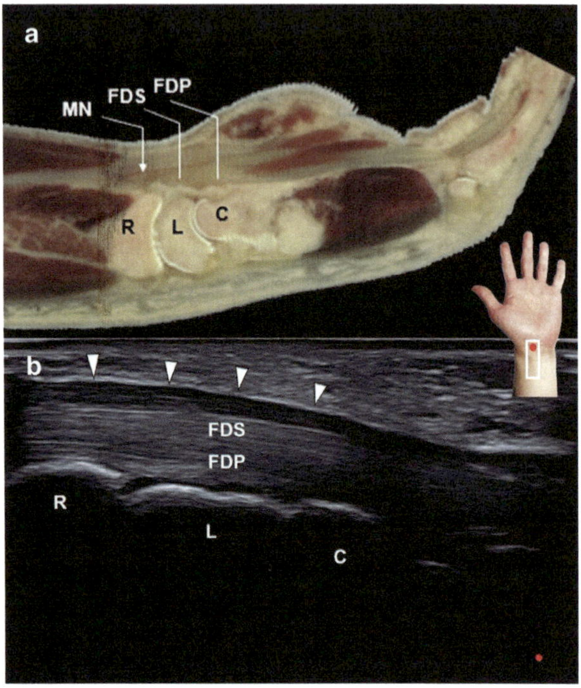

Fig. 11.7 The cadaveric cross-sectional imaging (**a**) and ultrasound imaging (**b**) of the carpal tunnel in the long axis. MN and white arrowheads: median nerve; FDS flexor digitorum superficialis; FDP flexor digitorum profundus; R radius; L lunate; C capitate

11.4 Ultrasound Diagnosis for Carpal Tunnel Syndrome

Electrodiagnostic studies have traditionally served as the gold standard for diagnosing carpal tunnel syndrome. This condition, characterized as a compressive neuropathy, leads to the enlargement of the portion of the median nerve proximal to the point of entrapment, resulting from the obstruction of axoplasmic flow [9]. When examined through ultrasound imaging, the distinctive honeycomb appearance of the median nerve may become less pronounced due to the presence of nerve fascicle edema.

Recently, ultrasound imaging has emerged as a valuable alternative to electrophysiological studies for diagnosing CTS, offering comparable accuracy with the added benefit of a comfortable, non-invasive examination. However, a range of ultrasound parameters and modes are available, each with distinct strengths and limitations for diagnosis. Ultrasound evaluation of CTS can be categorized into qualitative and quantitative assessments.

Qualitatively, the median nerve in affected wrists may lose its typical fascicular pattern at the carpal tunnel inlet (Fig. 11.8a), contrasting with the normal fascicular pattern in the proximal segment (Fig. 11.8b) in axial view. In long-axis views, focal compression of the median nerve by a thickened retinaculum can also be observed (Fig. 11.8c). For patients with previous carpal tunnel release, residual or recurrent symptoms may be due to hypertrophic scar tissue compressing the median nerve

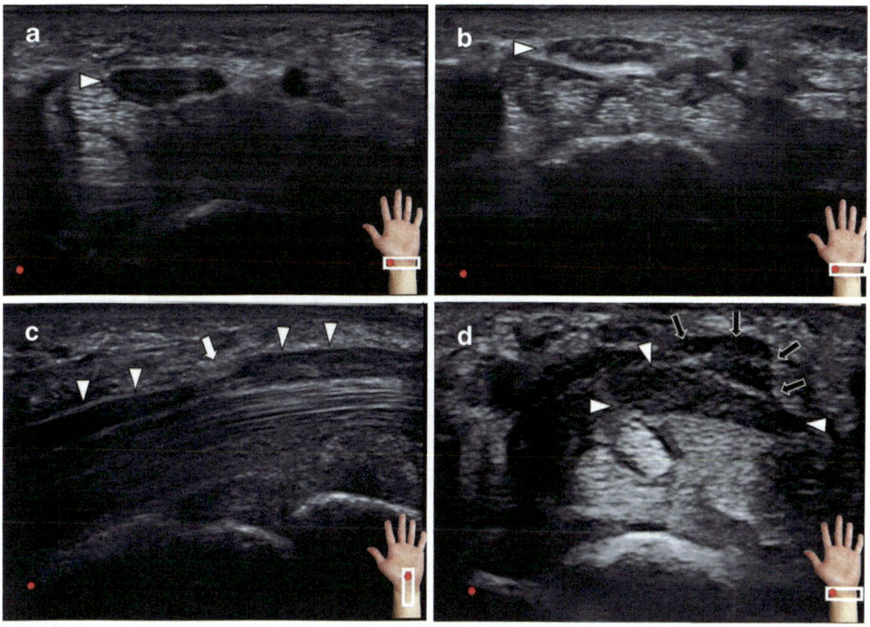

Fig. 11.8 In a case of carpal tunnel syndrome, the median nerve's fascicular pattern in the axial view is disrupted at the level of the carpal tunnel inlet (**a**), in contrast to the normal fascicular pattern observed proximal to the inlet (**b**). In the long-axis view, focal encroachment of the median nerve by the thickened flexor retinaculum (white arrow) is noted (**c**). In another case where the patient underwent carpal tunnel release but experienced no symptom improvement, a hypertrophic scar (black arrows) is observed compressing the median nerve, which appears flattened and enlarged (**d**). White arrowheads: median nerve

(Fig. 11.8d). Additionally, the recurrent motor branches of the median nerve often display increased cross-sectional area in carpal tunnel syndrome patients, as shown in observational studies like that of Picasso et al. [10] (short axis, Fig. 11.9a; long axis, Fig. 11.9b).

Crystal deposition, such as tophus (affected side, Fig. 11.10a; non-affected side, Fig. 11.10b), protein deposition, including amyloidosis (short axis, Fig. 11.11a; long axis, Fig. 11.11b), or thickening of the tendon sheath within the carpal tunnel (Fig. 11.12), can increase carpal tunnel pressure, resulting in CTS. Additionally, certain anatomical variants, such as a persistent median artery or bifid median nerve (Fig. 11.13a), may be associated with CTS. A meta-analysis by Asghar et al. [11] reported a 50% higher incidence of bifid median nerve in CTS patients compared to controls. This variant increases the mean cross-sectional area of the median nerve at the wrist by 1.5 mm^2. Furthermore, a case report by Kim et al. [12] highlighted the potential for thrombosis of a persistent median artery to trigger the acute onset of CTS. In some cases, the distal muscle bellies of the flexor digitorum superficialis may encroach on the already narrow carpal tunnel, exacerbating the condition (Fig. 11.13b). These pathologies and variants can be effectively visualized using

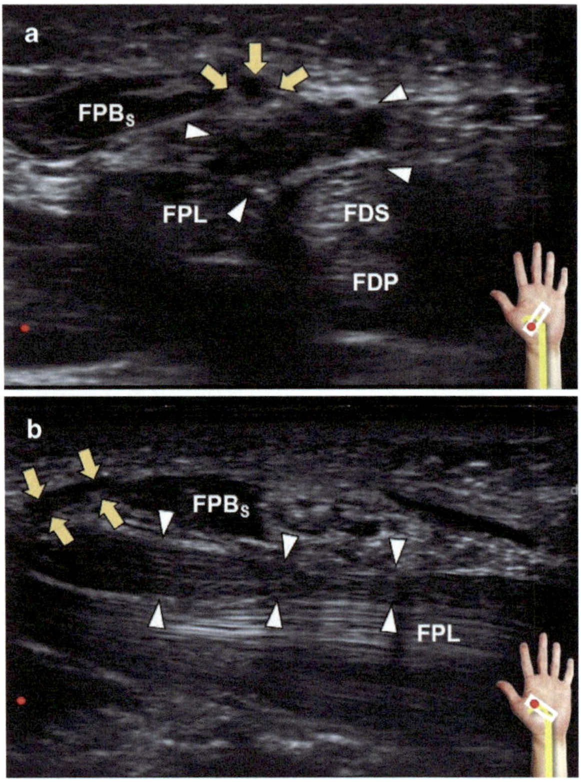

Fig. 11.9 Axial (**a**) and longitudinal (**b**) ultrasound views show an increased cross-sectional area of the recurrent motor branch (yellow arrows) of the median nerve in a patient with carpal tunnel syndrome. White arrowheads: proximal trunk of the median nerve; FPL flexor pollicis longus; FDS flexor digitorum superficialis; FDP flexor digitorum profundus; FPB$_S$ superficial head of the flexor pollicis brevis

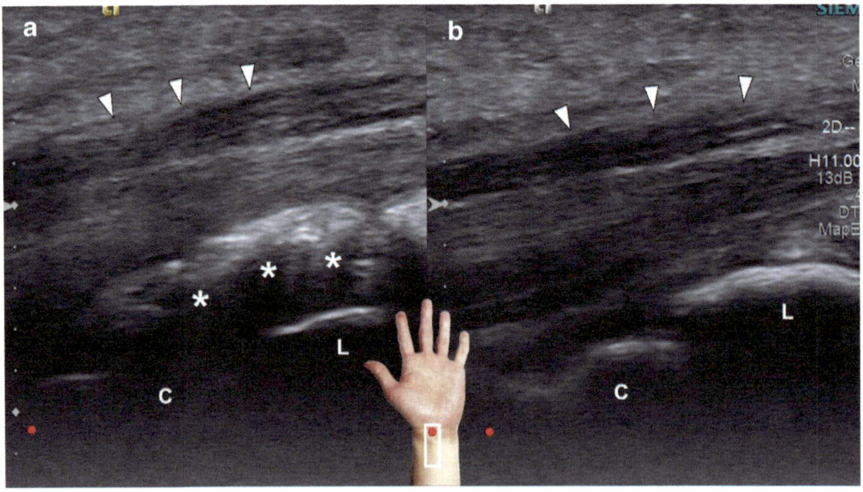

Fig. 11.10 Longitudinal ultrasound views show tophus deposition (asterisks) at the base of the carpal tunnel (**a**), compared to the normal side (**b**). White arrowheads: median nerve; C capitate; L lunate

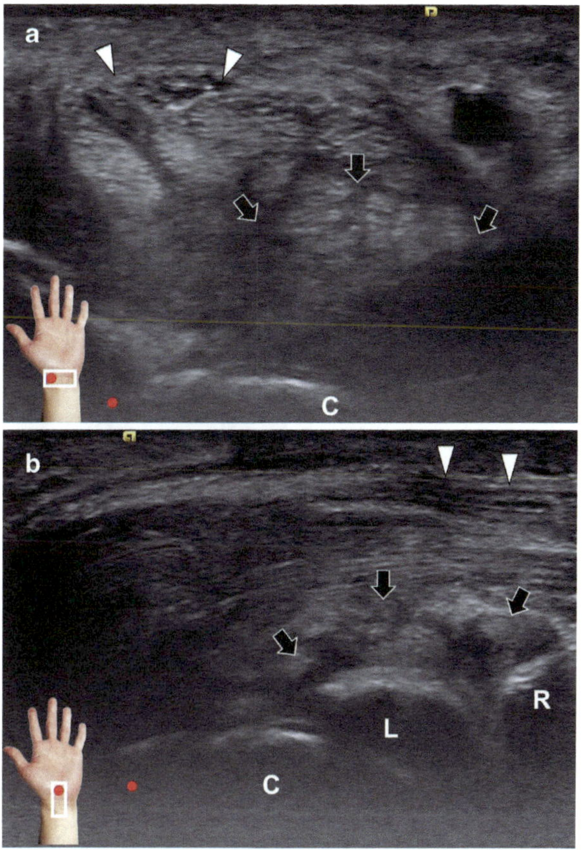

Fig. 11.11 Axial (**a**) and longitudinal (**b**) ultrasound views demonstrate amyloid deposition (black arrows) at the base of the carpal tunnel. White arrowheads: median nerve; C capitate; L lunate; R radius

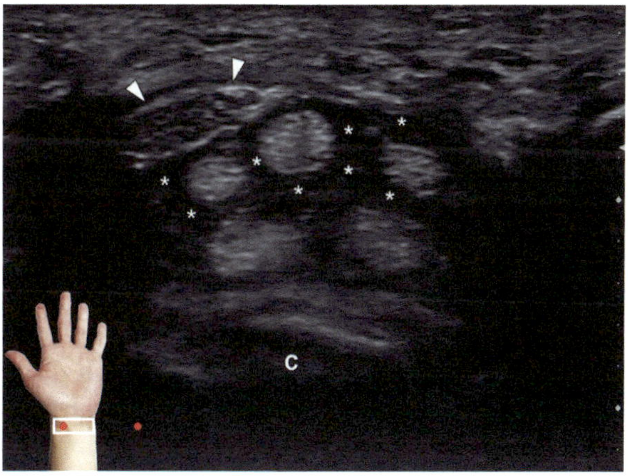

Fig. 11.12 Axial ultrasound view shows thickening of the finger flexor tendon sheath (asterisks) within the carpal tunnel. White arrowheads: median nerve; C capitate

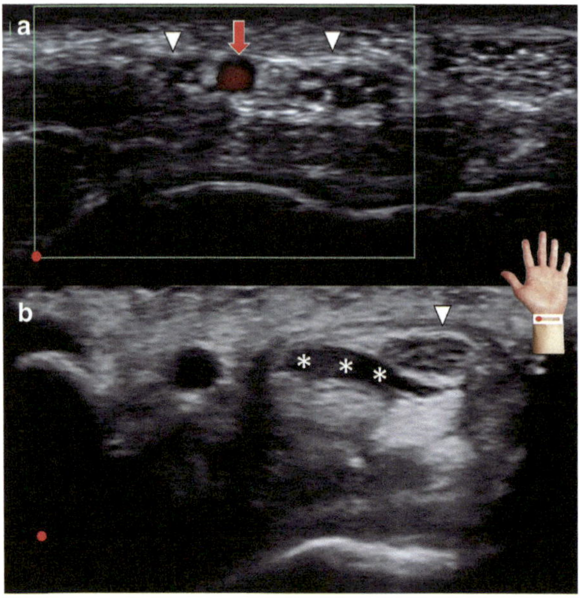

Fig. 11.13 Axial ultrasound images demonstrate a persistent median artery (red arrow) and a bifid median nerve, with two separate components of the median nerve (white arrows) (**a**), as well as distal muscle bellies of the flexor digitorum superficialis (asterisks) within the carpal tunnel (**b**)

qualitative ultrasound imaging. Beyond grayscale ultrasound's qualitative assessments, we explore quantitative parameters and advanced imaging techniques to improve the evaluation of CTS.

11.4.1 Nerve Cross-Sectional Area (CSA)

The cross-sectional area (CSA) is typically derived either indirectly through a mathematical formula or by directly tracing the median nerve. Various locations for CSA measurements have been proposed, particularly emphasizing the carpal tunnel inlet (pisiform level) and outlet (hamate level). The diagnostic efficacy of the inlet CSA appears to be superior to that of the outlet CSA. Additionally, the inlet CSA exhibits the strongest correlation with electrodiagnostic study outcomes. CSA measurement is usually performed in the nerve's axial view. In cases where the direct tracking method is applied, the tracking line is frequently drawn inside the epineurium, highlighting changes in the nerve fascicles rather than the surrounding connective tissues (Fig. 11.14). The cutoff value typically ranges between 9.5 and 10.5 mm^2 [13]. Importantly, an increase in the cutoff CSA value is linked to lower sensitivity and higher specificity. Furthermore, ultrasound has demonstrated efficacy in diagnosing carpal tunnel syndrome in patients with diabetes mellitus, even in the presence of existing polyneuropathy. It is worth noting that in the diabetic population, median nerves appear less enlarged in individuals with concurrent diabetic polyneuropathy than in those without it [14].

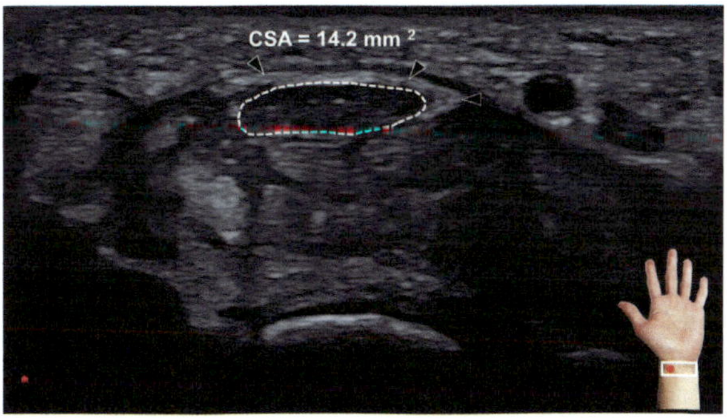

Fig. 11.14 The ultrasound imaging for the cross-sectional area (CSA, area within the dashed line) of the median nerve within the epineurium (black arrowheads) at the carpal tunnel inlet

11.4.2 Swelling Ratio

The swelling ratio was determined by dividing the CSA at various anatomical levels, such as wrist-to-forearm and inlet-to-outlet. The advantage of employing the swelling ratio is to mitigate the impact of diverse body sizes or statures. Despite the inlet-to-outlet ratio appearing to be the most dependable parameter within the swelling ratio, there exists conflicting evidence regarding whether individuals with carpal tunnel syndrome should exhibit a larger or smaller ratio [13].

11.4.3 Median Nerve Stiffness

Two primary methods have been utilized to evaluate median nerve stiffness: strain and shear wave sonoelastography. Strain sonoelastography provides qualitative insights into tissue elasticity via color elastograms, relying on the displacement determined by the operator through repeated compressions and decompressions with the transducer. In contrast, shear wave sonoelastography entails applying acoustic radiation force through the ultrasound beam to the tissue, with the ensuing propagation velocity correlating with tissue elasticity, measurable in either m/s or kPa (Fig. 11.15). Shear wave sonoelastography stands out as a more dependable measurement, exhibiting reduced susceptibility to manual compressive force variations from the transducer compared to strain sonoelastography. With a shear modulus threshold ranging from 38.38 to 70.00 kPa, shear wave sonoelastography demonstrates a pooled sensitivity and specificity of 94% and 80%, respectively, in diagnosing CTS [15]. Despite these promising results, there is a notable absence of a comparative study evaluating diagnostic performance between CSA and sonoelastography.

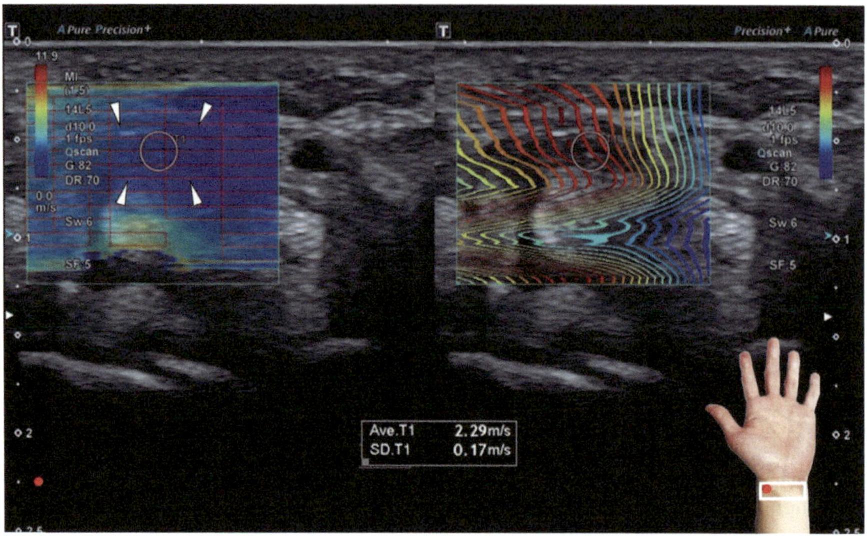

Fig. 11.15 Shear wave sonoelastography for measurement of the median nerve (arrowheads) stiffness. The average shear wave velocity inside the region of interest is 2.29 m/s with a standard deviation of 0.17 m/s

11.4.4 Vascularity Measurement

Color and power Doppler ultrasound are commonly utilized to assess the vascularity of the median nerve, particularly at the carpal tunnel inlet. In individuals without carpal tunnel syndrome, the previously mentioned conventional Doppler modes struggle to detect any flow within the median nerve. Conversely, in patients with CTS, venous congestion and neovascularization contribute to the visualization of increased intra-neural vascularity. Nevertheless, relying on intra-neural blood flow as the exclusive parameter for diagnosing CTS is less practical due to the challenges in accurately quantifying vascularity.

An innovative ultrasound technology, Superb Microvascular Imaging (SMI), has emerged to overcome the limitations of traditional color and power Doppler technologies. SMI addresses these issues by suppressing low-velocity components and retaining crucial low-flow elements, resulting in a more precise estimation of minute blood flow. Significantly, SMI enables the identification of small arterioles near the median nerve in asymptomatic individuals [16]. When employing the semi-quantitative method, SMI consistently reveals a higher vascularity score in patients with CTS compared to those without the condition. Enhanced sensitivity can be achieved by incorporating CSA measurements with SMI, providing a more comprehensive evaluation of vascularity in the diagnosis and management of CTS (Fig. 11.16).

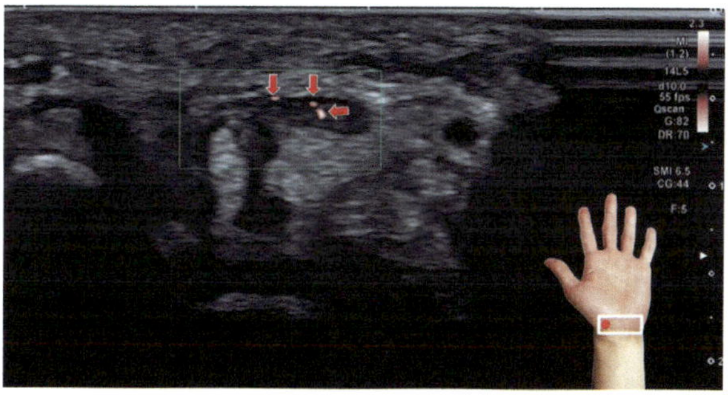

Fig. 11.16 Superb microvascular imaging for the median nerve, showing intra-neural vascularity (red arrows)

11.5 Ultrasound-Guided Injection for Carpal Tunnel Syndrome

Ultrasound-guided injection has proven to be an effective intervention for patients experiencing carpal tunnel syndrome resistant to non-invasive treatments, such as medication and physical therapy. Commonly utilized injectates include corticosteroid, 5% dextrose, and platelet-rich plasma. A network meta-analysis has demonstrated that 5% dextrose yields the most favorable outcomes in symptom relief, followed by platelet-rich plasma and corticosteroid [17]. To optimize efficacy, it is recommended that the volume of 5% dextrose reach a specified level, such as 4 mL [18], and recent research even suggests that 10 mL may be more effective than 5 mL [19]. Conversely, the volume of platelet-rich plasma is constrained to a range between 2 mL and 3 mL, contingent on variations in products/brands. Similar to 5% dextrose, a larger volume of corticosteroid mixture (exceeding 3 mL) is linked to a diminished rate of treatment failure within one year [20]. The dosage of corticosteroid, employing commonly used regimens like triamcinolone acetonide, typically ranges from 10 mg to 40 mg.

In the context of the ultrasound injection technique, it is recommended to employ hydro-dissection for the separation of the epineurium and subsynovium connective tissue to enhance the mobility of the median nerve during wrist movements. The optimal target level is the carpal tunnel inlet as viewed axially. To maximize the operational space, the use of a hockey-stick transducer is advised. During the in-plane approach, the needle should be introduced from the ulnar to radial direction, with careful attention to avoiding injury to the ulnar nerve and artery within Guyon's canal. The radial to ulnar approach is less preferable due to potential hindrance by the flexor carpi radialis tendon, limiting the window for needle insertion.

The sequence of needle insertion involves initial hydro-dissection between the median nerve and underlying finger flexors (Fig. 11.17a), followed by hydro-dissection between the median nerve and the overlying flexor retinaculum (Fig. 11.17b) [21]. This sequential approach helps prevent the injectate, containing crystalloid substances such as triamcinolone acetoacetate, from obstructing the visualization of underlying structures. Additionally, hydro-dissection along the long axis of the median nerve, situated between the flexor retinaculum and the nerve

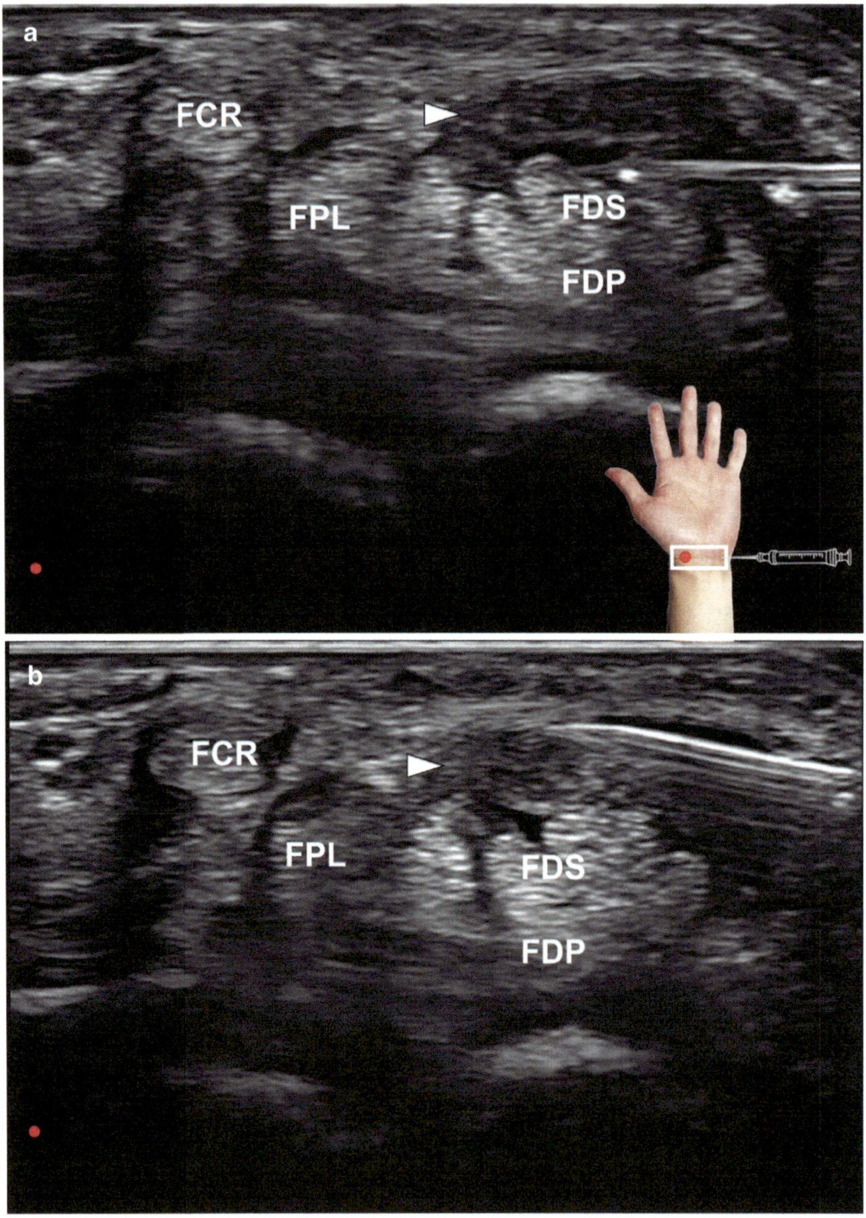

Fig. 11.17 Ultrasound-guided hydro-dissection between the median nerve (white arrowheads) and underlying finger flexors (**a**), followed by hydro-dissection between the median nerve and the overlying flexor retinaculum (**b**). FCR flexor carpi radialis; FPL flexor pollicis longus; FDS flexor digitorum superficialis; FDP flexor digitorum profundus

itself, is a feasible alternative. Its efficacy is comparable to classic hydrodissection through the axial plane [22].

11.6 Conclusion

High-resolution ultrasound facilitates the visualization of the carpal tunnel and its neural and tendinous structures. It proves valuable in diagnosing CTS, with a straightforward CSA measurement offering diagnostic accuracy on par with electrophysiological studies. Ultrasound guidance provides a safe avenue for nerve hydro-dissection, proving effective in treating CTS when non-invasive management proves ineffective.

Acknowledgments Images and illustrations adapted from cadaveric images provided by the Visible Human Project® of the National Library of Medicine. Excerpts featured in the VH Dissector are used with permission from Touch of Life Technologies Inc.

References

1. Feng B, Chen K, Zhu X, et al. Prevalence and risk factors of self-reported wrist and hand symptoms and clinically confirmed carpal tunnel syndrome among office workers in China: a cross-sectional study. BMC Public Health. 2021;21(1):57.
2. Guan W, Lao J, Gu Y, Zhao X, Rui J, Gao K. Case-control study on individual risk factors of carpal tunnel syndrome. Exp Ther Med. 2018;15(3):2761–6.
3. Cobb TK, Dalley BK, Posteraro RH, Lewis RC. Anatomy of the flexor retinaculum. J Hand Surg Am. 1993;18(1):91–9.
4. Fussey JM, Chin KF, Gogi N, Gella S, Deshmukh SC. An anatomic study of flexor tendon sheaths: a cadaveric study. J Hand Surg Eur. 2009;34(6):762–5.
5. Hodde FL, Ioannou CI, Altenmüller E. Mapping of finger fascicles within the flexor digitorum superficialis and profundus muscles. Muscle Nerve. 2019;60(5):579–82.
6. Wang JC, Wu WT, Chang KV, Chen LR, Nakashima Y, Özçakar L. Sonoanatomy and step-wise/systematic ultrasound examination of the extrinsic/intrinsic wrist ligaments. Diagnostics (Basel). 2021;11(10)
7. Chang KV, Mezian K, Naňka O, et al. Ultrasound imaging for the cutaneous nerves of the extremities and relevant entrapment syndromes: from anatomy to clinical implications. J Clin Med. 2018;7(11)
8. Wu WT, Chang KV, Hsu YC, et al. Ultrasound imaging and guidance for distal peripheral nerve pathologies at the wrist/hand. Diagnostics (Basel). 2023;13(11)
9. Chang KV, Wu WT, Özçakar L. Ultrasound imaging and guidance in peripheral nerve entrapment: hydrodissection highlighted. Pain Manag. 2020;10(2):97–106.
10. Picasso R, Zaottini F, Pistoia F, et al. Recurrent motor branch neuropathy in carpal tunnel syndrome: an ultrasound study. Muscle Nerve. 2023;68(2):184–90.
11. Asghar A, Patra A, Satish Ravi K, Tubbs RS, Kumar A, Naaz S. Bifid median nerve as an anatomical risk factor for carpal tunnel syndrome: a meta-analysis. Clin Anat. 2022;35(7):946–52.
12. Kim D, Park JW, Choi IC. Thrombosed persistent median artery with bifid median nerve causing acute carpal tunnel syndrome: a case report. ahm. 2017;22(4):256–60.

13. Lin TY, Chang KV, Wu WT, Özçakar L. Ultrasonography for the diagnosis of carpal tunnel syndrome: an umbrella review. J Neurol. 2022;269(9):4663–75.
14. Chen IJ, Chang KV, Lou YM, Wu WT, Özçakar L. Can ultrasound imaging be used for the diagnosis of carpal tunnel syndrome in diabetic patients? A systemic review and network meta-analysis. J Neurol. 2020;267(7):1887–95.
15. Lin CP, Chen IJ, Chang KV, Wu WT, Özçakar L. Utility of ultrasound elastography in evaluation of carpal tunnel syndrome: a systematic review and meta-analysis. Ultrasound Med Biol. 2019;45(11):2855–65.
16. Lin T-Y, Shen P-C, Chang K-V, Wu W-T, Özçakar L. Assessment of the carpal tunnel and associated neural structures with superb microvascular imaging: a scoping review. Expert Review of Medical Devices:1–7.
17. Lin CP, Chang KV, Huang YK, Wu WT, Ozcakar L. Regenerative injections including 5% dextrose and platelet-rich plasma for the treatment of carpal tunnel syndrome: a systematic review and network meta-analysis. Pharmaceuticals (Basel). 2020;13(3)
18. Lin MT, Liao CL, Hsiao MY, Hsueh HW, Chao CC, Wu CH. Volume matters in ultrasound-guided perineural dextrose injection for carpal tunnel syndrome: a randomized, double-blinded. Three-Arm Trial Front Pharmacol. 2020;11:625830.
19. Huang CY, Lai CY, Reeves KD, et al. Volume effect of nerve hydrodissection for carpal tunnel syndrome: a prospective, randomized, and single-blind study. J Ultrasound Med. 2024;43(1):161–9.
20. Evers S, Bryan AJ, Sanders TL, Gunderson T, Gelfman R, Amadio PC. Influence of injection volume on rate of subsequent intervention in carpal tunnel syndrome over 1-year follow-up. J Hand Surg Am. 2018;43(6):537–44.
21. Wang JC, Hsu PC, Wang KA, Chang KV. Ultrasound-guided triamcinolone acetonide hydrodissection for carpal tunnel syndrome: a randomized controlled trial. Front Med (Lausanne). 2021;8:742724.
22. Chen SR, Ho TY, Shen YP, et al. Comparison of short- and long-axis nerve hydrodissection for carpal tunnel syndrome: a prospective randomized, single-blind trial. Int J Med Sci. 2021;18(15):3488–97.

Chapter 12
Guyon Canal Unveiled

Ke-Vin Chang, Wei-Ting Wu, and Yuan-Yuan Tsai

12.1 Introduction

The Guyon canal represents a distinctive site vulnerable to compressive injury for the ulnar nerve, in contrast to the more common occurrence of ulnar nerve injuries at the elbow, referred to as cubital tunnel syndrome. Guyon canal syndrome is a relatively infrequent form of peripheral ulnar neuropathy characterized by damage to the ulnar nerve's distal portion within a narrow anatomical passageway at the wrist [1].

Various factors can contribute to the compression of the ulnar nerve within the Guyon canal, encompassing ganglion cysts, fractures, displacements of the hook of hamate, tumors, external compression from a cyclist's handlebar, aberrant abductor digiti minimi, hyperproliferation of fat tissue within the canal, or ulnar artery thrombosis or aneurysm. Among these causes, ganglion cysts and repetitive trauma are the most commonly reported contributors to Guyon canal syndrome [2].

The diagnosis of Guyon canal syndrome primarily relies on clinical evaluation, with signs and symptoms presenting as either purely motor, purely sensory, or a combination, contingent on the location of the distal ulnar nerve lesion. Motor-related complaints may include weakness or paralysis of the intrinsic hand muscles innervated by the ulnar nerve, resulting in diminished handgrip strength and clawing of the fourth and fifth digits [3]. Significantly, the preservation of the dorsal surface of the ulnar dermatome (dorsal medial hand and two fingers) serves as an indicative feature of Guyon canal syndrome, as this region is innervated by the dorsal ulnar cutaneous branch, originating approximately proximal to the Guyon canal entrance.

Compromise of the deep motor branch of the ulnar nerve within the Guyon canal can lead to weakness of the adductor pollicis muscle. Pathologically, a Froment sign

K.-V. Chang (✉) · W.-T. Wu · Y.-Y. Tsai
Bei-Hu Branch, National Taiwan University Hospital, Taipei, Taiwan

K.-V. Chang (ed.), *Ultrasonography of Musculoskeletal Pain*,
https://doi.org/10.1007/978-981-96-6787-1_12

may be observed, characterized by hyperflexion of the thumb interphalangeal joint (via the flexor pollicis longus tendon, innervated by the anterior interosseous nerve) compensating for the inability to adduct the thumb [4].

In recent times, ultrasound has gained widespread adoption as a valuable tool for assessing peripheral nerve neuropathies [5]. In the subsequent discussion, we aim to elaborate the anatomical aspects of the Guyon canal and explore the applications of ultrasound for diagnosing and treating its pathologies.

12.2 Regional Anatomy

Before entering the Guyon canal, the ulnar nerve gives off two cutaneous branches: the palmar ulnar cutaneous nerve (usually) from its radial side in the distal forearm [6], and the dorsal ulnar cutaneous nerve from its ulnar side, which crosses the pronator quadratus and extensor carpi ulnaris to reach the dorsal wrist (Fig. 12.1) [7]. The proximal segment of the Guyon canal is situated at the level of the pisiform. Its roof is formed by the palmar carpal ligament, while the floor is constituted by the transverse carpal ligament. The palmar carpal ligament attaches to the flexor carpi ulnaris tendon, and the transverse carpal ligament inserts onto the deep radial aspect of the pisiform. Within the Guyon canal, one can find the ulnar artery, ulnar nerve, and more distal branches, including the proper digital nerve of the little finger, the common digital nerve of the fourth web space, and the deep motor branch, along with accompanying veins [8] (Fig. 12.2). Compression of the nerve at this level

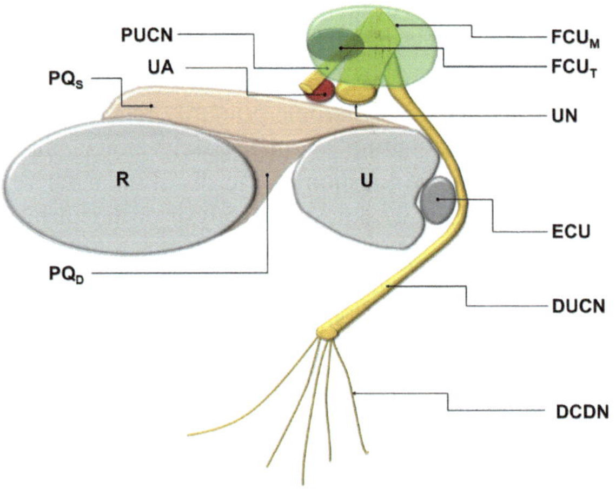

Fig. 12.1 The illustration shows the palmar and dorsal ulnar cutaneous nerves branching from the ulnar nerve. PUCN palmar ulnar cutaneous nerve; DUCN dorsal ulnar cutaneous nerve; DCDN dorsal common digital nerve; PQ_S superficial head of the pronator quadratus; PQ_D deep head of the pronator quadratus; FCU_M flexor carpi ulnaris muscle; FCU_T flexor carpi ulnaris tendon; UA ulnar artery; UN ulnar nerve; ECU extensor carpi ulnaris tendon; R radius; U ulna

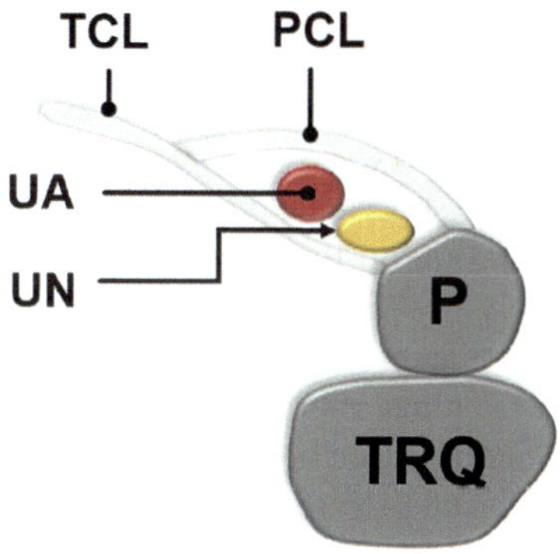

Fig. 12.2 The illustration depicts relevant anatomy of the Guyon canal at the inlet level. PCL palmar carpal ligament; TCL transverse carpal ligament; UA ulnar artery; UN ulnar nerve; P pisiform; TRQ triquetrum

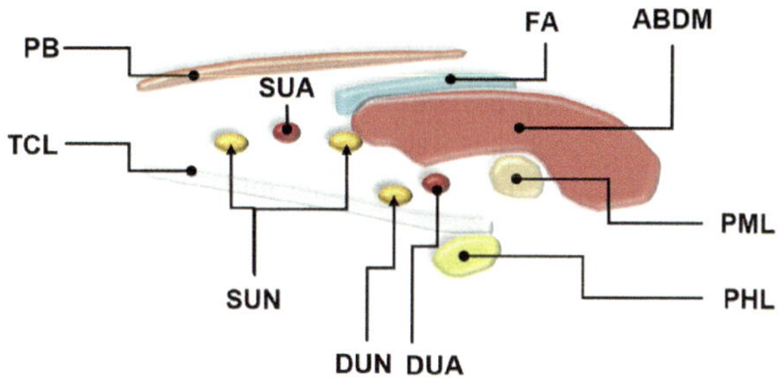

Fig. 12.3 The illustration depicts relevant anatomy of the middle segment of the Guyon canal. FA fibrous arch of the hypothenar muscles; ABDM abductor digiti minimi; PML pisometacarpal ligament; SUN superficial sensory branch of the ulnar nerve; DUN deep motor branch of the ulnar nerve; SUA superficial branch of the ulnar artery; DUA deep branch of the ulnar artery; TCL transverse carpal ligament; PHL pisohamate ligament; PB palmaris brevis

would result in motor weakness affecting all muscles innervated by the ulnar nerve in the hand, accompanied by a sensory deficit in the palmar surfaces of the hypothenar eminence and the fourth and fifth digits. Notably, sensation over the dorsum of the hand remains unaffected, as this area is innervated by the dorsal ulnar cutaneous nerve.

In the middle segment of the Guyon canal, it spans between the pisiform and the hook of hamate. The floor of this segment consists of the ulnar aspect of the transverse carpal ligament and the pisohamate ligament. Meanwhile, the roof is formed by the fascia and fibrous arch of the hypothenar muscles, which connects to the proximal portion of the palmaris brevis muscle, with the abductor digiti minimi muscle defining the ulnarmost border. Directly beneath the abductor digiti minimi muscle lies the pisometacarpal ligament (Fig. 12.3).

Within this section, the primary trunk of the ulnar nerve branches into the superficial sensory branch, including the proper digital nerve of the little finger and the common digital nerve of the fourth web space, and the deep motor branch [8]. These branches are arranged from radial to ulnar aspects, positioned atop or besides the pisohamate ligament. In the distal region, the motor branch lies beneath the two sensory branches and supplies the hypothenar muscles, deep head of the flexor pollicis brevis, and adductor pollicis (Fig. 12.4). On the other hand, the superficial head of the flexor pollicis brevis is innervated by the recurrent motor branch of the median nerve.

The superficial branch of the ulnar artery and the deep branch of the ulnar artery contribute to the development of the superficial and deep palmar arches, respectively [9] (Fig. 12.5). The superficial branch of the ulnar artery follows a radial course in proximity to the sensory branch of the ulnar nerve, while the deep branch of the ulnar artery intersects the superficial branch of the ulnar nerve in a radial-to-ulnar direction before running alongside the deep branch of the ulnar nerve.

Distal to the hamate, which marks the outlet of the Guyon canal, the fibrous arch of the hypothenar muscles serves as the anatomical landmark for delineating the superficial and deep hiatuses (Fig. 12.6). The superficial hiatus contains the superficial branches of the ulnar arteries and nerves. The deep hiatus, also referred to as the pisohamate hiatus, is traversed by the deep branch of the ulnar artery and nerve. Moving further distally, the deep branch of the ulnar artery and nerve courses from the ulnar to radial aspects, penetrates the opponens digiti minimi, and subsequently innervates the palmar/dorsal interosseous muscles and the adductor pollicis muscles.

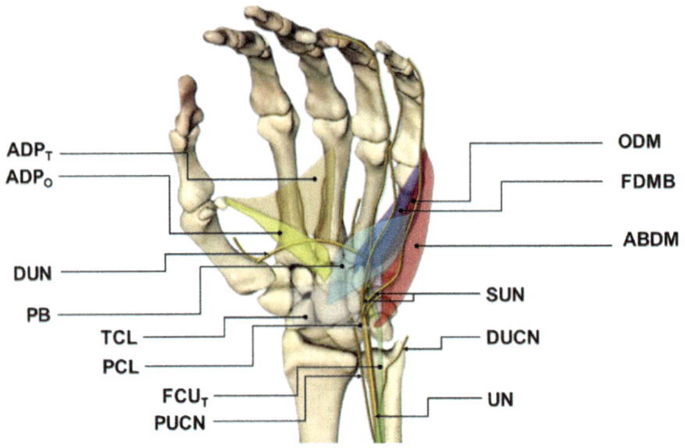

Fig. 12.4 The illustration depicts branches of the ulnar nerve and their relationship to hypothenar muscles. UN ulnar nerve; PUCN palmar ulnar cutaneous nerve; DUCN dorsal ulnar cutaneous nerve; SUN superficial sensory branch of the ulnar nerve; DUN deep motor branch of the ulnar nerve; ADP$_T$ transverse head of the adductor pollicis; ADP$_O$ oblique head of the adductor pollicis; ABDM abductor digiti minimi; FDMB flexor digiti minimi brevis; ODM opponens digiti minimi; PB palmaris brevis; FCU$_T$ flexor carpi ulnaris tendon; PCL palmar carpal ligament; TCL transverse carpal ligament

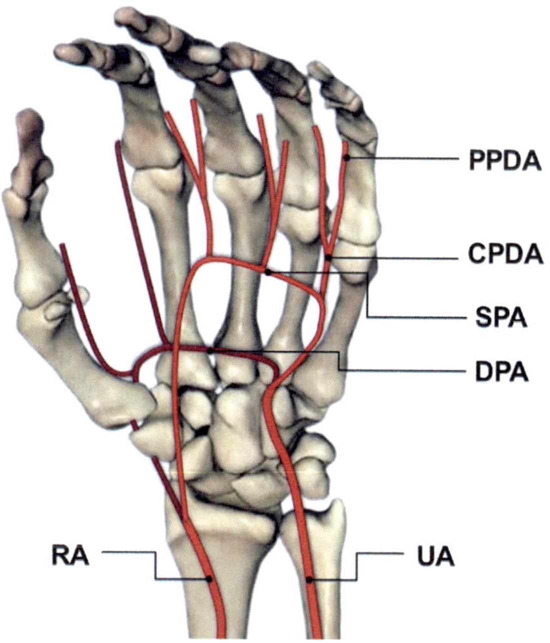

Fig. 12.5 The illustration depicts the deep and superficial palmar arches of the ulnar artery and their branches. RA radial artery; UA ulnar artery; DPA deep palmar arch; SPA superficial palmar arch; CPDA common palmar digital artery; PPDA proper palmar digital artery

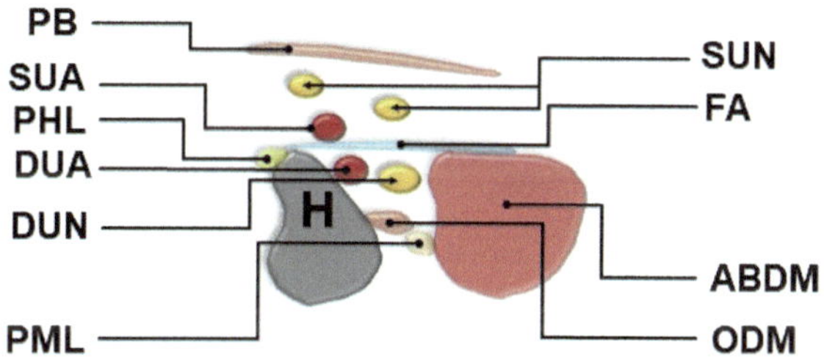

Fig. 12.6 The illustration depicts relevant anatomy of Guyon canal at the outlet level. PB palmaris brevis; FA fibrous arch of the hypothenar muscles; ABDM abductor digiti minimi; ODM opponens digiti minimi; PHL pisohamate ligament; PML pisometacarpal ligament; SUN superficial sensory branch of the ulnar nerve; DUN deep motor branch of the ulnar nerve; DUA deep branch of the ulnar artery; SUA superficial branch of the ulnar artery; H hamate

12.3 Sonoanatomy

12.3.1 *Proximal to the Guyon Tunnel Inlet*

The transducer is initially positioned over the ulnar aspect of the distal forearm in the axial plane. The primary trunk of the ulnar nerve lies beneath the flexor carpi ulnaris muscle, alongside the ulnar artery. As the transducer is moved distally, the palmar ulnar cutaneous nerve on the radial side becomes visible first (Fig. 12.7a, b), followed by the dorsal ulnar cutaneous nerve, which emerges from the ulnar aspect of the ulnar nerve (Fig. 12.8a, b). The palmar cutaneous nerve supplies sensation to the ulnar aspect of the palm, while the dorsal ulnar cutaneous nerve innervates the dorsal ulnar one and a half fingers and the corresponding region of the dorsal wrist.

Upon reaching the pisiform, the flexor carpi ulnaris muscle transforms into a tendon attaching to the pisiform. Radially adjacent to the pisiform, the ulnar nerve is observed, followed by the ulnar artery. Superficially, the palmar carpal ligament

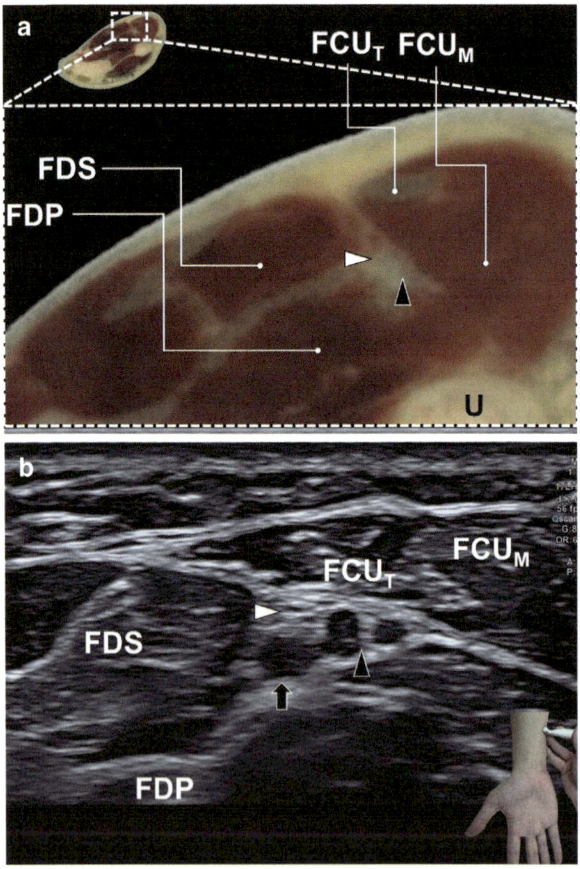

Fig. 12.7 The cadaveric image (**a**) and corresponding sonoanatomy (**b**) depict the palmar ulnar cutaneous nerve, emerging from the radial aspect of the ulnar nerve. White arrowheads: palmar ulnar cutaneous nerve; black arrowheads: ulnar nerve; black arrow: ulnar artery; FCU_T flexor carpi ulnaris tendon; FCU_M flexor carpi ulnaris muscle; FDS flexor digitorum superficialis; FDP flexor digitorum profundus; U ulna

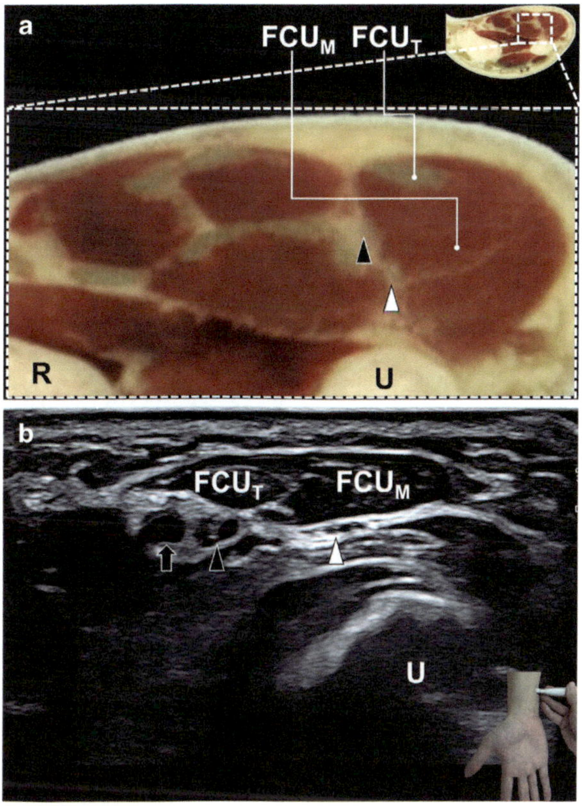

Fig. 12.8 The cadaveric image (**a**) and corresponding sonoanatomy (**b**) depict the dorsal ulnar cutaneous nerve, emerging from the ulnar aspect of the ulnar nerve. White arrowheads: dorsal ulnar cutaneous nerve; black arrowheads: ulnar nerve; black arrow: ulnar artery; FCU$_T$ flexor carpi ulnaris tendon; FCU$_M$ flexor carpi ulnaris muscle; R radius; U ulna

and, deeper, the transverse carpal ligament, intervene between the ulnar artery and nerve (Fig. 12.9a, b).

12.3.2 Within the Guyon Tunnel

Once the transducer is advanced distal to the pisiform, the pisohamate ligament assumes the role of the floor for the ulnar neurovascular bundle, whereas the piso-metacarpal ligament directs to the ulnar side as the floor for the hypothenar muscles. For a comprehensive view, the transducer can be rotated to align with the long axis of the palm. This rotation reveals the pisohamate ligament as a hyperechoic fibrillary linear structure connecting the pisiform and hamate (Fig. 12.10a, c). The distal end of the transducer can be rotated ulnarly towards the fifth metacarpal bone to investigate the long axis of the pisometacarpal ligament. (Fig. 12.10b, d).

Returning to the axial view of the Guyon tunnel, three nerve fascicles can be clearly identified: two superficial sensory branches and one deep motor branch at this level (Fig. 12.11a, b) [10]. The sensory branches include the proper digital

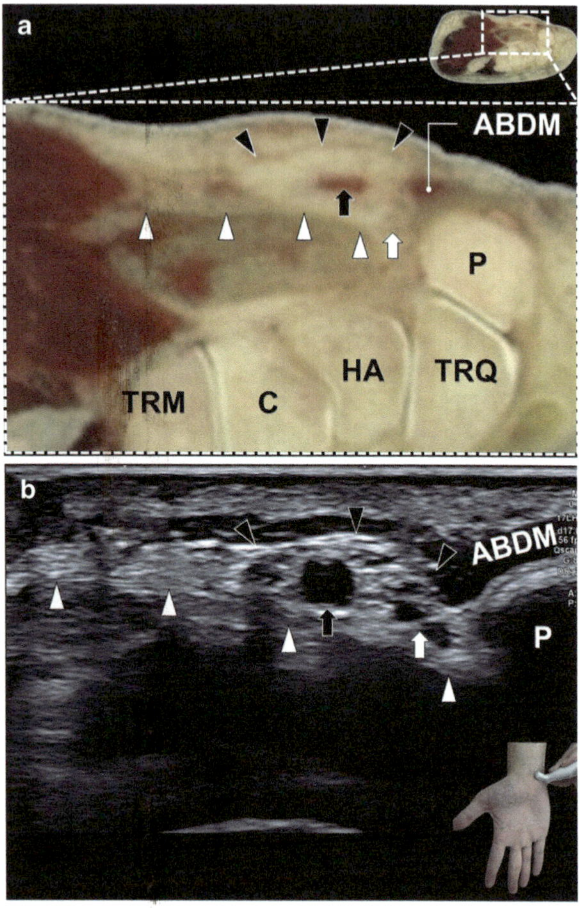

Fig. 12.9 The cadaveric image (**a**) and corresponding somoanatomy (**b**) demonstrate the inlet of the Guyon canal. White arrows: ulnar nerve; black arrows: ulnar artery; white arrowheads: transverse carpal ligament; black arrowheads: palmar carpal ligament; ABDM abductor digiti minimi; TRM trapezium; C capitate; HA hamate; TRQ triquetrum; P pisiform

nerve of the little finger on the ulnar aspect and the common digital nerve of the fourth web space on the radial aspect. Additionally, a small muscular branch emerges from the deep motor branch of the ulnar nerve to innervate the abductor digiti minimi. Simultaneously, the ulnar artery bifurcates into superficial and deep branches, with the latter coursing alongside the deep motor branch of the ulnar nerve. Continuing the distal movement of the transducer, the hamate comes into view. The deep motor branch of the ulnar nerve dives beneath the abductor digiti minimi when it travels towards the more ulnar aspect. When positioning the transducer over the hamate or just distal to it, the deep motor branch of the ulnar nerve, along with the deep branch of the ulnar artery, are segregated from the superficial sensory branch of the ulnar nerve and the superficial branch of the ulnar artery by the fibrous arch of the hypothenar muscles (Fig. 12.12a, b).

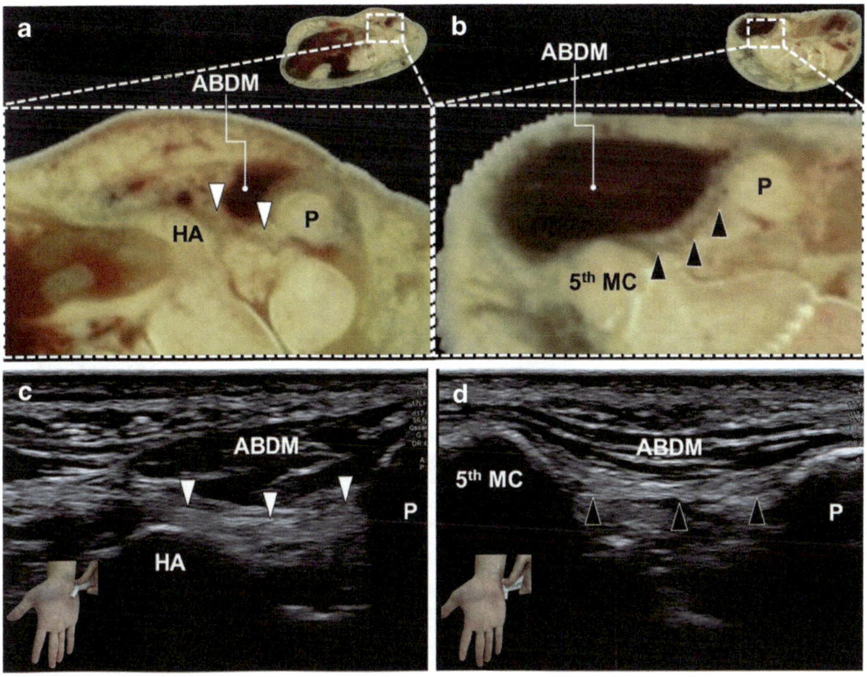

Fig. 12.10 The cadaveric image (**a**) and corresponding sonoanatomy (**c**) illustrate the pisohamate ligament, while the cadaveric image (**b**) and corresponding sonoanatomy (**d**) show the pisometacarpal ligament, both displayed in their long axes. White arrowheads: pisohamate ligament; black arrowheads: pisometacarpal ligament; ABDM abductor digiti minimi; HA hamate: P pisiform; 5th MC fifth metacarpal

12.3.3 Distal to the Guyon Canal

At this particular level, the palmaris brevis serves as a roof over the superficial sensory branch of the ulnar nerve and the superficial branch of the ulnar artery. As the transducer moves distally, the palmaris brevis shifts to the ulnar side of these structures (Fig. 12.13a, b). As the transducer is moved further distally, the deep motor branch traverses through the opponens digiti minimi, then shifts radially to travel amidst the tendons of the flexor digitorum profundus and the palmar interosseous muscles before penetrating the adductor pollicis muscle (Fig. 12.14a, b).

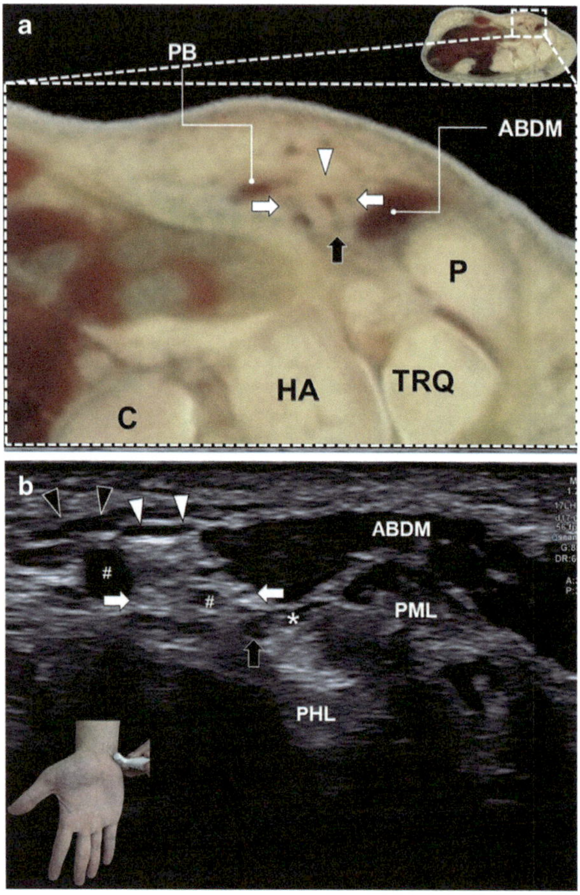

Fig. 12.11 The cadaveric image (**a**) and corresponding sonoanatomy (**b**) depict the intracanal level of the Guyon canal. Black arrowheads and PB palmaris brevis; white arrowheads: fibrous arch of the hypothenar muscles; white arrows: superficial sensory branch of the ulnar nerve; black arrows: deep motor branch of the ulnar nerve; white asterisk: deep ulnar artery; white hashtags: superficial ulnar artery; PHL pisohamate ligament; PML pisometacarpal ligament; ABDM abductor digiti minimi; P pisiform; TRQ triquetrum; HA hamate; C capitate

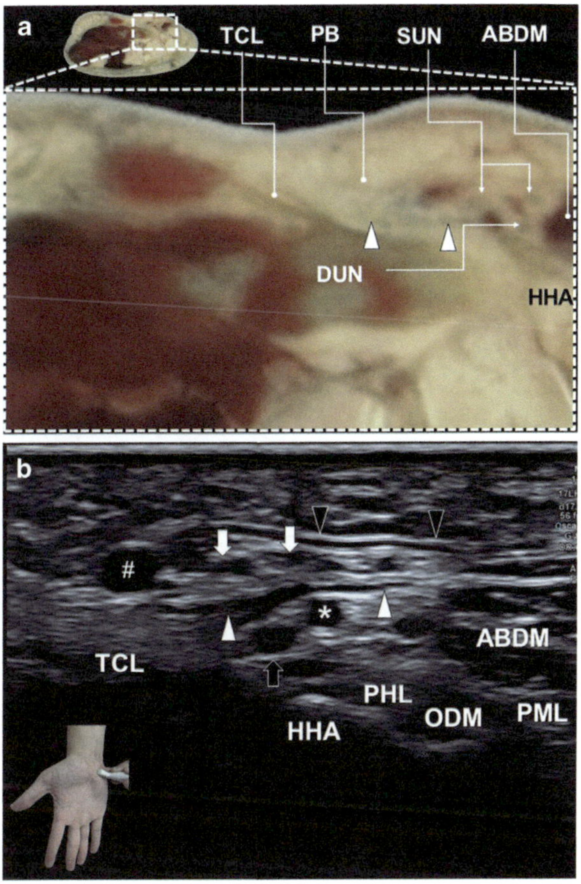

Fig. 12.12 The cadaveric image (**a**) and corresponding sonoanatomy (**b**) depict the outlet of the Guyon canal. PB and black arrowheads: palmaris brevis; white arrowheads: fibrous arch of the hypothenar muscles; SUN and white arrows: superficial sensory branch of ulnar nerve; DUN and black arrow: deep motor branch of ulnar nerve; white asterisk: deep ulnar artery; white hashtag: superficial ulnar artery; TCL transverse carpal ligament; PHL pisohamate ligament; PML pisometacarpal ligament; ABDM abductor digiti minimi; ODM opponens digiti minimi; HHA hook of the hamate

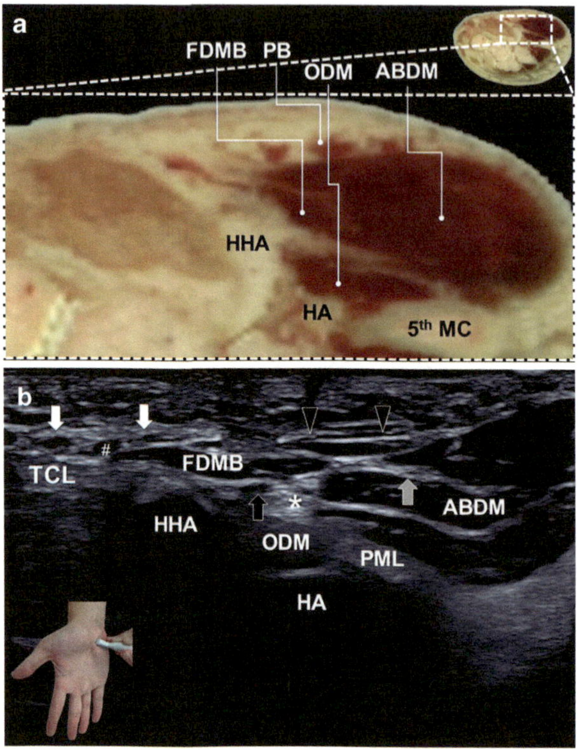

Fig. 12.13 The cadaveric image (**a**) and corresponding sonoanatomy (**b**) at a level just distal to the Guyon canal outlet show the origins of the opponens digiti minimi and flexor digiti minimi brevis. White arrows: superficial sensory branch of the ulnar nerve; gray arrow: motor branch of the ulnar nerve to abductor digiti minimi; black arrow: deep motor branch of the ulnar nerve; white hashtag: superficial ulnar artery; white asterisk: deep ulnar artery; black arrowheads and PB: palmaris brevis; 5th MC fifth metacarpal; PML pisometacarpal ligament; TCL transverse carpal ligament; ABDM abductor digiti minimi; ODM opponens digit minimi; FDMB flexor digiti minimi brevis; HHA hook of the hamate; HA hamate

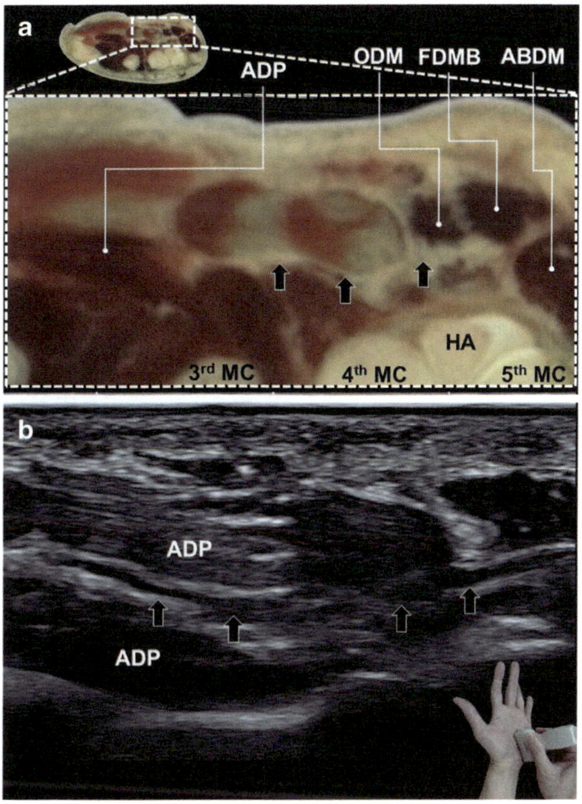

Fig. 12.14 The cadaveric image (**a**) and corresponding sonoanatomy (**b**) show the deep motor branch of the ulnar nerve (black arrows) in the long axis. ADP adductor pollicis; ODM opponens digiti minimi; FDMB flexor digiti minimi brevis; ABDM abductor digiti minimi; 3rd MC third metacarpal; 4th MC fourth metacarpal; 5th MC fifth metacarpal; HA hamate

12.4 Normal Variants and Pathologies

Injuries to the ulnar nerve and dorsal ulnar cutaneous nerve in the distal forearm can result from trauma or entrapment by suture material following surgery. In such cases, proximal to the Guyon canal, an indistinct border, hypoechoic appearance, fascicular swelling, and hyperechoic sutures may be visible (short axis, Fig. 12.15a; long axis, Fig. 12.15b). The dorsal ulnar cutaneous nerve may become entrapped as it passes through the myofibrous orifice between the flexor carpi ulnaris and pronator quadratus (short axis, Fig. 12.16a, b; long axis, Fig. 12.16c), or in the presence of a ganglion cyst (short axis, Fig. 12.17a; long axis, Fig. 12.17b).

At the level of the Guyon tunnel inlet, the presence of a hypoechoic structure superficial to the palmar carpal ligament may indicate the accessory abductor digiti minimi muscle. This accessory abductor digiti minimi is the most commonly encountered accessory hypothenar muscle, with a reported prevalence ranging from 22% to 35% [11]. The accessory digiti minimi can have a fascial origin either from the antebrachial fascia or the flexor retinaculum (short axis, Fig. 12.18a, b; long axis, Fig. 12.18c). Ultrasound images may reveal a well-defined mass with internal striations resembling muscle tissue. The presence of this accessory muscle has the

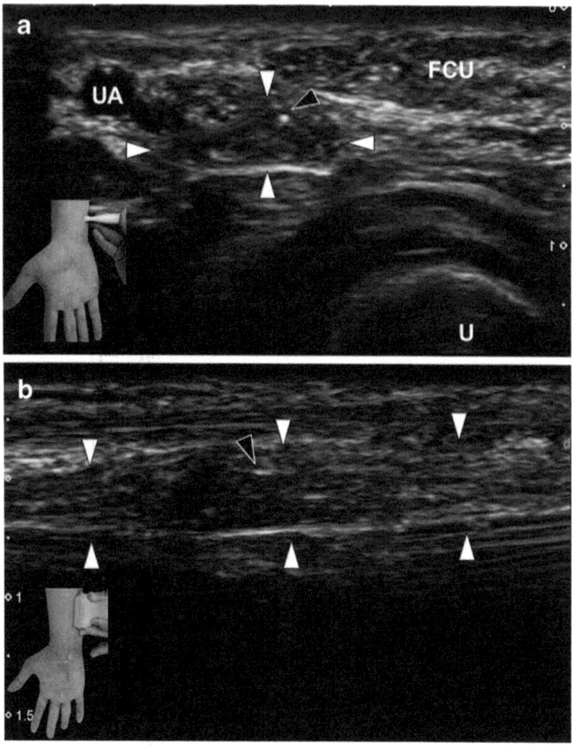

Fig. 12.15 The ultrasonography reveals a hypoechoic and swollen ulnar nerve (white arrowheads) caused by entrapment of suture material (black arrowheads) in the short-axis (**a**) and long-axis (**b**) views of the forearm following surgery. UA ulnar artery; FCU flexor carpi ulnaris; U ulna

potential to increase crowding within the narrow Guyon canal, possibly leading to compression of the ulnar nerve and artery.

Hypothenar hammer syndrome is a rare condition marked by injury and thrombosis of the distal ulnar artery [12], stemming from repetitive blunt trauma to the hypothenar area. Predominantly affecting middle-aged men with occupations that expose their hands to frequent trauma, individuals with this syndrome often exhibit signs and symptoms reflective of diminished blood flow to the digits served by ulnar artery branches. Ultrasound imaging of the distal ulnar artery may reveal a region of mixed echogenicity within the vessel lumen, extending from the ulnar-carpal junction into the hypothenar area, suggestive of an occlusive thrombus. Notably, this thrombotic segment exhibits an inability to compress under the pressure of the transducer. Confirmation of impaired blood flow at the suspected thrombotic site is achieved with Color Doppler, which shows a lack of vascular flow in the affected region compared to the patent flow in the non-affected site (Fig. 12.19).

Compression of the ulnar nerve within the Guyon canal can be attributed to a space-occupying lesion, such as a ganglion cyst, possibly originating from the underlying pisotriquetrum joint. Another potential pathology is a schwannoma, a typically benign tumor composed solely of Schwann cells and arising from the nerve sheath [13] (short axis, Fig. 12.20a; long axis, Fig. 12.20b). Ultrasound imaging may reveal a hypoechoic mass lesion proximal, within or distal to the Guyon

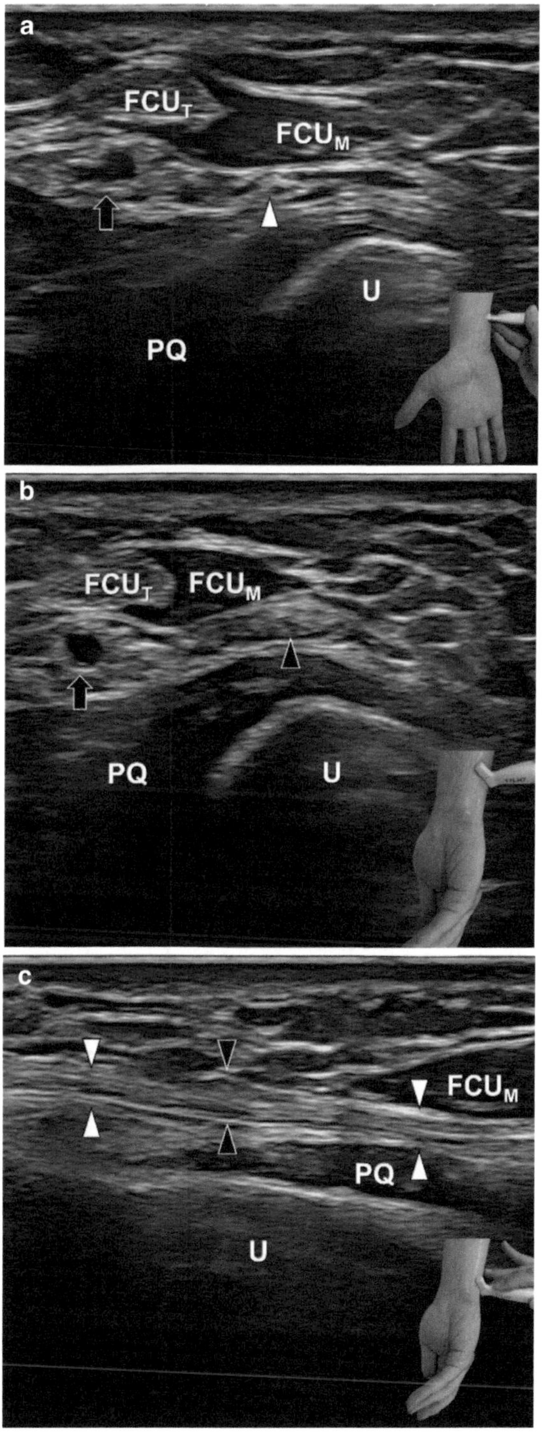

Fig. 12.16 The ultrasonography shows focal swelling of the dorsal ulnar cutaneous nerve from the proximal (**a**) to distal level (**b**) in both short and long axes (**c**) of the forearm, located between the flexor carpi ulnaris and pronator quadratus. Black arrows: main trunk of the ulnar nerve; white arrowheads: normal segment of the dorsal ulnar cutaneous nerve; black arrowheads: swollen segment of the dorsal ulnar cutaneous nerve; PQ pronator quadratus; FCU_M flexor carpi ulnaris muscle; FCU_T flexor carpi ulnaris tendon; U ulna

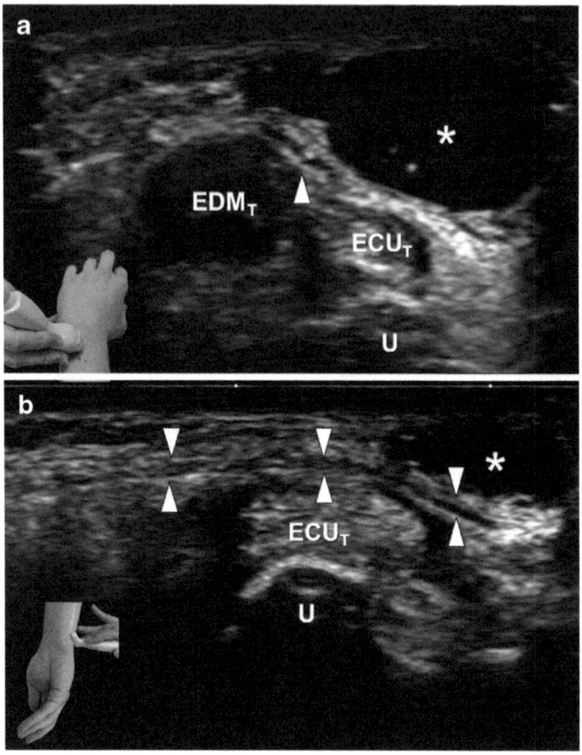

Fig. 12.17 The ultrasonography reveals entrapment of the dorsal ulnar cutaneous nerve (white arrowheads) caused by a ganglion cyst (asterisks), along with swelling of the extensor digiti minimi tendon in the short axis (**a**) and oblique-long axis (**b**) of the forearm. ECU_T extensor carpi ulnaris tendon; EDM_T extensor digiti minimi tendon; U ulna

canal, which serves as a direct extension of the ulnar nerve. Notably, if the deep motor ulnar branch is affected, muscles innervated by it, such as the palmar interosseous muscles, may exhibit thinning and atrophy compared to the contralateral hand.

Lipomatosis of nerve, also referred to as fibrolipomatous hamartoma of the nerve [14], lipofibromatous hamartoma, or neural fibrolipoma, is a non-cancerous growth affecting nerves. It occurs due to abnormal growth of fibroadipose tissue enclosed by the epineurium, leading to the expansion of the nerve and separation of nerve fascicles. This condition can often be detected within the Guyon canal. Ultrasound examination typically shows a distinctive hypoechoic cable-like neural fascicle, surrounded by hyperechoic fat (short axis, Fig. 12.21a; long axis, Fig. 12.21b).

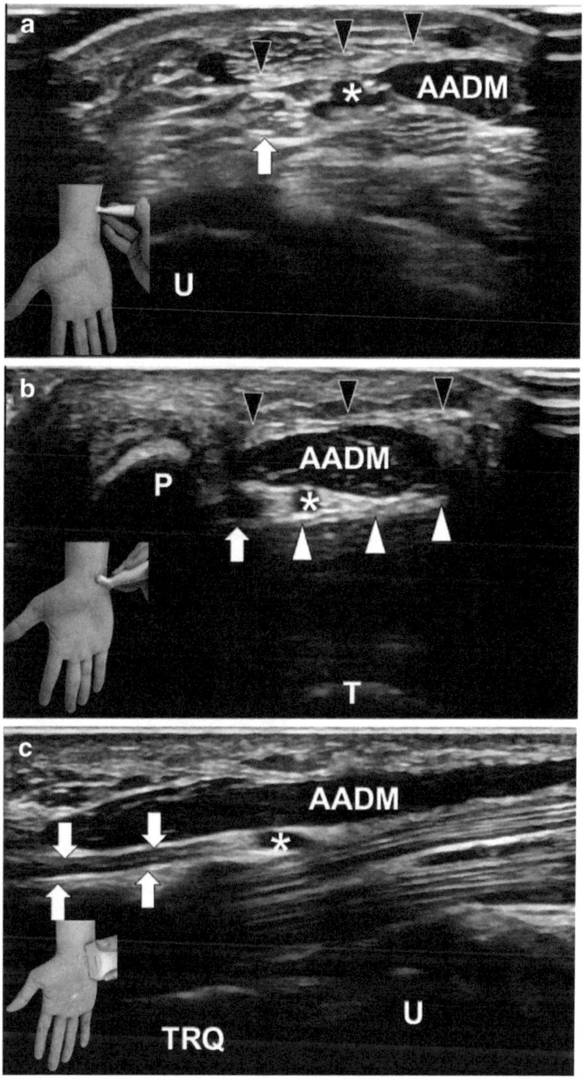

Fig. 12.18 The ultrasonography reveals the accessory abductor digiti minimi (AADM) muscle proximal to (**a**) and within (**b**) the Guyon canal in the short axis. Ultrasound imaging of the muscle in the long axis is shown in (**c**). Black arrowheads: palmar carpal ligament; white arrowheads: transverse carpal ligament; white arrows: ulnar nerve; asterisks: ulnar artery; U ulna; P pisiform; TRQ triquetrum

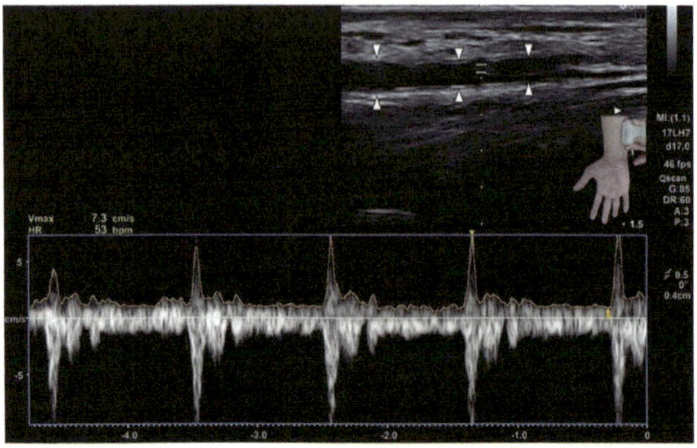

Fig. 12.19 The spectral Doppler images aligned with the ulnar artery (white arrowheads) in the long axis display a triphasic waveform, indicating normal arterial flow

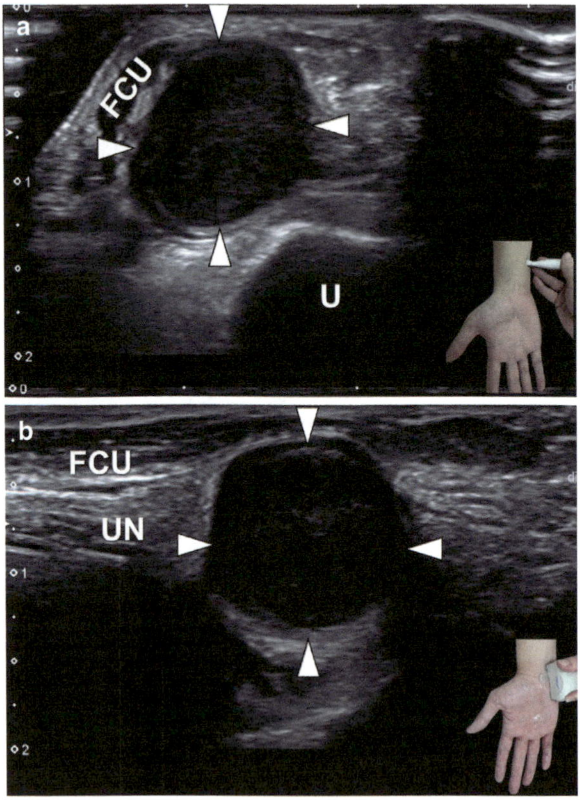

Fig. 12.20 The ultrasonography reveals a solid mass with a well-defined border and a homogeneous, hypoechoic pattern. These findings are indicative of a Schwannoma (white arrowheads) of the ulnar nerve proximal to the Guyon canal, as shown in both the short axis (**a**) and long axis (**b**) of the forearm. UN ulnar nerve; FCU flexor carpi ulnaris; U ulna

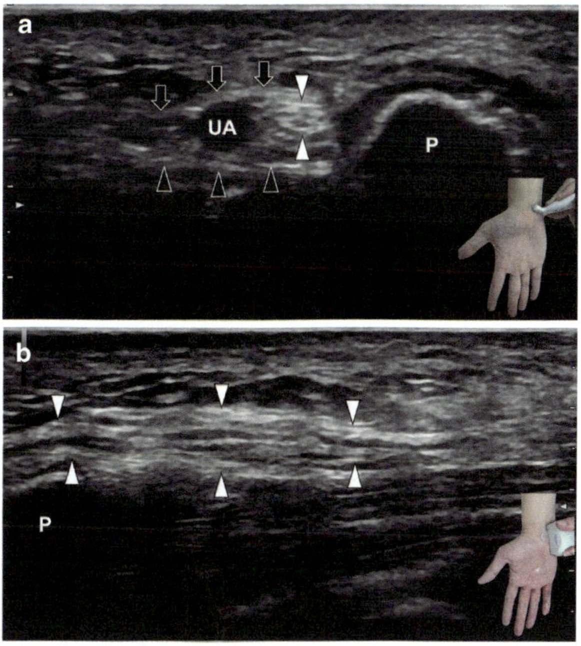

Fig. 12.21 The ultrasonography reveals the fibrolipomatous hamartoma (white arrowheads) in the short-axis (**a**) and long-axis (**b**) views. Black arrows: palmar carpal ligament; black arrowheads: transverse carpal ligament; UA ulnar artery; P pisiform

12.5 Ultrasound-Guided Injection

While the practice of injecting structures, primarily the ulnar nerve, is not commonplace, ultrasound guidance proves beneficial for accurately delivering injectates, such as corticosteroids, around the ulnar nerve. In a study conducted by Meng et al. [15], ultrasound-guided injections were performed using a 22-gauge, 50 mm length injection needle. The ultrasound transducer was aligned parallel to the axial plane, and the injection needle was advanced from the ulnar skin into the Guyon canal at an angle of approximately 45 degrees. The needle traversed the radial side of the pisiform, entering the Guyon canal, with the needle tip positioned just outside the epineurium of the ulnar nerve (Fig. 12.22). Great care was taken to avoid puncturing the ulnar artery and veins. A mixture of 1 mL of India ink with physiologic saline solution was administered until the injected ink formed a clearly visible hypoechoic rim around the ulnar nerve. Upon subsequent dissection, it was observed that the injected ink selectively stained only the perineural sheaths of the nerves in all specimens.

In 2021, Chang et al. [16] presented a case involving a 63-year-old woman who underwent conservative treatment for a left thalamic intracerebral hemorrhage. Following the treatment, she experienced spasticity in the muscles of her right hand, leading to restrictions in the extension of the metacarpophalangeal joints of the fingers and the extension and abduction of the thumb. To alleviate the spasticity, ethyl alcohol was injected around the motor branch of the right ulnar nerve, located at the distal end of Guyon canal. This injection, guided by ultrasound, took place

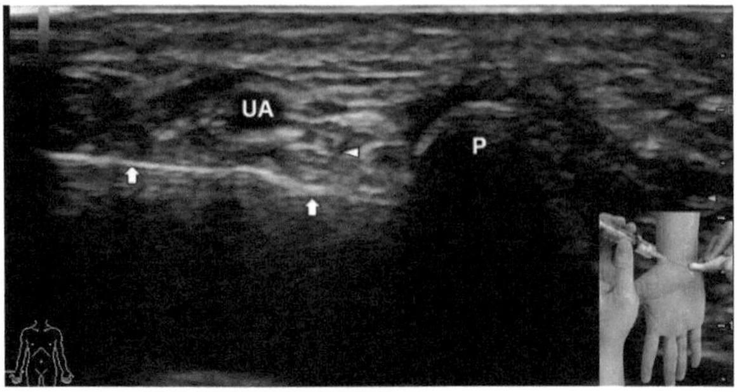

Fig. 12.22 The ultrasound-guided injection, performed using an in-plane approach from the radial to ulnar aspect, is administered into the Guyon canal, following the technique described by Meng et al. [15]. White arrows: needle; white arrowhead: ulnar nerve; UA ulnar artery; P pisiform

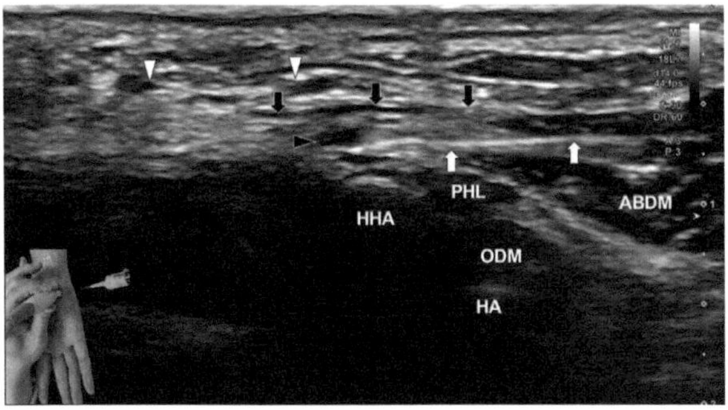

Fig. 12.23 The ultrasound-guided injection, using the in-plane approach, is administered to the deep motor branch of the ulnar nerve from ulnar to radial, similar to the method described by Chang et al. [16]. White arrows: needle; black arrowhead: deep motor branch of the ulnar nerve; white arrowheads: superficial sensory branch of the ulnar nerve; black arrows: fibrous arch of the hypothenar muscles; PHL pisohamate ligament; ABDM abductor digiti minimi; ODM opponens digiti minimi; HHA hook of the hamate; HA hamate

with the patient in a supine position and the right hand in a supinated posture. The injection site was targeted precisely at the location where the fibrous arch of the hypothenar muscles separated the superficial and deep branches (Fig. 12.23). A month after the injection, a notable reduction in hand spasticity was observed.

12.6 Conclusion

Ultrasound facilitates the visualization of the Guyon canal and the neurovascular structures within. The bifurcation/trifurcation of the ulnar nerve and artery occurs within the confines of the Guyon canal, adding complexity to its sonoanatomy. While nerve entrapment syndrome at this location is uncommon, ultrasound guidance is crucial to prevent potential ulnar artery injury associated with the procedure.

Acknowledgments Images and illustrations adapted from cadaveric images provided by the Visible Human Project® of the National Library of Medicine. Excerpts featured in the VH Dissector are used with permission from Touch of Life Technologies Inc.

References

1. Aleksenko D, Varacallo M. Guyon Canal Syndrome. In: StatPearls. StatPearls Publishing. Copyright © 2024, StatPearls Publishing LLC.: Treasure Island (FL) ineligible companies. Disclosure: Matthew Varacallo declares no relevant financial relationships with ineligible companies; 2024.
2. Kwak KW, et al. Ulnar nerve compression in Guyon's canal by ganglion cyst. J Korean Neurosurg Soc. 2011;49(2):139–41.
3. Lane R, Nallamothu SV. Claw hand. In: StatPearls. StatPearls Publishing. Copyright © 2024, StatPearls publishing LLC.: Treasure Island (FL) ineligible companies. Disclosure: Shivajee Nallamothu declares no relevant financial relationships with ineligible companies; 2024.
4. Bains S, Rocha Cabrero F. *Electrodiagnostic evaluation of ulnar neuropathy*. In: *StatPearls*. StatPearls Publishing. Copyright © 2024, StatPearls publishing LLC.: Treasure Island (FL) ineligible companies. Disclosure: Franklyn Rocha Cabrero declares no relevant financial relationships with ineligible companies; 2024.
5. Wu W-T, et al. Ultrasound imaging and guidance for distal peripheral nerve pathologies at the wrist/hand. Diagnostics. 2023;13(11):1928.
6. Tubbs RS, et al. Anatomy of the palmar branch of the ulnar nerve: application to ulnar and median nerve decompressive surgery. J Neurosurg. 2011;114(1):263–7.
7. Puna R, Poon P. The anatomy of the dorsal cutaneous branch of the ulnar nerve. J Hand Surg Eur. 2010;35(7):583–5.
8. Maroukis BL, et al. Guyon canal: the evolution of clinical anatomy. J Hand Surg Am. 2015;40(3):560–5.
9. Gellman H, et al. Arterial patterns of the deep and superficial palmar arches. Clin Orthop Relat Res. 2001;383:41–6.
10. Bianchi S, Beaulieu JY, Poletti PA. Ultrasound of the ulnar-palmar region of the wrist: normal anatomy and anatomic variations. J Ultrasound. 2020;23(3):365–78.
11. Rixey A, et al. Accessory abductor digiti minimi muscle, less muscular than thought: an update on prevalence, morphology, and review of the literature. Skeletal Radiol. 2021;50(8):1687–95.
12. Queiroz MMM, et al. Hypothenar hammer syndrome: case report and literature review. Rev Bras Ortop. 2013;48(1):104–7.
13. Khajeh R, et al. Guyon canal syndrome due to schwannomas of zone 3 ulnar nerve without neurologic symptoms: a case report. Arch Bone Jt Surg. 2021;9(5):598–600.
14. Gilet A, Jeremy M, Gould E. Fibrolipomatous hamartoma of the median nerve. Radiol Case Rep. 2008;3(3):195.
15. Meng S, et al. Ultrasound-guided Perineural injection at Guyon's tunnel: an anatomic feasibility study. Ultrasound Med Biol. 2015;41(8):2119–24.
16. Chang MC, Boudier-Revéret M. Management of hand spasticity with ultrasound-guided ethyl alcohol injection to the deep branch of the ulnar nerve. J Med Ultrasound. 2021;29(3):207–8.

Chapter 13
Ulnar Wrist Pain with a Focus on Triangular Fibrocartilage Complex

Ke-Vin Chang, Wei-Ting Wu, Yuan-Yuan Tsai, and Shao-Yu Chi

13.1 Introduction

In a systematic review conducted in 2014 [1], it was demonstrated that the prevalence of triangular fibrocartilage complex (TFCC) abnormalities increases with age. Among patients under 30 years old, the prevalence was 27%, while in those aged 70 and older, it rose to 49%. This escalation was supported by an odds ratio (OR) of 2.7 and a 95% confidence interval (CI) of 1.9–3.8. Even among asymptomatic individuals, TFCC abnormalities were significant, increasing from 15% to 49% across the same age groups, with an OR of 5.4 and a 95% CI of 3.3–8.9. Symptomatic patients aged 50–69 years old exhibited a prevalence ranging from 39% to 70%, with an OR of 3.6 and a 95% CI of 1.3–9.9. Consequently, the authors concluded that TFCC abnormalities are common in both symptomatic and asymptomatic wrists, with a clear trend of increasing prevalence with age.

Furthermore, patients with TFCC injury typically present with ulnar-sided wrist pain, often accompanied by clicking or point tenderness between the pisiform and the ulnar head. The pathophysiology indicates that positive ulnar variation can make the TFCC susceptible to injury [2]. Various diagnostic tools, including magnetic resonance imaging and arthrography, have been utilized to evaluate TFCC conditions.

Subsequently, in 2019, a pictorial review was published [3], providing detailed insights into ultrasound scanning techniques and the ultrasound classification of TFCC injuries. This chapter aims to revisit the anatomy and sonoanatomy of the TFCC while also exploring ultrasound-guided techniques specific to the relevant region.

K.-V. Chang (✉) · W.-T. Wu · Y.-Y. Tsai · S.-Y. Chi
Bei-Hu Branch, National Taiwan University Hospital, Taipei, Taiwan

K.-V. Chang (ed.), *Ultrasonography of Musculoskeletal Pain*,
https://doi.org/10.1007/978-981-96-6787-1_13

13.2 Anatomy

The point of origin of the radioulnar ligament from the base of the ulnar styloid is noticeably narrower than its origin from the fovea. Fibers from the ulnar fovea and base of the ulnar styloid curve distally and extend toward the radius. Some central fibers merge with the proximal edge of the fibrocartilaginous disc on the coronal central plane [4]. Peripheral fibers branch dorsally and palmarly before attaching to the radius, enveloping the proximal side of the articular disc. Histologically, a few chondrocytes or chondroid cells are visible at the origin points in the fovea and at the base of the ulnar styloid. The ulnolunate and ulnotriquetral ligaments seem to originate from the palmar aspect of the TFCC [4] (Fig. 13.1).

Vertically oriented fibers extend from the fibrocartilage at the tip of the ulnar styloid to contribute to the extensor carpi ulnaris subsheath along the dorsal edge of the TFCC (Fig. 13.2). This region also features a dense matrix of hyaline-like fibrocartilage with numerous chondrocytes, spanning from the middle to the tip of the ulnar styloid process. From this cartilage site, vertically oriented fibers extend toward the triquetrum, forming part of a thickened ulnar joint capsule.

Some loose fibers oriented in the radioulnar direction spread outward and merge into the distal ulnar side of the disc, corresponding to its meniscus homologue. The fibers of the thickened ulnar joint capsule merge with those of the meniscus homologue, collectively forming the ulnar wall of the distal aspect of the TFCC. Above the sigmoid notch of the radius, the insertion of the TFCC into the radius reveals an increase in cartilage cells and a decrease in fibers as the fibrocartilaginous disc merges with the hyaline cartilage of the sigmoid notch (Fig. 13.3). Additionally,

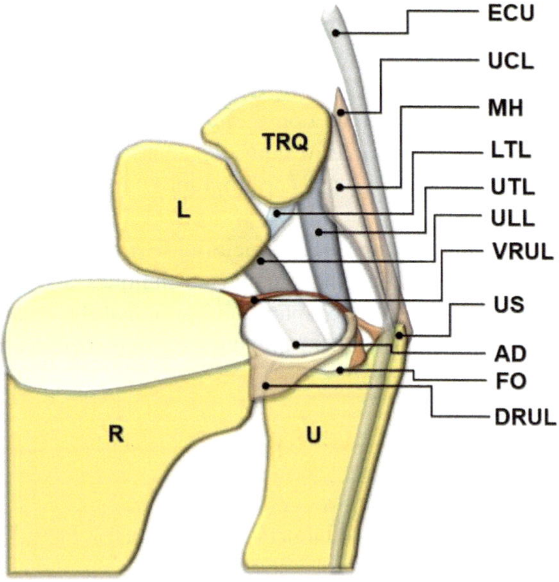

Fig. 13.1 The illustration of the triangular fibrocartilage complex. ECU extensor carpi ulnaris tendon; DRUL dorsal radioulnar ligament; PRUL palmar radioulnar ligament; LTL lunotriquetral ligament; ULL ulnolunate ligament; UTL ulnotriquetral ligament; UCL ulnar collateral ligament; AD articular disc; MH meniscus homologue; FO fovea of the ulna; US ulnar styloid; L lunate; TRQ triquetrum; R radius; U ulna

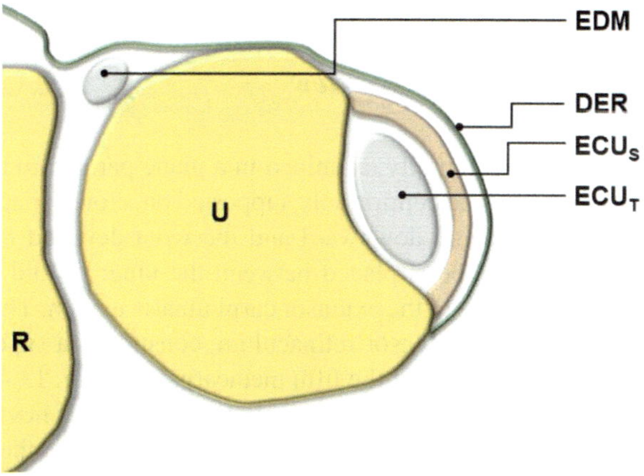

Fig. 13.2 The illustration of the extensor carpi ulnaris and its subsheath. DER dorsal extensor retinaculum; ECU$_S$ extensor carpi ulnaris subsheath; ECU$_T$ extensor carpi ulnaris tendon; EDM extensor digiti minimi tendon; R radius; U ulna

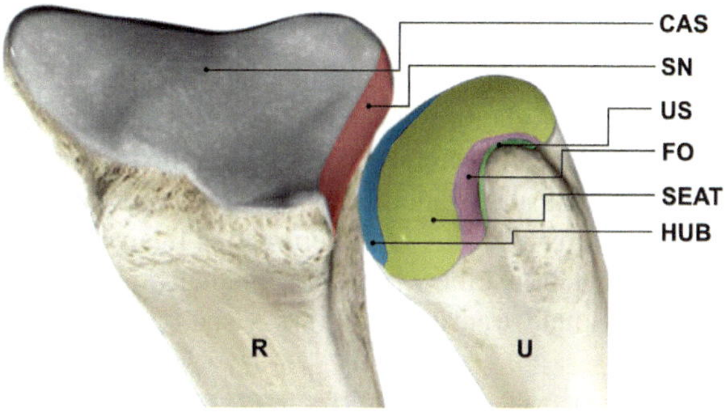

Fig. 13.3 The illustration of the bony components of the distal radioulnar joint. CAS carpal articular surface of the radius; US ulnar styloid; FO fovea of the ulna; SEAT seat of the ulna; HUB hub of the ulna; U ulna; SN sigmoid notch of the radius; R radius

sagittal sections through the sigmoid notch reveal fibrous insertions into the most dorsal and palmar areas of the hyaline cartilage [4].

Histologically, the thickened joint capsule inserting into the triquetrum displays a collagen matrix that is loosely arranged, gradually transitioning into hyaline cartilage towards the ulnar side. Originating from the palmar edge of the TFCC, the ulnolunate and ulnotriquetral ligaments insert into the lunate and triquetrum, respectively, forming substantial bundles that extend from the palmar radiocarpal joint capsule.

The blood supply to the TFCC originates from the soft tissues surrounding the ulnocarpal joint. Vessels from the peripheral capsular and synovial tissue penetrate the TFCC toward the radial aspect and are directed toward the center of the TFCC. No vessels enter the TFCC from its radial attachment. The fibrocartilage of the TFCC blends with the articular cartilage of the radius. The articular cartilage of the radius appears to act as a barrier, preventing vessels from the subchondral bone of the radius from entering the TFCC at its radial attachment [5].

13.3 Sonoanatomy

13.3.1 Long-Axis View

The TFCC is initially examined in a plane parallel to the long axis of the forearm. The wrist can be comfortably supported on a towel, pad, or pillow, with the forearm positioned facing downward and the wrist deviated towards the thumb side. The ultrasound probe is placed between the ulnar styloid process and the triquetrum, aligned parallel to the extensor carpi ulnaris tendon. This tendon, surrounded by the subsheath and extensor retinaculum, constitutes a superficial barrier of the TFCC, linking to the base of the fifth metacarpal [3] (Fig. 13.4a, b).

Within the TFCC, the hypoechoic articular disc lies between the ulna and radius, stabilized by the radioulnar ligament. Occasionally, the shadow of the ulnar styloid process may obscure parts of these structures (Fig. 13.5a). In certain instances, a fluid-filled space known as the prestyloid recess might be visible between the disc and the meniscus homologue, contributing to wrist stability (Fig. 13.5b). However, this space is discernible only in the presence of effusion. Additionally, the ulnar collateral ligament, a bright, fibrous band connecting the ulna to the hamate and fifth metacarpal, is visible between the extensor carpi ulnaris sheath and the radioulnar ligament.

The lunate and triquetrum bones are covered by a thin layer of dark cartilage and connected by a prominent interosseous ligament. During ultrasound evaluation of ligament stability, the wrist can be maneuvered either ulnarly or radially. Adjusting the ultrasound transducer allows visualization of the ulnar fovea, a small bony

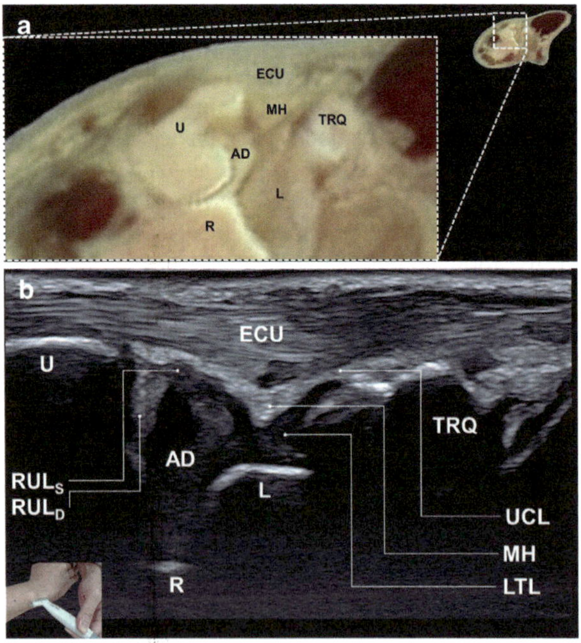

Fig. 13.4 The cadaveric image (**a**) and corresponding sonoanatomy (**b**) of the triangular fibrocartilage complex in the coronal long-axis plane. ECU extensor carpi ulnaris tendon; AD articular disc; MH meniscus homologue; LTL lunotriquetral ligament; RUL$_S$ superficial limb of the radioulnar ligament; RUL$_D$ deep limb of the radioulnar ligament; UCL ulnar collateral ligament; TRQ triquetrum; L lunate; R radius; U ulna

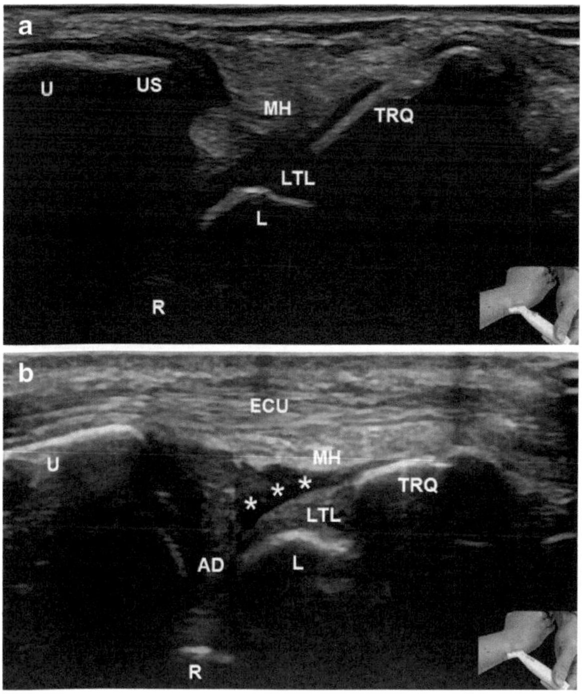

Fig. 13.5 The sonographic image of the triangular fibrocartilage complex with the ulnar styloid and its shadow (**a**), and in another case, show prestyloid recess effusion (asterisks) (**b**) in the coronal long-axis plane. ECU extensor carpi ulnaris tendon; AD articular disc; MH meniscus homologue; LTL lunotriquetral ligament; TRQ triquetrum; L lunate; R radius; US ulnar styloid; U ulna

concavity on the ulna. This adjustment facilitates examination of the attachment of the radioulnar ligament to the ulna. Its superficial portion links the radius and ulna, while its deeper segment encircles the disc. The deeper segment may appear darker due to the angle of the sound waves, known as anisotropy [6].

13.3.2 Short-Axis View

To examine the TFCC in the short-axis view, the transducer is positioned at the ulnar wrist, perpendicular to the extensor carpi ulnaris tendon (Fig. 13.6a). When dealing with a narrow ulnocarpal space, visualizing the TFCC is aided by tilting the wrist towards the thumb side. For investigating pathologies near the ulnar fovea, the transducer is situated in the axial plane slightly distal to the ulnar styloid process, and then angled towards the distal ulna (Fig. 13.6b). This positioning allows for observation of the ulnar fovea's bony cortex, the proximal attachment of the ulnar collateral ligament, and both the superficial and deep limbs of the radioulnar ligament.

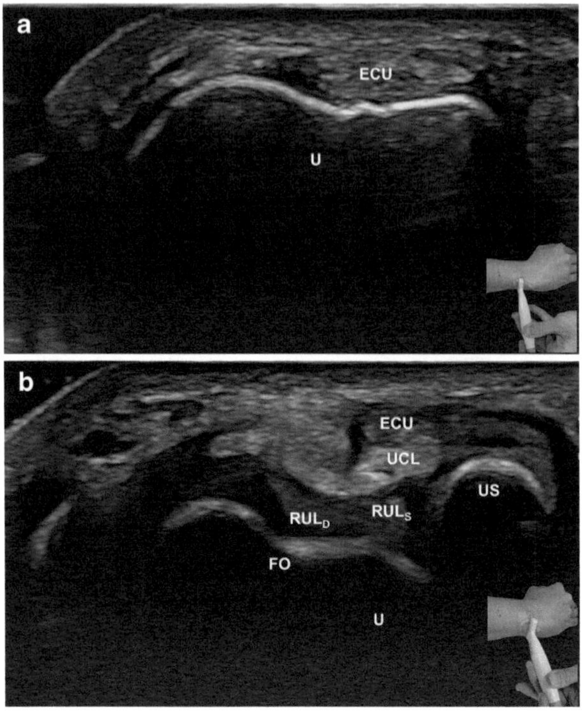

Fig. 13.6 Ultrasound examination of the ulnar fovea demonstrates the corresponding sonoanatomy from the ulnar styloid process (**a**) to the fovea (**b**) in the axial plane, moving from proximal to distal. ECU extensor carpi ulnaris tendon; RUL_S superficial limb of the radioulnar ligament; RUL_D deep limb of the radioulnar ligament; UCL ulnar collateral ligament; FO fovea of the ulna; US ulnar styloid; U ulna

Moving the transducer gradually from proximal to distal reveals the circular-shaped articular disc besides the sigmoid notch, located on the ulnar aspect of the distal radius (Fig. 13.7a). Progressing further distally, the meniscus homologue and the underlying interosseous ligaments become visible (Fig. 13.7b). The interosseous ligament appears less echogenic than the meniscus homologue due to the steep angle of the sound waves on its oblique fibers. Adjusting the angle enables visualization of the entire course of the dorsal and palmar radioulnar ligaments wrapping around the articular disc from the dorsal (Fig. 13.8a) or palmar (Fig. 13.8b) aspect of the ulnar wrist.

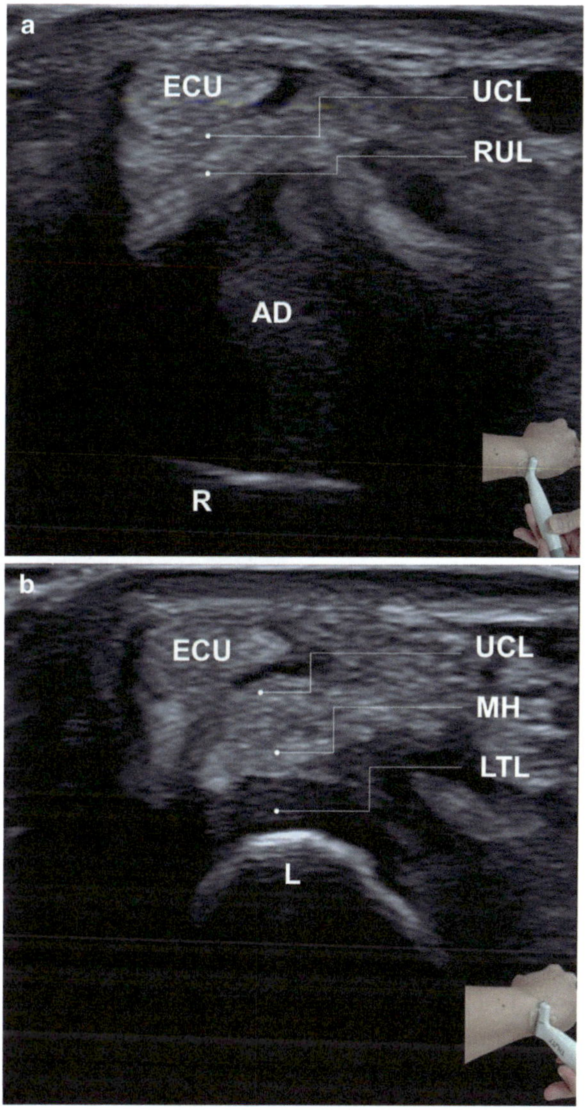

Fig. 13.7 Sonoanatomy at the level of (**a**) the articular disc and (**b**) the meniscus homologue of the triangular fibrocartilage complex in the axial plane. ECU extensor carpi ulnaris tendon; RUL radioulnar ligament; UCL ulnar collateral ligament; LTL lunotriquetral ligament; AD articular disc; MH meniscus homologue; L lunate; R radius

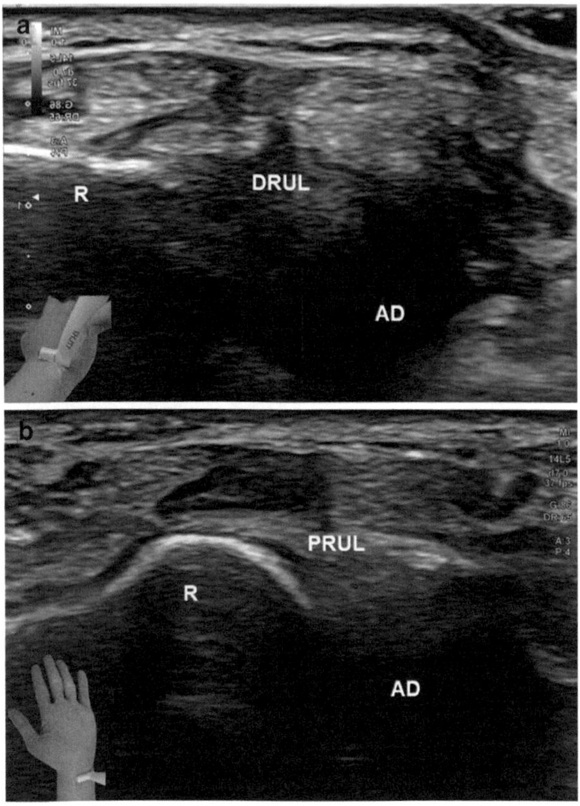

Fig. 13.8 The sonoanatomy of the entire course of the dorsal (**a**) and palmar (**b**) radioulnar ligaments wrapping around the articular disc in the axial plane. AD articular disc; DRUL dorsal radioulnar ligament; PRUL palmar radioulnar ligament; R radius

13.4 Pathology

Typically, the Doppler signal is not detected within the TFCC, although small vessels may be present in nearby ligaments. Acute injuries often exhibit increased vascularity within the TFCC. TFCC lesions include various conditions such as ruptures of the articular disc or meniscus homologue, disruption of the juxta-articular ligaments, and extensor carpi ulnaris tendinopathy. Consequently, we introduced a modified classification based on ultrasound findings, adapting from the Palmer classification, primarily relying on MRI findings [7] (Table 13.1). In our classification, TFCC lesions are divided into two main groups:

Class 1 (Trauma)
Class 1A–D injuries involve articular disc ruptures. Class 1A features central tears visible on ultrasound as a hypoechoic cleft without affecting the entire disc diameter (illustration of pathology, Fig. 13.9a; long axis, Fig. 13.9b; short axis, Fig. 13.9c). Class 1B includes tears at the distal ulnar insertion (illustration of pathology, Fig. 13.10a; long axis, Fig. 13.10b; short axis, Fig. 13.10c), possibly associated with ulnar styloid fractures (illustration of pathology, Fig. 13.11a; long axis, Fig. 13.10b;

Table 13.1 Ultrasonographic classification for triangular fibrocartilage complex lesions

Class 1 (Traumatic)
(A) Central tear of the articular disc
(B) Ulnar attachment tear of the articular disc
(C) Radial attachment tear of the articular disc
(D) Horizontal tear of the articular disc
(E) Injury of the triangular fibrocartilage component other than the articular disc, i.e., meniscus homologue, radioulnar, lunotriquetral, and ulnar collateral ligaments; or extensor carpi ulnaris tendon subsheath
Class 2 (Degenerative)
(A) Articular disc wear
(B) Class 2A plus chondromalacia of the lunate or the ulna
(C) Class 2B plus articular disc rupture
(D) Class 2C plus lunotriquetral ligament rupture and cartilage abnormalities
(E) Class 2D plus ulnocarpal/radioulnar arthritis

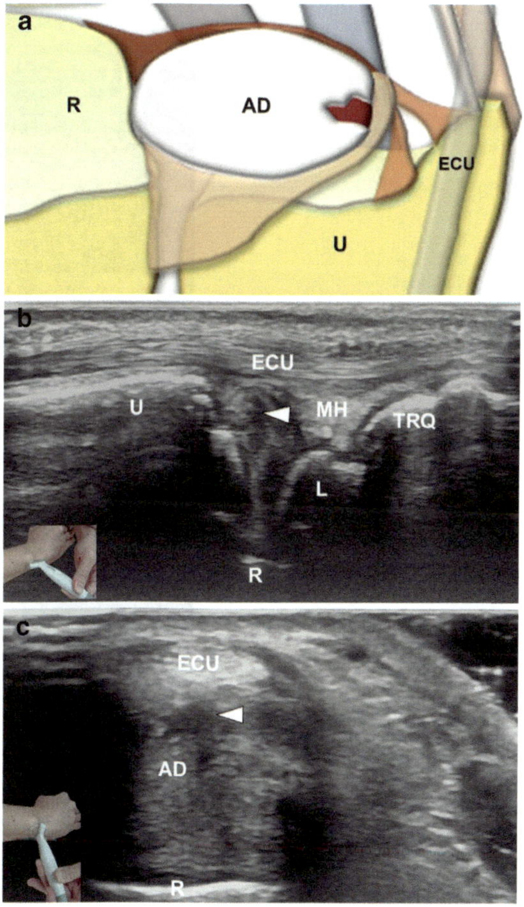

Fig. 13.9 The illustration (**a**) and ultrasonography images show a central tear (white arrowheads) of the articular disc in both the coronal (**b**) and axial (**c**) planes. ECU extensor carpi ulnaris tendon; AD articular disc; MH meniscus homologue; L lunate; TRQ triquetrum; R radius; U ulna

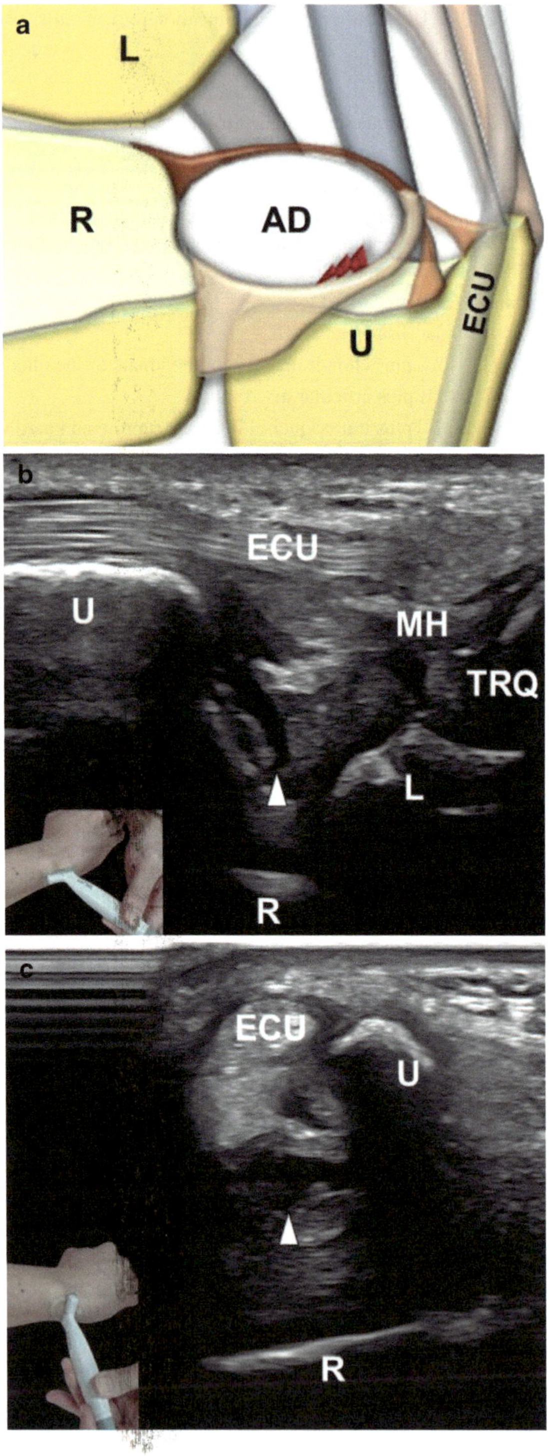

Fig. 13.10 The illustration (**a**) and ultrasonography images depict a tear at the ulnar attachment of the articular disc (white arrowheads) in both coronal (**b**) and axial (**c**) planes. ECU extensor carpi ulnaris tendon; AD articular disc; MH meniscus homologue; L lunate; TRQ triquetrum; R radius; U ulna

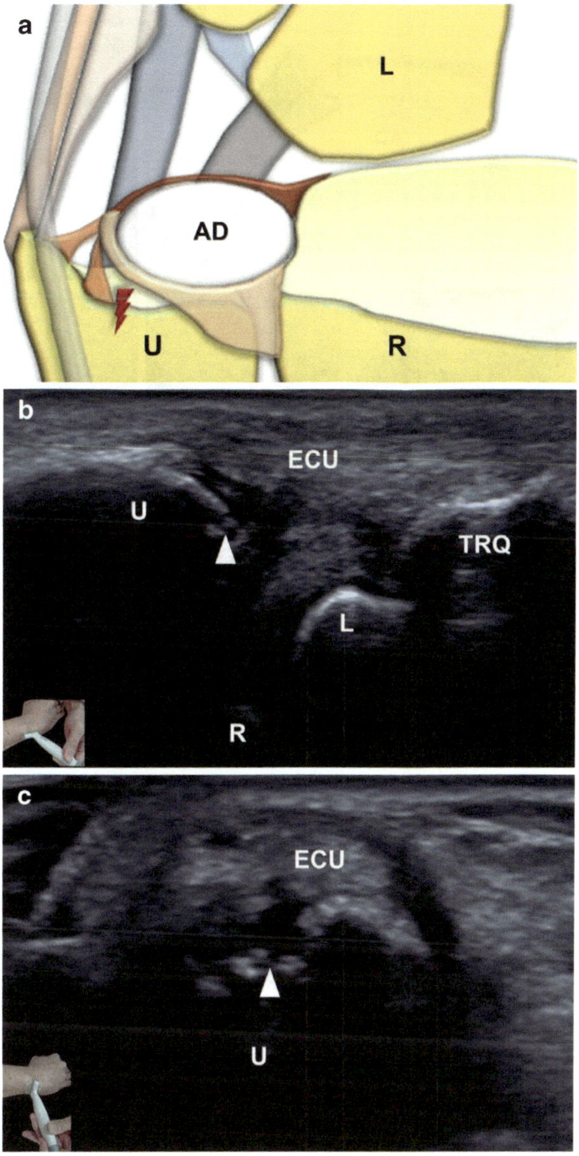

Fig. 13.11 The illustration (**a**) and ultrasonography images demonstrate a small ulnar fracture (white arrowheads) with cortical irregularity in both the coronal (**b**) and axial (**c**) planes. ECU extensor carpi ulnaris tendon; AD articular disc; MH meniscus homologue; L lunate; TRQ triquetrum; R radius; U ulna

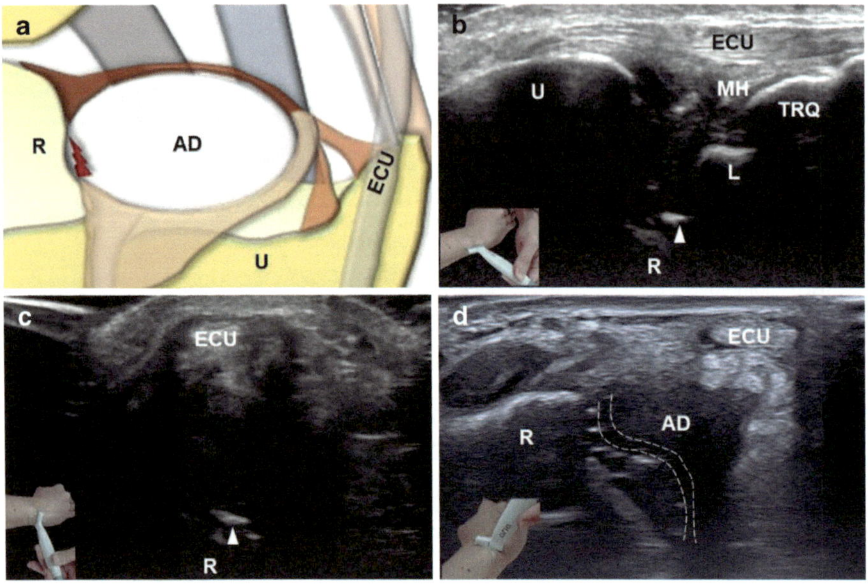

Fig. 13.12 The illustration (**a**) and ultrasonography images depict the avulsion (white arrowheads) of the sigmoid notch of the radius in both the coronal (**b**) and axial (**c**) planes, along with the radial attachment tear (dashed lines) of the articular disc in the axial plane (**d**). ECU extensor carpi ulnaris tendon; AD articular disc; MH meniscus homologue; L lunate; TRQ triquetrum; R radius; U ulna

short axis, Fig. 13.10c). Class 1C indicates radial attachment tears, characterized by a hypoechoic slit on ultrasound (illustration of pathology, Fig. 13.12a; long axis, Fig. 13.12b; short axis, Fig. 13.12c, d). Class 1D signifies tears extending through the entire disc depth (illustration of pathology, Fig. 13.13a; short axis, Fig. 13.13b; long axis, Fig. 13.13c).

Class 1E denotes TFCC involvement beyond the articular disc, including injuries to the meniscus homologue (illustration of pathology, Fig. 13.14a; long axis, Fig. 13.14b), the ulnar collateral ligament (illustration of pathology, Fig. 13.14c;

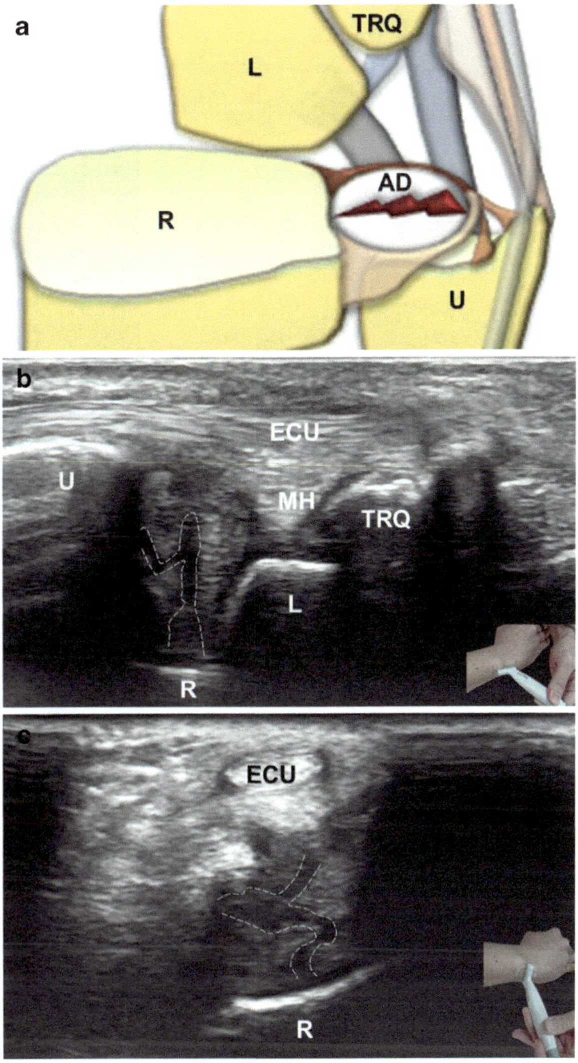

Fig. 13.13 The illustration (**a**) and ultrasonography images depict a horizontal tear (dashed lines) of the articular disc extending through the entire disc in both the coronal (**b**) and axial (**c**) planes. ECU extensor carpi ulnaris tendon; AD articular disc; MH meniscus homologue; L lunate; TRQ triquctrum; R radius; U ulna

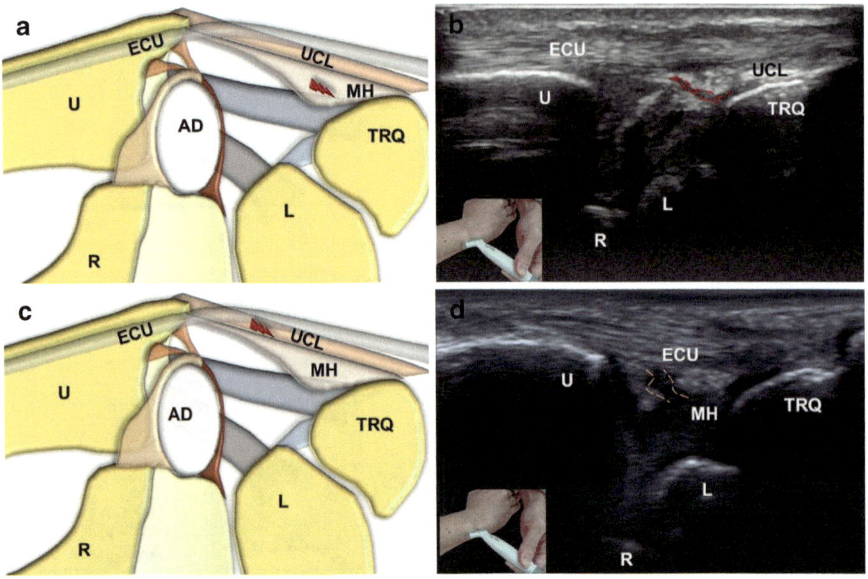

Fig. 13.14 The illustration (**a**) and ultrasonography images show a tear (red dashed lines) of the meniscus homologue (**b**) in the coronal plane. Similarly, the illustration (**c**) and ultrasonography images demonstrate a tear (brown dashed lines) of the ulnar collateral ligament (**d**) in the coronal plane. ECU extensor carpi ulnaris tendon; UCL ulnar collateral ligament; AD articular disc; MH meniscus homologue; L lunate; TRQ triquetrum; R radius; U ulna

long axis, Fig. 13.14d), the radioulnar ligament (illustration of pathology, Fig. 13.15a and Fig. 13.15c; Doppler imaging in long axis, Fig. 13.15b; gray-scale imaging in short axis, Fig. 13.15d), the lunotriquetral ligament (illustration of pathology, Fig. 13.16a; long axis, Fig. 13.16b; short axis, Fig. 13.16c), and ulnar fovea injuries (illustration of pathology, Fig. 13.17a; affected side, Fig. 13.17b; illustration of normal anatomy, Fig. 13.17c; healthy side, Fig. 13.17d), which may appear heterogeneous on ultrasound due to anisotropy. Similarly, the ECU tendon, its tendon sheath, and subsheath may be involved in Class 1E injuries (illustration of pathology, Fig. 13.18a; long axis, Fig. 13.18b; short axis, Fig. 13.18c). In patients with subsheath rupture, a dynamic examination using wrist supination and pronation can confirm tendon instability (illustration of pathology, Fig. 13.19a; short axis, Fig. 13.19b).

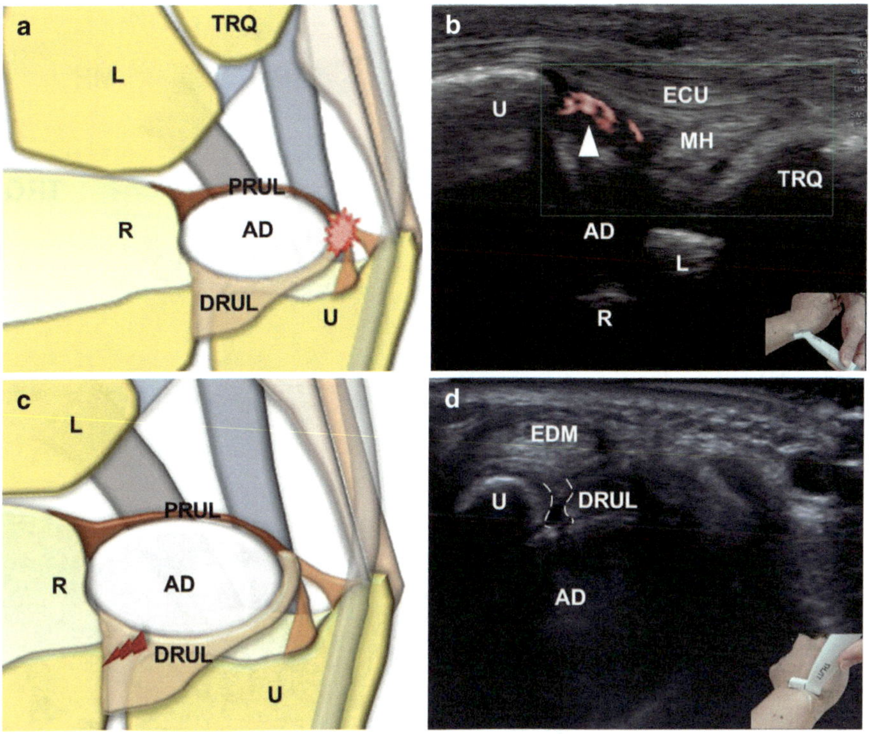

Fig. 13.15 The illustration (**a**) and corresponding ultrasound image (**b**) demonstrate inflammation (white arrowhead) of the radioulnar ligament. In contrast, the illustration (**c**) and corresponding ultrasound image (**d**) show a tear (dashed line) of the dorsal radioulnar ligament. DRUL dorsal radioulnar ligament; PRUL palmar radioulnar ligament; EDM extensor digiti minimi; ECU extensor carpi ulnaris tendon; AD articular disc; MH meniscus homologue; L lunate; TRQ triquetrum; R radius; U ulna

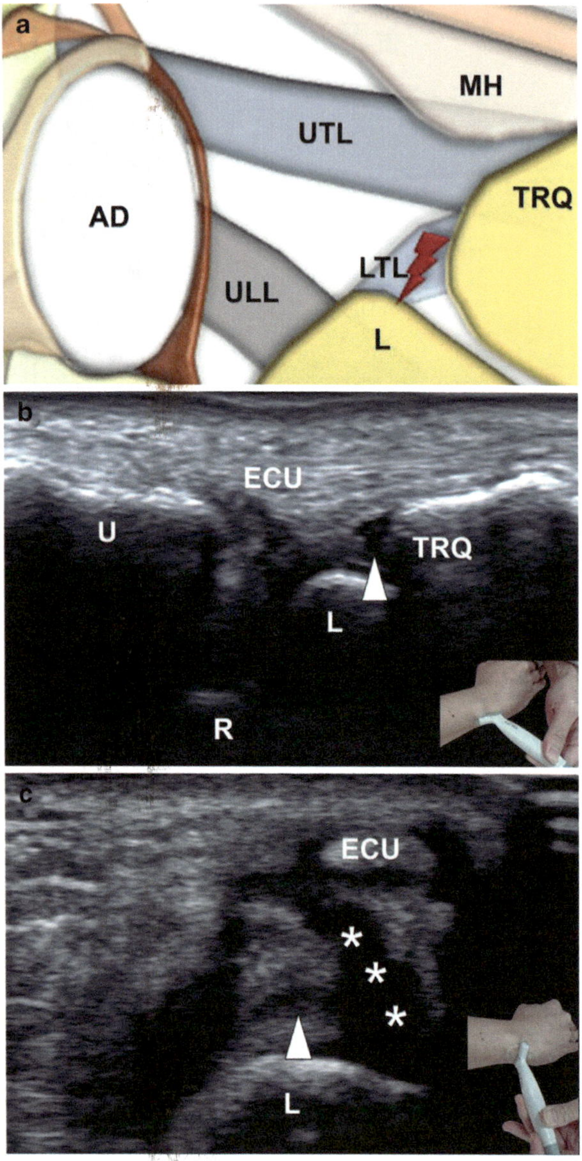

Fig. 13.16 Illustration (**a**) and the corresponding ultrasound images reveal a tear (white arrowheads) of the lunotriquetral ligament accompanied by periligamentous effusion (asterisks) in both coronal (**b**) and axial (**c**) planes. LTL lunotriquetral ligament; ULL ulnolunate ligament; UTL ulnotriquetral ligament; ECU extensor carpi ulnaris tendon; AD articular disc; MH meniscus homologue; L lunate; TRQ triquetrum; R radius; U ulna

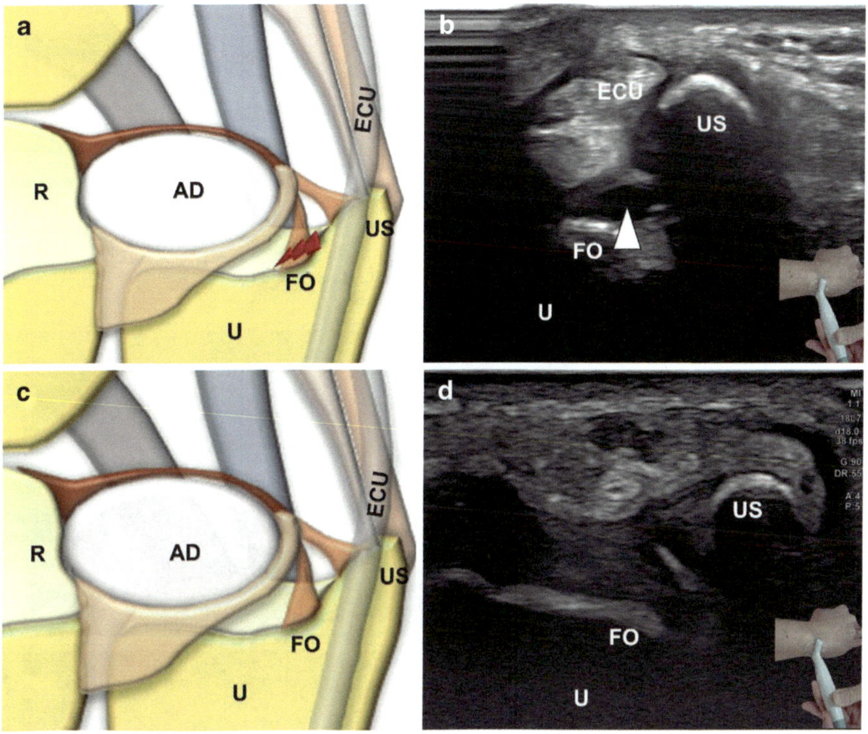

Fig. 13.17 The illustration (**a**) and ultrasonography image (**b**) depict an ulnar fovea injury (white arrowhead) in the short axis, compared to the illustration (**c**) and ultrasonography image (**d**) of the healthy side. ECU extensor carpi ulnaris tendon; AD articular disc; US ulnar styloid; FO fovea of the ulna; R radius; U ulna

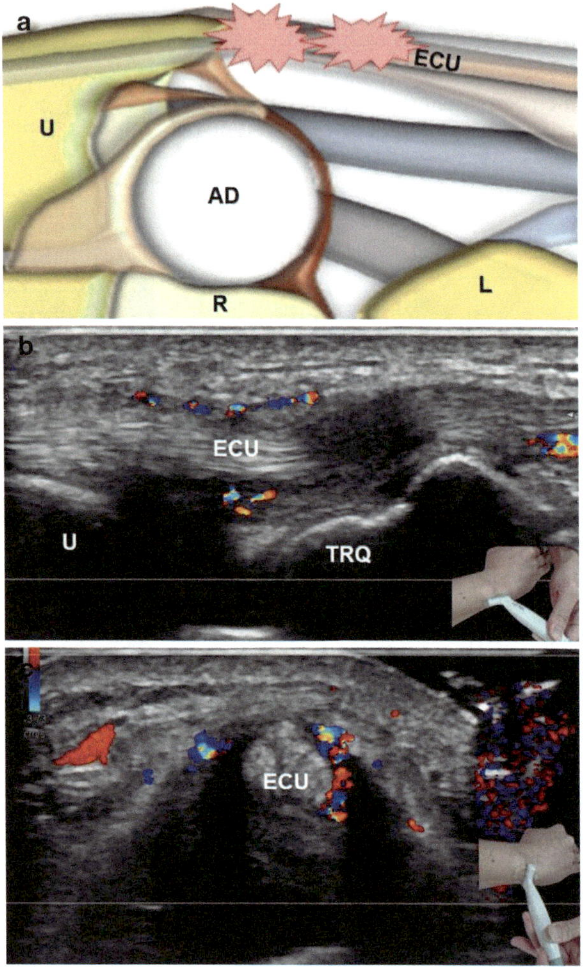

Fig. 13.18 The illustration (**a**) and ultrasonography images depict a subsheath injury with hypervascularity of the extensor carpi ulnaris (ECU) tendon in the coronal (**b**) and axial (**c**) planes. AD articular disc; L lunate; TRQ triquetrum; R radius; U ulna

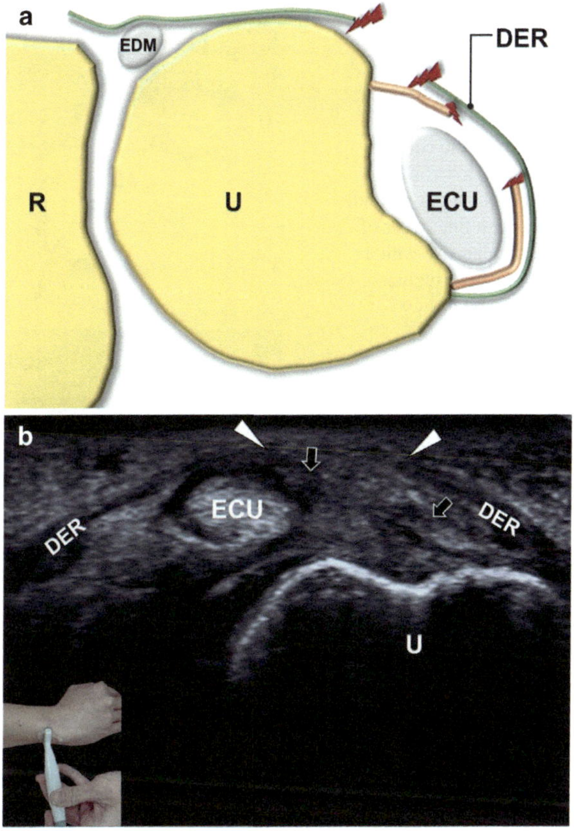

Fig. 13.19 The illustration (**a**) and ultrasonography image (**b**) show subluxation of the extensor carpi ulnaris tendon, a tear of the dorsal extensor retinaculum (white arrowheads), and a tear of the subsheath of the extensor carpi ulnaris (black arrows). DER dorsal extensor retinaculum; EDM extensor digiti minimi tendon; ECU extensor carpi ulnaris tendon; R radius; U ulna

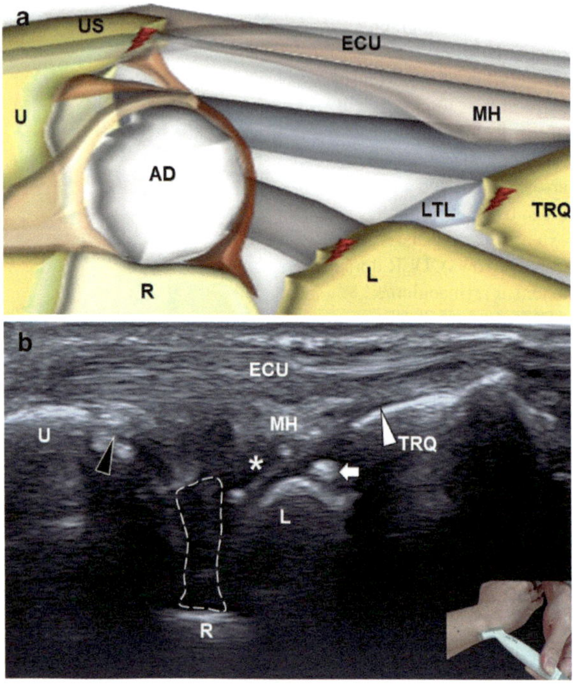

Fig. 13.20 The illustration (**a**) and ultrasonography image (**b**) depict class 2A degeneration of the triangular fibrocartilage complex in the coronal plane. Black arrowhead: spurs of the ulnar styloid; white dash line: wear of the articular disc with a thinning and irregular border; white arrow: calcification of the lunotriquetral ligament; white arrowhead: degeneration of the overlying cartilage; asterisk: effusion; ECU extensor carpi ulnaris tendon; AD articular disc; MH meniscus homologue; L lunate; LTL lunotriquetral ligament; TRQ triquetrum; US ulnar styloid; R radius; U ulna

Class 2 (Degeneration)

Class 2 injuries signify TFCC degeneration with or without preceding trauma, progressing from Class 2A to 2E. Class 2A denotes articular disc wear, observed as thinning with irregular borders on ultrasound. Class 2B indicates disc wear with adjacent chondromalacia, evidenced by thinning and irregularities of surrounding cartilage and carpal bones (Fig. 13.20). Class 2C resembles 2B but may progress to disc rupture. Class 2D involves additional lunotriquetral ligament ruptures, while Class 2E suggests arthritis and synovitis with a large disc tear.

13.5 Ultrasound-Guided Intervention

To perform an ultrasound-guided injection of the TFCC using the out-of-plane approach, the wrist should be positioned on a pillow with the forearm fully pronated and the wrist radially deviated. The linear transducer is placed parallel to the extensor carpi ulnaris tendon between the ulnar styloid process and the triquetrum. Then, a 25-gauge needle is introduced toward the radial aspect, deeper to the extensor carpi ulnaris tendon, until it reaches the target site (Fig. 13.21a).

For conducting in-plane US-guided injection, the linear transducer is placed over the dorsal wrist in a horizontal plane, and a 25-gauge needle is advanced toward the radial aspect, deep to the extensor carpi ulnaris tendon, to target the TFCC

(Fig. 13.21b). The TFCC is predominantly innervated by the dorsal ulnar cutaneous nerve [8, 9] and receives its blood supply from the ulnar artery and branches of the anterior or posterior interosseous artery (Fig. 13.22). It is essential to clearly identify these structures and prevent any collateral injury during the injection process.

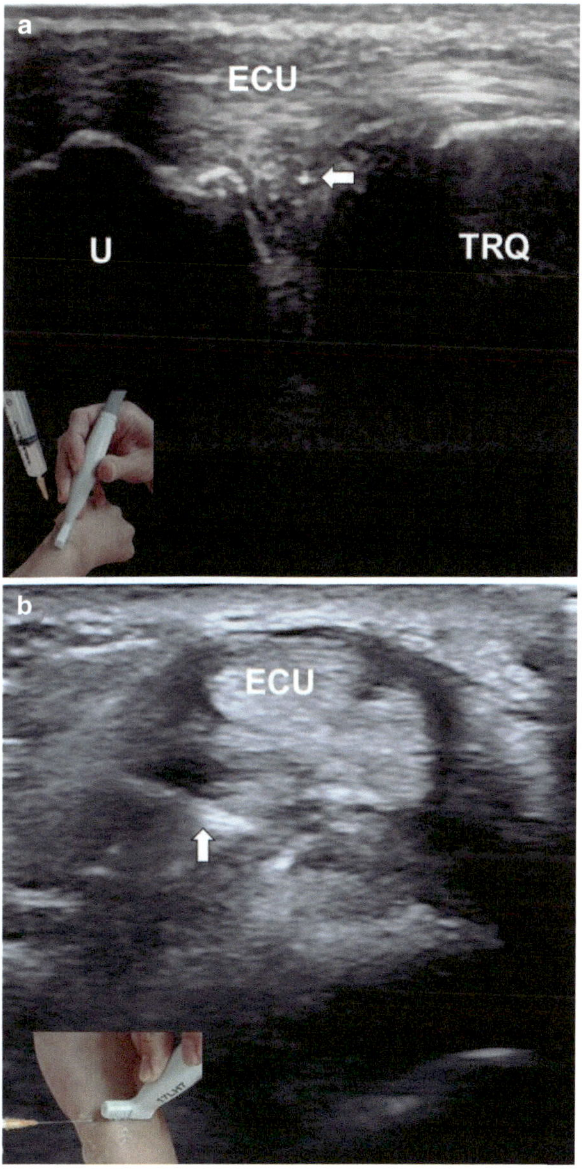

Fig. 13.21 Ultrasound-guided injections for the triangular fibrocartilage complex are administered using the out-of-plane (**a**) and in-plane (**b**) approaches. White arrows: needle tip/shaft; ECU extensor carpi ulnaris tendon; TRQ triquetrum; U ulna

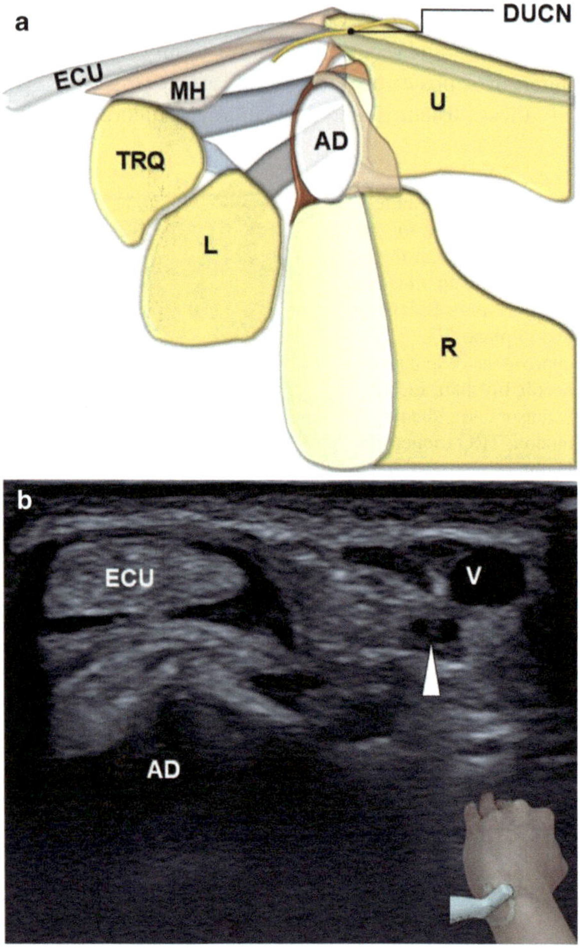

Fig. 13.22 The illustration (**a**) and ultrasonography image (**b**) depict the triangular fibrocartilage complex and its relationship to the dorsal ulnar cutaneous nerve (white arrowhead and DUCN). ECU extensor carpi ulnaris tendon; AD articular disc; MH meniscus homologue; L lunate; TRQ triquetrum; V vessel; R radius; U ulna

13.6 Conclusion

Using a systematic approach, ultrasound can effectively depict the various components of the TFCC and outline lesions affecting the articular disc, meniscus homologue, and juxta-articular ligaments. In cases of TFCC disorders, ultrasound can also assist in delivering injectables accurately to the affected areas, thereby reducing the risk of unintended harm to nearby neurovascular structures.

Acknowledgments Images and illustrations adapted from cadaveric images provided by the Visible Human Project® of the National Library of Medicine. Excerpts featured in the VH Dissector are used with permission from Touch of Life Technologies Inc.

References

1. Chan JJ, Teunis T, Ring D. Prevalence of triangular fibrocartilage complex abnormalities regardless of symptoms rise with age: systematic review and pooled analysis. Clin Orthop Relat Res. 2014;472(12):3987–94.
2. Scigliano NM, McSweeny KF, Garcia Fleury I, Buckwalter JA. Ulnar variance in athletes: a scoping review. Sports Health. 2023;16:19417381231195527.
3. Wu WT, Chang KV, Mezian K, et al. Ulnar wrist pain revisited: ultrasound diagnosis and guided injection for triangular fibrocartilage complex injuries. J Clin Med. 2019;8(10):1540.
4. Nakamura T, Takayama S, Horiuchi Y, Yabe Y. Origins and insertions of the triangular fibrocartilage complex: a histological study. J Hand Surg Br. 2001;26(5):446–54.
5. Thiru RG, Ferlic DC, Clayton ML, McClure DC. Arterial anatomy of the triangular fibrocartilage of the wrist and its surgical significance. J Hand Surg Am. 1986;11(2):258–63.
6. Wu WT, Chang KV, Hsu YC, Hsu PC, Ricci V, Özçakar L. Artifacts in musculoskeletal ultrasonography: from physics to clinics. Diagnostics (Basel). 2020;10(9):645.
7. Cody ME, Nakamura DT, Small KM, Yoshioka H. MR imaging of the triangular fibrocartilage complex. Magn Reson Imaging Clin N Am. 2015;23(3):393–403.
8. Poublon AR, Kraan G, Lau SP, Kerver AL, Kleinrensink GJ. Anatomical study of the dorsal cutaneous branch of the ulnar nerve (DCBUN) and its clinical relevance in TFCC repair. J Plast Reconstr Aesthet Surg. 2016;69(7):983–7.
9. Wu WT, Chang KV, Hsu YC, et al. Ultrasound imaging and guidance for distal peripheral nerve pathologies at the wrist/hand. Diagnostics (Basel). 2023;13(11):1928.

Chapter 14
Intrinsic and Extrinsic Wrist Ligaments Unmasked

Ke-Vin Chang, Wei-Ting Wu, and Yuan-Yuan Tsai

14.1 Introduction

Commonly used imaging methods to investigate wrist pain include plain radiographs, wrist arthrography, and magnetic resonance imaging, which has gained increased prominence recently. However, ultrasound has become increasingly valuable in assessing musculoskeletal disorders, especially with advancements in high-resolution probe technology. Its exceptional resolution enables thorough examination of superficial structures and accurate diagnosis of wrist pathologies.

Within the wrist, intrinsic and extrinsic ligaments are essential for stabilizing carpal bones during movement, facilitating interactions with forearm bones and metacarpals, and transmitting motion between carpal bones [1]. These ligaments, categorized as intracapsular and extrasynovial, are named based on their origins and insertions, following a pattern from proximal to distal and radial to ulnar directions [2].

The identification of individual carpal bones can be challenging due to the non-parallel alignment of the radiocarpal, midcarpal, and carpometacarpal joints. Consequently, wrist ligaments are often not included in basic wrist scanning protocols [3]. However, precise visualization of these ligaments relies on accurate recognition of carpal bones. Therefore, this chapter aims to elucidate the sonoanatomy of the carpal bones and present a systematic approach for identifying both intrinsic and extrinsic wrist ligaments, relevant pathologies, and injection techniques.

K.-V. Chang (✉) · W.-T. Wu · Y.-Y. Tsai
Bei-Hu Branch, National Taiwan University Hospital, Taipei, Taiwan

K.-V. Chang (ed.), *Ultrasonography of Musculoskeletal Pain*,
https://doi.org/10.1007/978-981-96-6787-1_14

14.2 Anatomy

The wrist comprises two distinct categories of ligaments: intrinsic and extrinsic. Intrinsic ligaments are exclusive attachments to the carpal bones, while extrinsic ligaments extend to surrounding structures such as the forearm, retinacula, or tendon sheaths. In terms of biomechanics, intrinsic ligaments possess greater elasticity, allowing for more elongation before enduring deformation, whereas extrinsic ligaments are characterized by increased rigidity [4].

14.2.1 Intrinsic Carpal Ligament

Intrinsic ligaments are categorized into two main types: interosseous ligaments, located between adjacent carpal bones, and intrinsic capsular ligaments, which attach to the carpal bones, sometimes spanning across three carpal bones [2]. Proximal interosseous ligaments encompass the scapholunate and lunotriquetral ligaments, while distal interosseous ligaments include the trapeziotrapezoid, trapezocapitate, and capitohamate ligaments in the dorsal (Fig. 14.1) and palmar (Fig. 14.2) regions. The palmar ligaments that bridge proximal and distal carpal rows consist of the scaphotrapeziotrapezoidal, scaphocapitate, and triquetrocapitate ligaments [2].

The scapholunate ligament is comprised of three distinct components: volar, dorsal, and proximal interosseous (Fig. 14.3a, b) [5]. While the volar and dorsal components are authentic ligaments, the proximal interosseous component is primarily composed of fibrocartilage and lacks collagen connections and neurovascular bundles. Typically, the volar aspect exhibits an oblique orientation, whereas the dorsal component aligns transversely to the lunate and scaphoid, closely associated with the joint capsule. In the sagittal plane, the scapholunate ligament forms a C-shape (Fig. 14.3c), with the dorsal region being the thickest.

Three distinct distal interosseous ligament complexes connect the trapezium, trapezoid, capitate, and hamate bones (Fig. 14.4a). Each ligament complex comprises at least a dorsal and a palmar region. The dorsal and palmar trapeziotrapezoid ligaments extend across nearly the whole dorsal and palmar edges of the joint. Similarly, the dorsal and palmar trapezocapitate ligaments are like the trapeziotrapezoid ligaments. However, because the capitate bone has a neck and head that extend proximally, these ligaments only connect to the distal body part of the capitate bone. Additionally, a robust deep trapezocapitate ligament traverses the central region of the joint. Likewise, the dorsal and palmar capitohamate ligaments mimic the trapeziotrapezoid and trapezocapitate ligaments, respectively, but they only cross the distal half of the joint due to the proximal extension of the hamate's pole and the head and neck of the capitate.

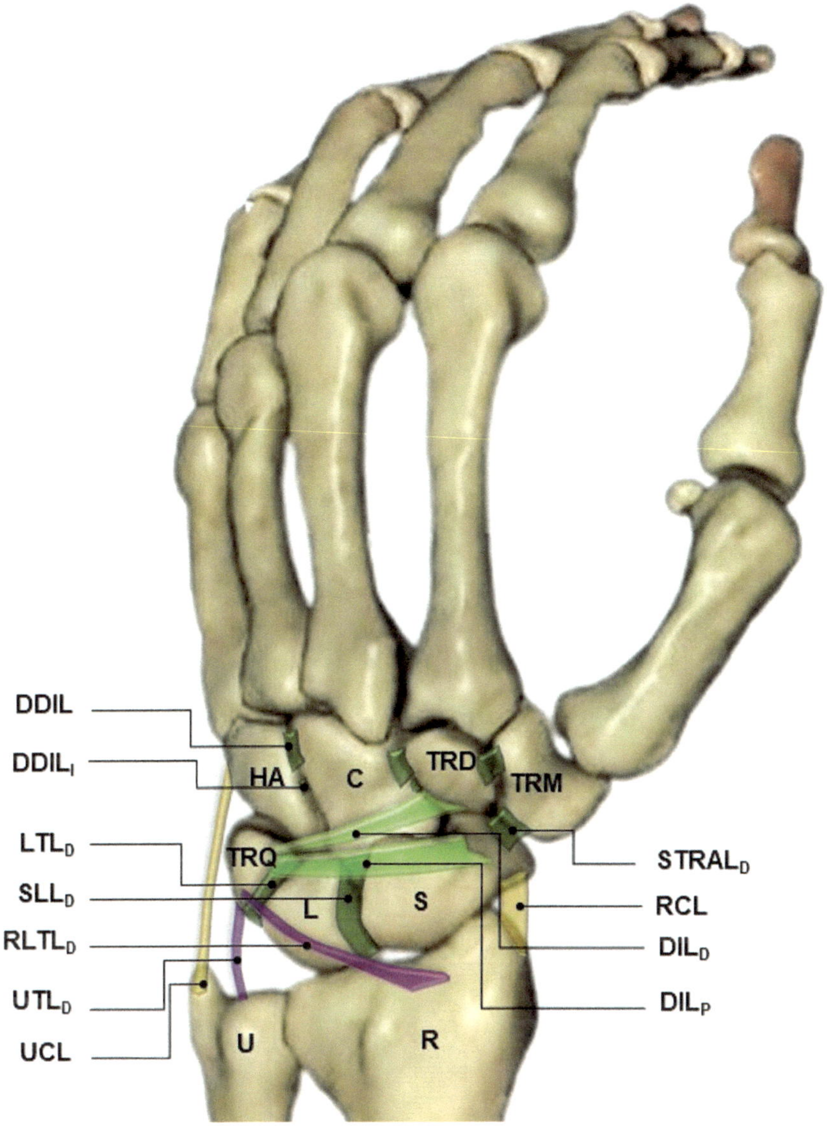

Fig. 14.1 The illustration shows the extrinsic and intrinsic ligaments of the dorsal wrist. RCL radial collateral ligament; UCL ulnar collateral ligament; RLTL$_D$ dorsal radiolunotriquetral ligament; UTL$_D$ dorsal ulnotriquetral ligament; SLL$_D$ dorsal scapholunate ligament; LTL$_D$ dorsal lunotriquetral ligament; DIL$_P$ proximal band of the dorsal intercarpal ligament; DIL$_D$ distal band of the dorsal intercarpal ligament; STRAL$_D$ dorsal scaphotrapezial ligament; DDIL dorsal distal interosseous ligament; DDIL$_I$ interosseous portion of dorsal distal interosseous ligament; S scaphoid; L lunate; TRQ triquetrum; C capitate; HA hamate; TRM trapezium; TRD trapezoid; R radius; U ulna

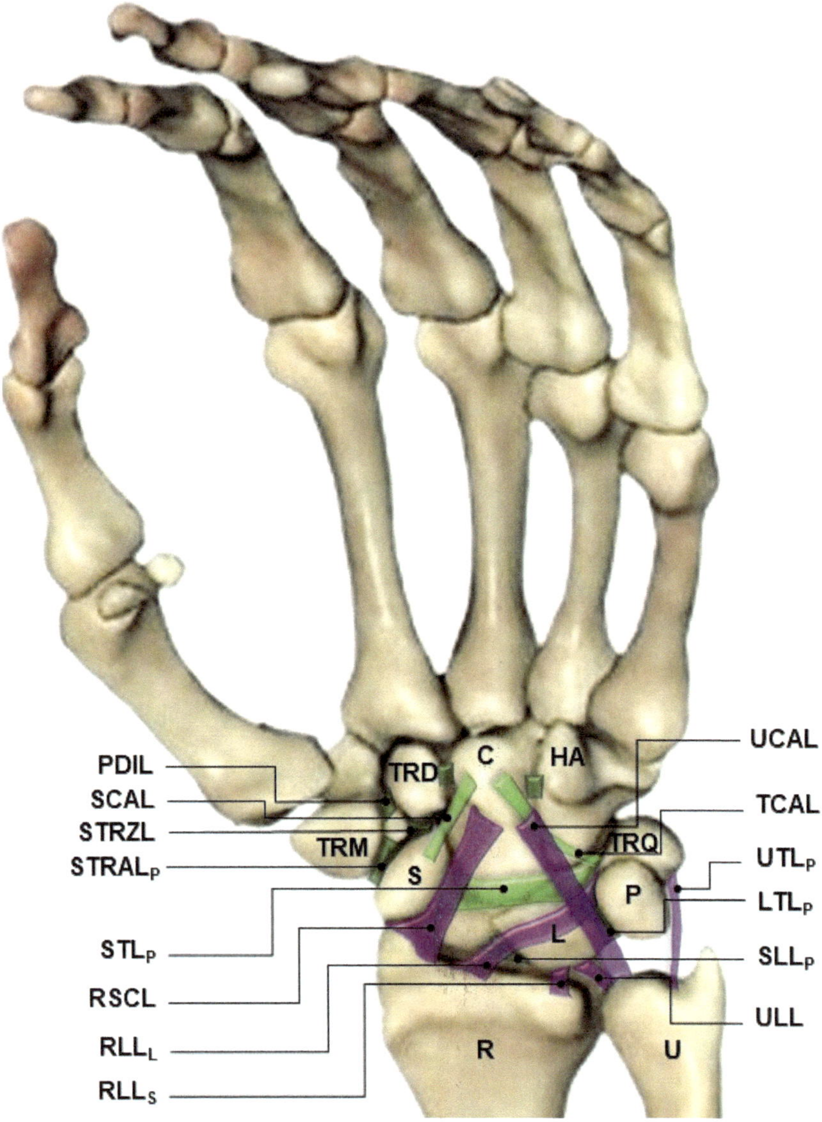

Fig. 14.2 The illustration shows the extrinsic and intrinsic ligaments of the palmar wrist. RSCL radioscaphocapitate ligament; RLL_L long radiolunate ligament; RLL_S short radiolunate ligament; UTL_P palmar ulnotriquetral ligament; UCAL ulnocapitate ligament; ULL ulnolunate ligament; SLL_P palmar scapholunate ligament; LTL_P palmar lunotriquetral ligament; STL_P palmar scaphotriquetral ligament; SCAL scaphocapitate ligament; TCAL triquetrocapitate ligament; $STRAL_P$ palmar scaphotrapezial ligament; STRZL scaphotrapezoid ligament; PDIL palmar distal interosseous ligament; S scaphoid; L lunate; TRQ triquetrum; TRM trapezium; TRD trapezoid; C capitate; HA hamate; R radius; U ulna

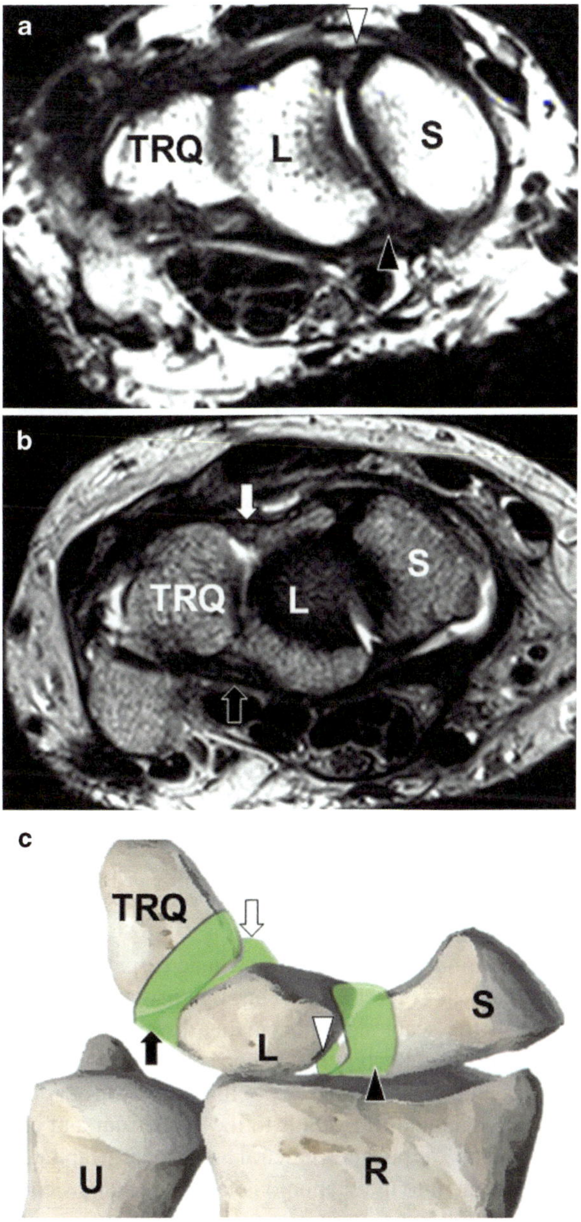

Fig. 14.3 The magnetic resonance images show the dorsal and palmar portions of the scapholunate (**a**) and lunotriquetral (**b**) ligaments, corresponding to the schematic illustration (**c**). White arrowheads: dorsal scapholunate ligament; black arrowheads: palmar scapholunate ligament; white arrows: dorsal lunotriquetral ligament; black arrows: palmar lunotriquetral ligament; S scaphoid; L lunate; TRQ triquetrum; R radius; U ulna

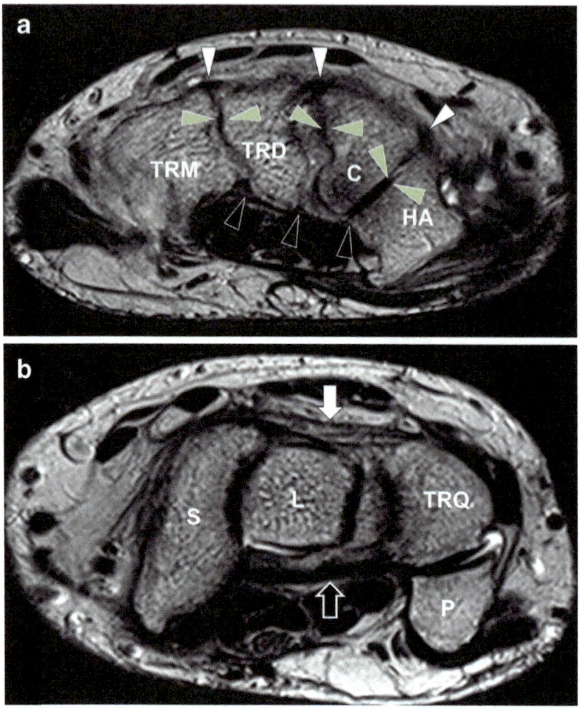

Fig. 14.4 The magnetic resonance imaging demonstrates the distal interosseous ligament complexes (**a**), while the second image highlights the proximal band of the dorsal intercarpal ligament and the palmar scaphotriquetral ligament (**b**). White arrowheads: dorsal distal interosseous ligament complexes; green arrowheads: interosseous portion of distal interosseous ligament complexes; black arrowheads: palmar distal interosseous ligament complexes; white arrow: proximal band of dorsal intercarpal ligament; black arrow: palmar scaphotriquetral ligament; S scaphoid; L lunate; TRQ triquetrum; P pisiform; C capitate; HA hamate; TRM trapezium; TRD trapezoid

Furthermore, a significant intrinsic carpal ligament is the palmar scaphotriquetral ligament (Fig. 14.4b). This ligament courses almost horizontally across the waist of the scaphoid and remains distinct from the capitate by a synovial fold, indicating no attachment to the capitate. Positioned within the joint capsule, it resides on the palmar surface of the head of the capitate, dorsal to the radioscaphocapitate ligament. It extends to the triquetrum and occupies the space between the attachments of the lunotriquetral and triquetrocapitate ligaments. On the radial side, its attachment to the scaphoid is fan-shaped and slender.

Another important ligament is the dorsal intercarpal ligament, which connects to the dorsal tubercle of the triquetrum and extends radially in two bands. The proximal band attaches to the dorsal ridge and radial surface of the distal pole of the scaphoid, while the distal band attaches to the dorsal cortex of the trapezoid. The proximal band is referred to as the dorsal scaphotriquetral fascicle, while the distal band is known as the trapezoidtriquetral fascicle. Notably, the proximal band is thicker than the distal band (Fig. 14.5).

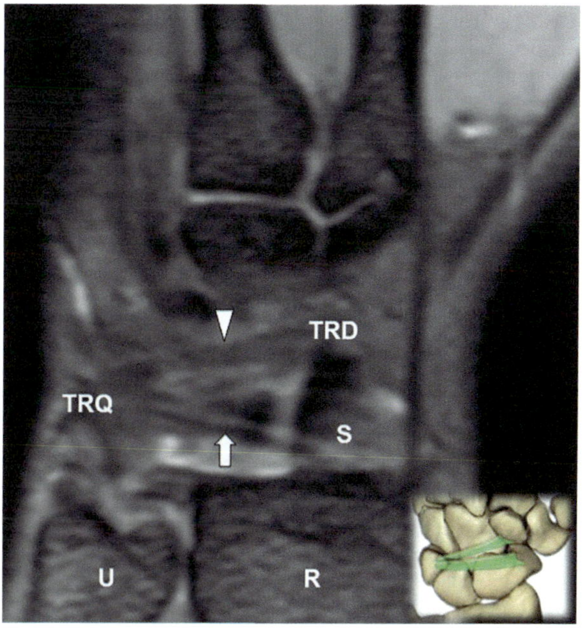

Fig. 14.5 The coronal magnetic resonance imaging shows the proximal and distal bands of the dorsal intercarpal ligaments. White arrow: proximal band of the dorsal intercarpal ligament (dorsal scaphotriquetral fascicle); white arrowhead: distal band of the dorsal intercarpal ligament (trapezoidtriquetral fascicle); TRQ triquetrum; TRD trapezoid; S scaphoid; R radius; U ulna

14.2.2 Extrinsic Carpal Ligament

There are three major palmar radiocarpal ligaments, each with a proximal attachment to the radius. The most radial ligament is the radioscaphocapitate ligament, which extends from the radial styloid process to the middle of the scaphoid fossa (Fig. 14.6a). Some of its fibers insert into the volar aspect of the capitate body. Adjacent to the radioscaphocapitate ligament, towards the ulnar side, is the long radiolunate ligament (Fig. 14.6b). This ligament arises from the volar edge of the radius, covering the remaining aspect of the scaphoid fossa, and traverses the radiocarpal joint volar to the proximal pole of the scaphoid before attaching to the lunate. Further ulnar lies the short radiolunate ligament (Fig. 14.6c), which originates proximally from the entire width of the lunate fossa region of the distal radius. It attaches distally onto the radial half of the palmar cortex of the lunate.

Three ulnocarpal ligaments have been identified, bridging the gap between the distal ulna and the carpus on the volar and ulnar aspects. Among them, the ulnocapitate ligament stands out for its direct attachment to the ulnar fovea region, a slight depression at the base of the ulnar styloid process. From there, it extends distally, passing just volar to the junction between the other ulnocarpal ligaments, until reaching the capitate (Fig. 14.6a). The other two ligaments are the ulnolunate (Fig. 14.7a) and ulnotriquetral ligaments (Fig. 14.7b). The boundary between the ulnolunate and ulnotriquetral ligaments is not clearly delineated, with the distinction primarily made by their distal attachments. Both ligaments originate proximally from the palmar radioulnar ligament, indirectly attaching to the ulna.

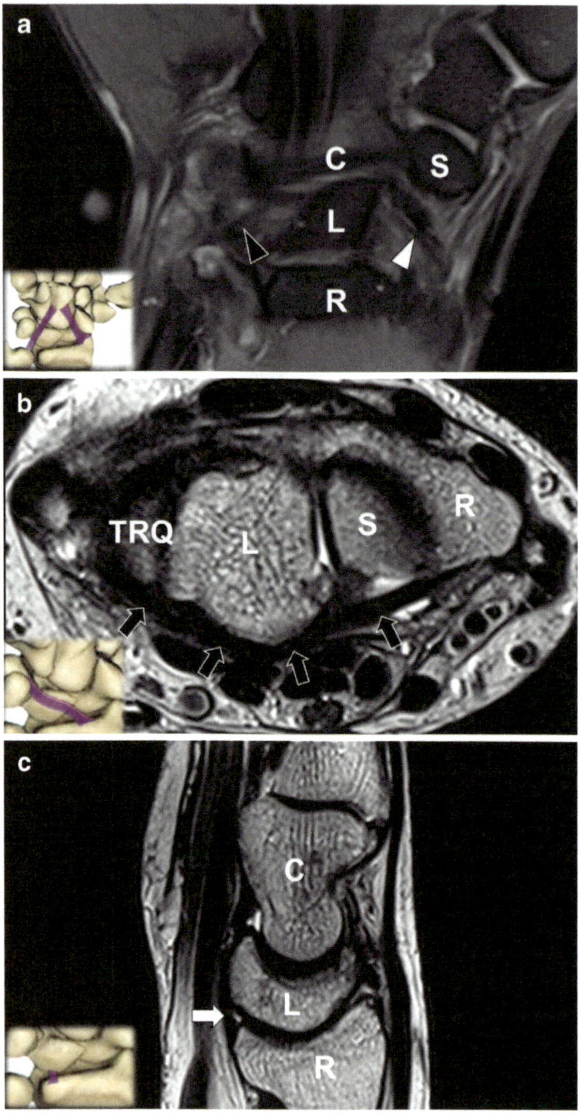

Fig. 14.6 The coronal magnetic resonance imaging shows the radioscaphocapitate ligament and ulnocapitate ligament (**a**). The axial magnetic resonance imaging illustrates the long radiolunate ligament (**b**), while the sagittal magnetic resonance imaging demonstrates the short radiolunate ligament (**c**). White arrowhead: radioscaphocapitate ligament; black arrowhead: ulnocapitate ligament; black arrows: long radiolunate ligament (radiolunotriquetral ligament); white arrow: short radiolunate ligament; TRQ triquetrum; S scaphoid; L lunate; C capitate; R radius

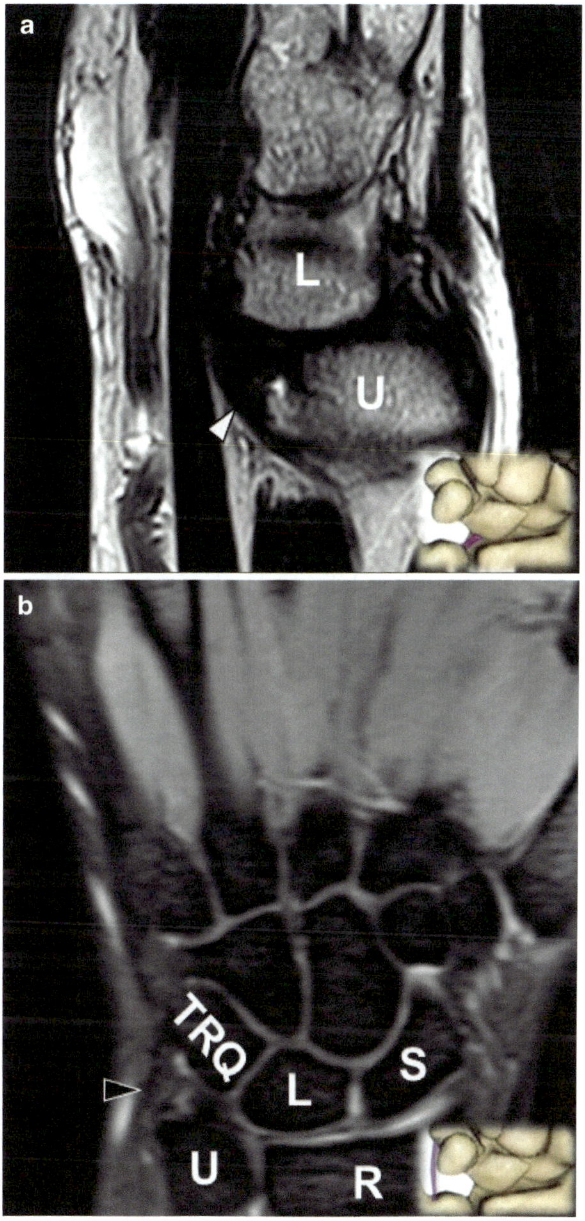

Fig. 14.7 The sagittal magnetic resonance imaging shows the ulnolunate ligament (**a**), while the coronal magnetic resonance imaging shows the ulnotriquetral ligament (**b**). White arrowhead: ulnolunate ligament; black arrowhead: ulnotriquetral ligament; S scaphoid; L lunate; TRQ triquetrum; R radius; U ulna

Additionally, the ulnolunate ligament is connected to the short radiolunate ligament, while the ulnotriquetral ligament attaches to the proximal and ulnar surfaces of the triquetrum.

The dorsal radiocarpal ligament originates from the dorsal margin of the distal radius, just ulnar and distal to Lister's tubercle, and extends obliquely and distally to the ulnar aspect. Its radial fibers attach to the dorsal ulnar aspect of the lunate and the dorsal distal region of the lunotriquetral ligament. Subsequently, the dorsal radiocarpal ligament inserts onto the dorsal tubercle of the triquetrum (Fig. 14.8a). Notably, there are no attachments to the scaphoid for the dorsal radiocarpal ligament. The radial collateral ligament (Fig. 14.8b) and ulnar collateral ligament (Fig. 14.8c) are essential stabilizing structures of the wrist joint that provide support during various movements. The radial collateral ligament is located on the radial side of the wrist, extending from the radial styloid process to the scaphoid and trapezium bones, where it provides lateral stability and prevents excessive ulnar deviation. Conversely, the ulnar collateral ligament is situated on the ulnar side of the wrist, originating from the ulnar styloid process and attaching to the triquetrum and pisiform bones, playing a critical role in resisting excessive radial deviation. Working in tandem, the radial collateral ligament and ulnar collateral ligament ensure the wrist's stability and maintain proper alignment during motion.

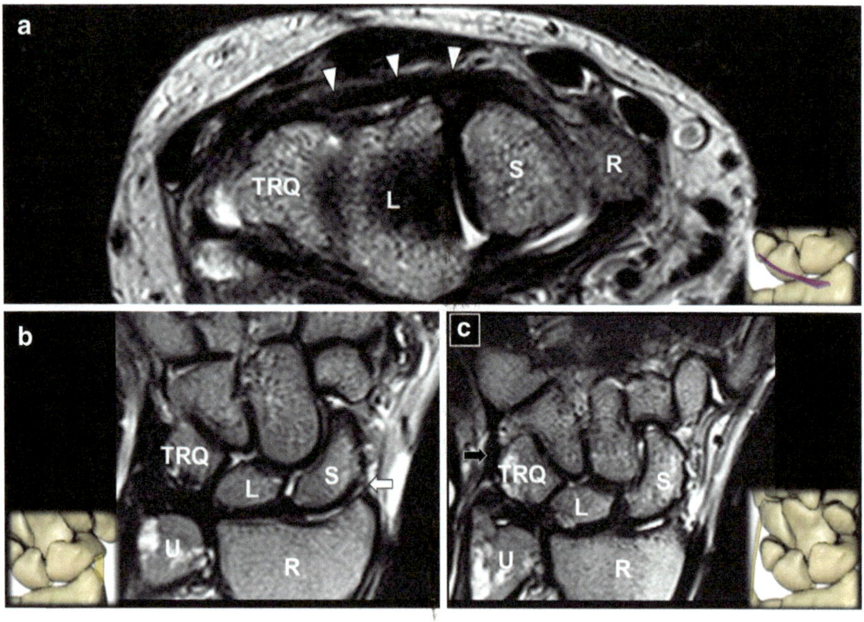

Fig. 14.8 The axial magnetic resonance image (**a**) shows the dorsal radiolunotriquetral ligament, while the coronal magnetic resonance images show the radial collateral ligament (**b**) and the ulnar collateral ligament (**c**). White arrowheads: dorsal radiolunotriquetral ligament; white arrow: radial collateral ligament; black arrow: ulnar collateral ligament; S scaphoid; L lunate; TRQ triquetrum; R radius; U ulna

14.3 Sonoanatomy

14.3.1 Volar Extrinsic Carpal Ligament Linking to the Capitate

The technique utilized for scanning wrist ligaments is derived from our previously published systematic scanning protocol [6]. Initially, we focus on identifying the volar extrinsic carpal ligaments, particularly those connecting to the capitate, such as the radioscaphocapitate (Fig. 14.9a) and ulnocapitate ligaments. The transducer is placed towards the radial aspect, ensuring its center aligns with the midpoint of the distal radius in the axial plane (Fig. 14.9b). Following this, the transducer is rotated 90° along the forearm's long axis and moved distally to visualize the proximal scaphoid at the center of the screen (Fig. 14.9c). To visualize the capitate, the distal part of the transducer is tilted 30° towards the midline. Notably, the radioscaphocapitate ligament extends across the radial styloid process, scaphoid, and capitate (Fig. 14.9d).

For scanning the ulnocapitate ligament (Fig. 14.10a), the transducer is situated slightly distal to the distal radioulnar joint in the axial plane (Fig. 14.10b), with the lunate positioned centrally on the screen (Fig. 14.10c). The radial end of the transducer is then tilted 60° towards the second finger to highlight the capitate. The ulnocapitate ligament extends over the distal ulna, lunate, and capitate, and can thus be visualized effectively (Fig. 14.10d).

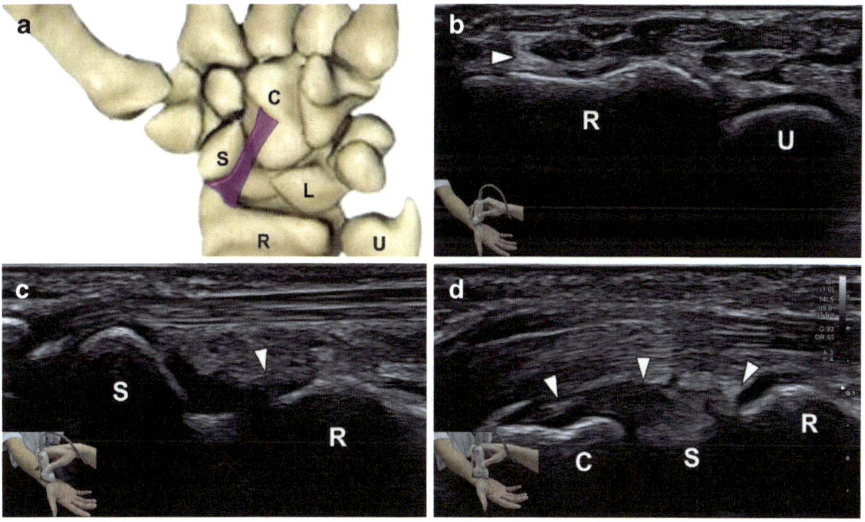

Fig. 14.9 The illustration depicts the radioscaphocapitate ligament (**a**). The transducer is first placed on the distal radius in the axial plane (**b**). Then, it is rotated 90° and moved distally to visualize the scaphoid (**c**). The distal part of the transducer is then tilted 30° towards the midline to visualize the capitate, allowing observation of the radioscaphocapitate ligament extending across the radial styloid (**d**). White arrowheads: radioscaphocapitate ligament; S scaphoid; L lunate; C capitate; R radius; U ulna

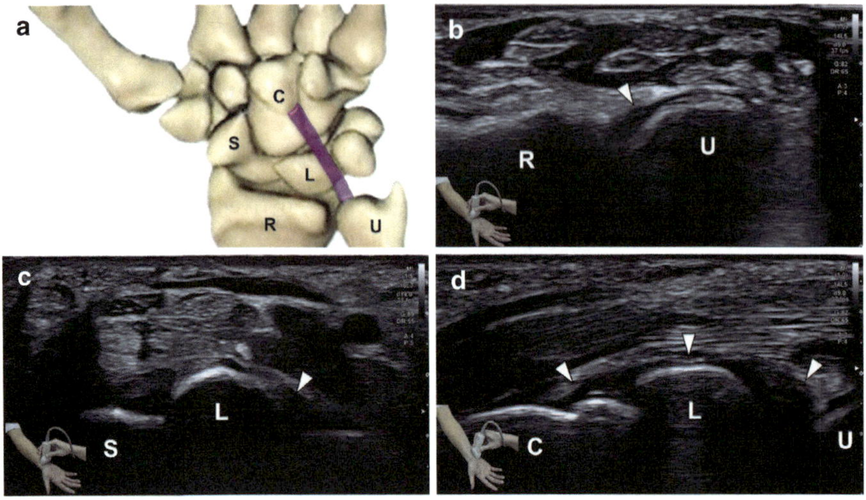

Fig. 14.10 The illustration depicts the ulnocapitate ligament (**a**). The transducer is initially positioned distal to the radioulnar joint (**b**), and then the lunate is identified in the axial plane (**c**). The radial end of the transducer is subsequently tilted 60° towards the capitate to visualize the ulnocapitate ligament (**d**). White arrowheads: ulnocapitate ligament; S scaphoid; L lunate; C capitate; R radius; U ulna

14.3.2 Volar Extrinsic Carpal Ligament Linking to the Lunate

Three volar extrinsic carpal ligaments, namely the long radiolunate, short radiolunate, and ulnolunate ligaments, attach to the lunate bone (Fig. 14.11a). To visualize the long radiolunate ligament, the transducer is initially positioned transversely over the distal radius. Subsequently, a 20° rotation is applied with the radial end as the pivot, facilitating the visualization of the lunate. This ligament extends between the distal radius and lunate, with some fibers reaching towards the triquetrum, hence, it is also known as the radiolunotriquetral ligament (Fig. 14.11b). For the short radiolunate ligament, the transducer's center point is placed over the ulnar aspect of the distal radius in a transverse orientation. Following this, the transducer is rotated to align with the forearm's longitudinal axis to achieve a clear view of the lunate. The short radiolunate ligament serves as a connecting structure between the radius and lunate (Fig. 14.11c). To observe the ulnolunate ligament, the scanning process begins by positioning the transducer over the distal radioulnar joint in a transverse plane. As the transducer moves distally, the lunate becomes visible, and then the ulnar aspect is rotated to fixate on the ulnar styloid. This ligament is discernible as a bridge between the ulna and lunate (Fig. 14.11d).

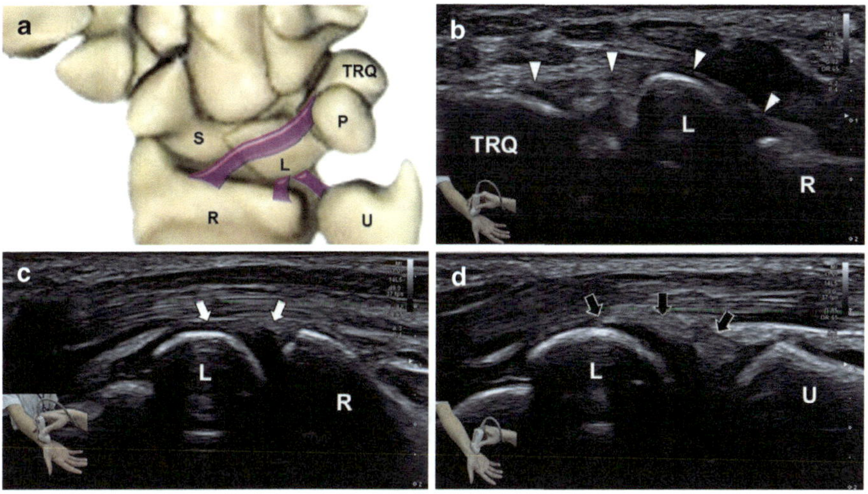

Fig. 14.11 The illustration (**a**) and the corresponding sonoanatomy show the long radiolunate ligament (white arrowheads) (**b**), short radiolunate ligament (white arrows) (**c**), and ulnolunate ligament (black arrows) (**d**) in the long-axis views. S scaphoid; L lunate; TRQ triquetrum; P pisiform; R radius; U ulna

14.3.3 Volar Extrinsic Carpal Ligament Linking to the Triquetrum

The primary extrinsic carpal ligament, connecting to the triquetrum, is known as the ulnotriquetral ligament (Fig. 14.12a), forming the boundary of the triangular fibrocartilage complex. The ligament can be observed by initially positioning the transducer over the distal radioulnar joint. The transducer is then rotated by 90° to intersect the triquetrum along the ulnar side of the pisiform bone. This adjustment allows visualization of the ulnotriquetral ligament spanning between the distal ulna and the triquetrum (Fig. 14.12b).

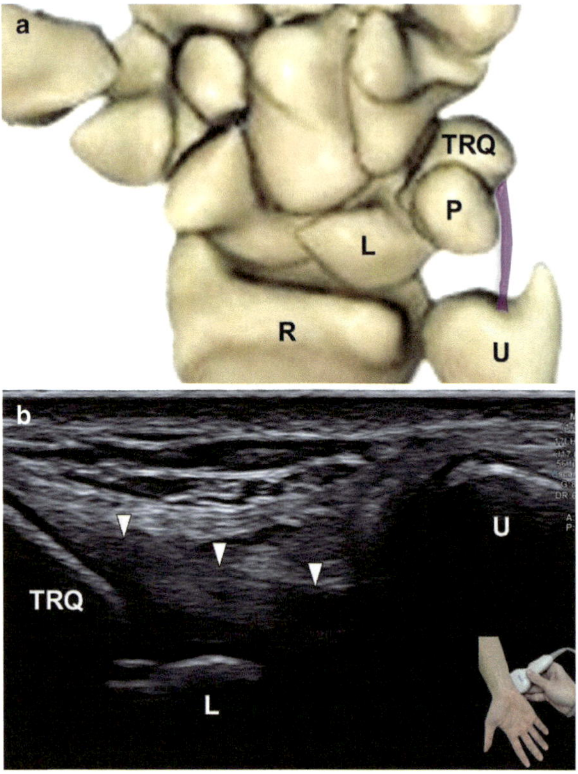

Fig. 14.12 The illustration (**a**) and corresponding sonoanatomy (**b**) depict the ulnotriquetral ligament in the long-axis view. White arrowheads: ulnotriquetral ligament; L lunate; TRQ triquetrum; P pisiform; R radius; U ulna

14.3.4 Volar Intrinsic Carpal Ligaments

We concentrate exclusively on the scapholunate and lunotriquetral ligaments due to their significant clinical relevance (Fig. 14.13a). Therefore, if the examiner can accurately identify the carpal bones, visualizing corresponding intrinsic ligaments such as the volar scapholunate and lunotriquetral ligaments should be relatively straightforward. When aiming to visualize these compact volar intrinsic ligaments, it is vital for the sonographer to align the scanning plane with the joint line, rather than parallel to the wrist crease. Specifically, when examining the scapholunate ligament, the radial end of the transducer should be slightly angled toward the scaphoid tubercle (Fig. 14.13b). Likewise, for imaging the lunotriquetral ligament, the ulnar end of the transducer should be directed toward the pisiform, positioned atop the distal triquetrum (Fig. 14.13c). The scaphotriquetral ligament is another volar intrinsic carpal ligament that spans multiple carpal bones. Its attachment to the scaphoid creates a broad connection. To visualize this ligament, the transducer is positioned near the wrist crease in the axial plane. It is visible connecting the scaphoid tubercle with the triquetrum, tucked beneath the pisiform's shadow, and passing over the capitate and hamate bones (Fig. 14.13d).

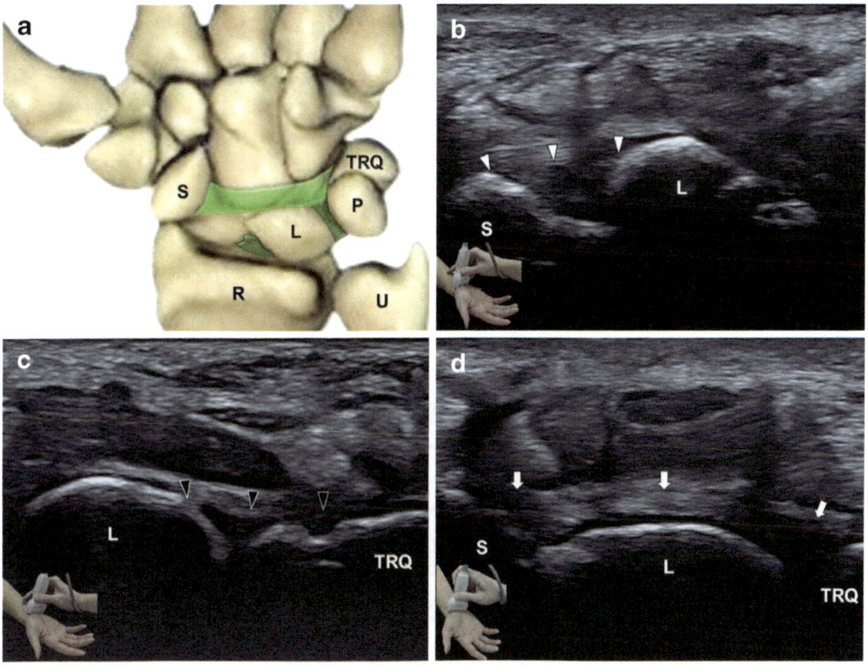

Fig. 14.13 The illustration (**a**) and corresponding sonoanatomy demonstrate the palmar scapholunate ligament (**b**), palmar lunotriquetral ligament (**c**), and palmar scaphotriquetral ligament (**d**) in the long-axis views. White arrowheads: palmar scapholunate ligament; black arrowheads: palmar lunotriquetral ligament; white arrows: palmar scaphotriquetral ligament; S scaphoid; L lunate; TRQ triquetrum; P pisiform; R radius; U ulna

14.3.5 Dorsal Extrinsic Carpal Ligaments

Two dorsal extrinsic carpal ligaments, referred to as the dorsal radiocarpal and dorsal ulnotriquetral ligaments, are attached to the triquetrum (Fig. 14.14a). The former is also known as the dorsal radiolunotriquetral ligament. When scanning, the transducer should be positioned on the distal radius in the axial plane, with the ulnar end pivoted towards the triquetrum. Once the lunate emerges in the center of the screen, the dorsal radial carpal ligament spanning over the distal radius, lunate, and triquetrum can be identified (Fig. 14.14b). To examine the dorsal ulnotriquetral ligament, the transducer is positioned over the distal radioulnar joint in the axial plane, with its midpoint aligned atop the distal ulna. The transducer is subsequently rotated to align with the long axis of the forearm until the triquetrum becomes visible on the screen. The dorsal ulnotriquetral ligament is depicted as a thickened section of the capsule rather than a distinct ligament (Fig. 14.14c).

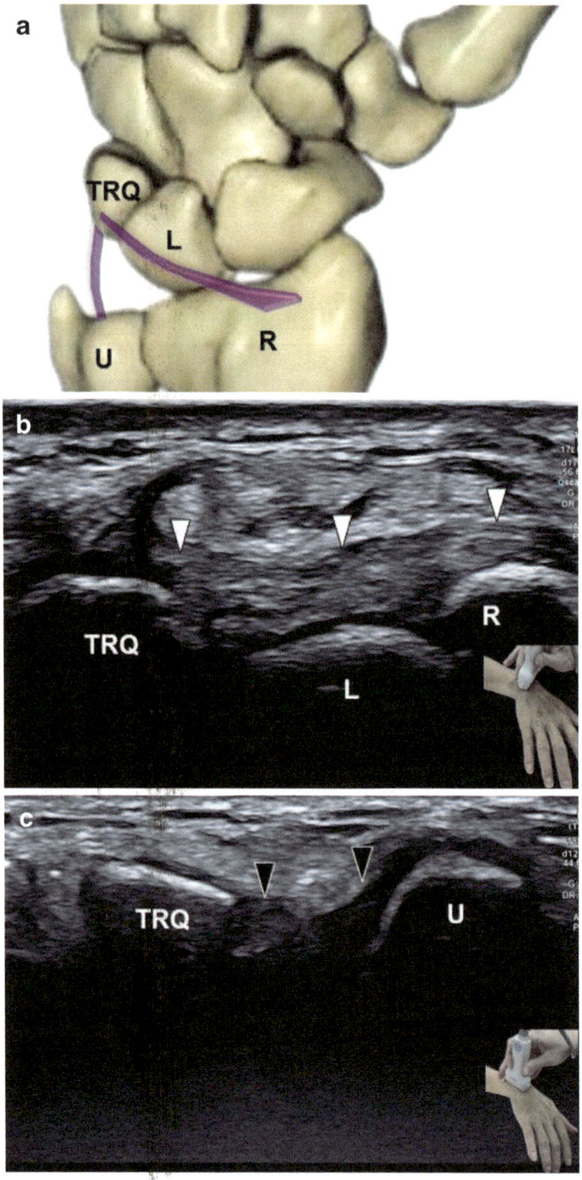

Fig. 14.14 The illustration (**a**) and corresponding sonoanatomy demonstrate the dorsal radiolunotriquetral ligament (white arrowheads) (**b**) and dorsal ulnotriquetral ligament (black arrowheads) (**c**) in the long-axis views. L lunate; TRQ triquetrum; R radius; U ulna

14.3.6 Dorsal Intrinsic Carpal Ligament

The dorsal intrinsic carpal ligaments, such as the dorsal scapholunate and lunotriquetral ligaments (Fig. 14.15a), are positioned between neighboring carpal bones, akin to the examination approach used for the volar intrinsic ligaments. To enhance visualization, a padded support can be utilized to maintain wrist flexion, facilitating clearer observation of these ligaments when they are under tension (Fig. 14.15b, c).

The dorsal intercarpal ligament spans across multiple carpal bones (Fig. 14.16a). The ulnar end of the transducer is initially positioned on the triquetrum in the axial plane. From this position, the ligament's origin from the triquetrum can be visualized as it passes over the lunate, with two bony attachments on its radial side: the proximal band attaching to the scaphoid (Fig. 14.16b) and the distal band attaching to the trapezoid and trapezium (Fig. 14.16c). Both radial attachments can be identified by rotating the radial end of the transducer.

The distal interosseous ligament complexes in the dorsal and palmar regions are located in the distal carpal row between adjacent bones (Fig. 14.17a). After identifying the dorsal scapholunate ligament in the proximal row, the transducer is moved distally to locate the capitate in the axial plane. The transducer is then rotated to align with the long axis of the distal carpal row to visualize the ligaments between the trapezium and trapezoid, trapezoid and capitate, and capitate and hamate (Fig. 14.17b and Fig. 14.17c). To examine the deep interosseous ligament, the transducer can be moved to the central region of the capitate near its head or neck (Fig. 14.17d). Full wrist flexion is recommended to widen the gap between adjacent distal row of carpal bones.

14.3.7 Wrist Collateral Ligament

The wrist possesses collateral ligaments on both its radial and ulnar aspects (Fig. 14.18a). Specifically, the radial collateral ligament serves as a link between the distal radius and the scaphoid bone. To observe this ligament, the transducer is positioned in the coronal plane beneath the first extensor compartment of the dorsal wrist. Originating broadly from the radial aspect, the ligament extends over the scaphoid side. A gentle ulnar deviation of the wrist aids in achieving clearer visualization (Fig. 14.18b). On the other hand, the ulnar collateral ligament connects the distal ulna and the triquetrum. Placing the transducer in the coronal plane, adjacent to the extensor carpal ulnar tendon, allows for its observation, typically situated above the triangular fibrocartilage complex. Slight radial deviation of the wrist facilitates the identification of this ligament (Fig. 14.18c).

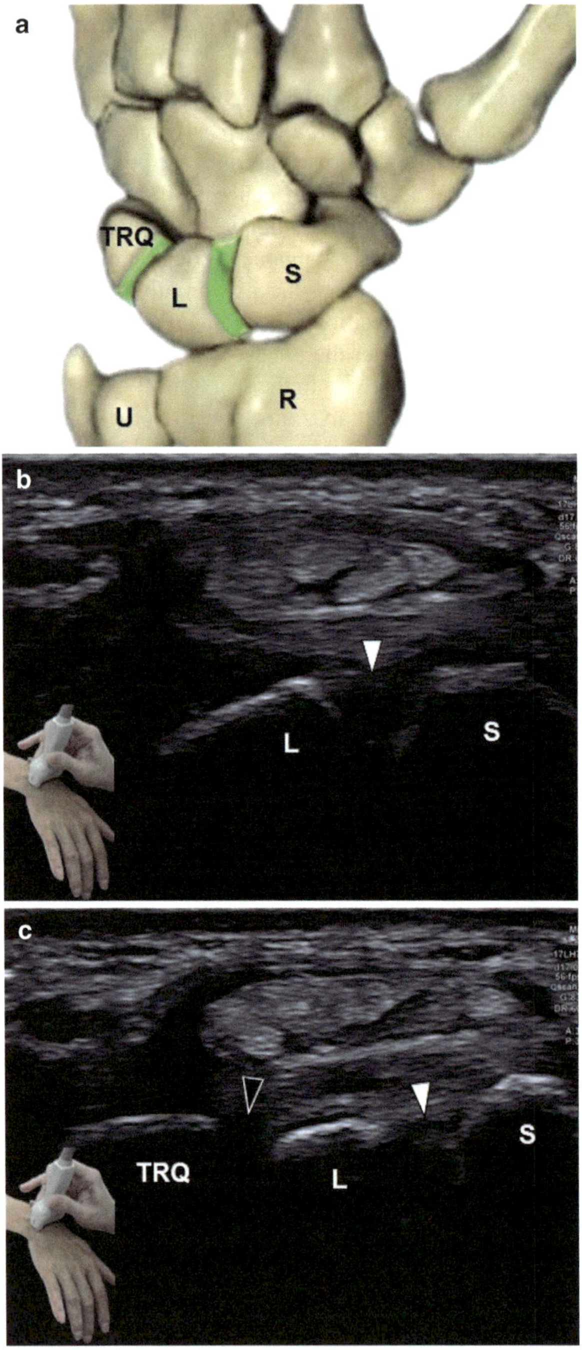

Fig. 14.15 The illustration (**a**) and the corresponding sonoanatomy demonstrate the dorsal scapholunate ligament (white arrowheads) (**b**) and the dorsal lunotriquetral ligament (black arrowhead) (**c**) in the long-axis views. S scaphoid; L lunate; TRQ triquetrum; R radius; U ulna

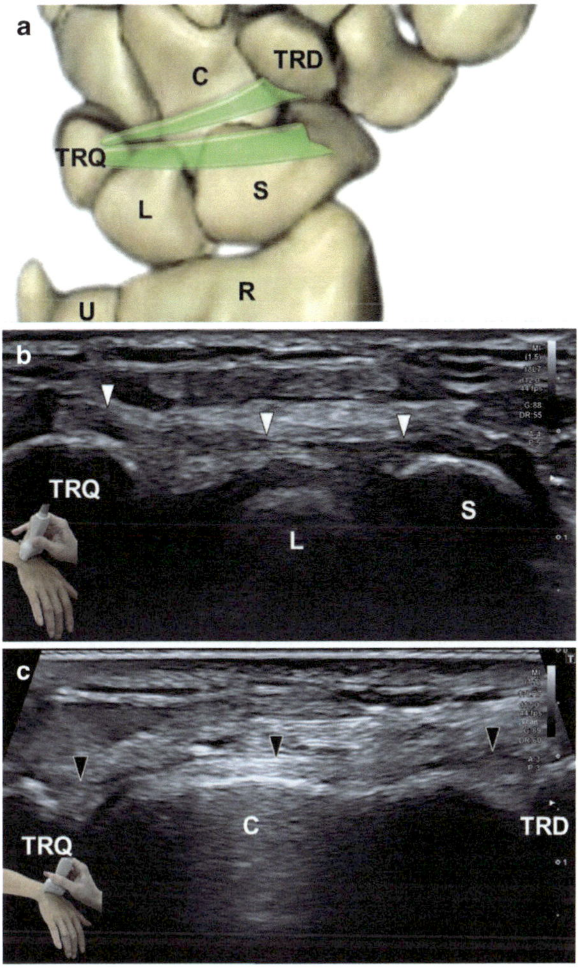

Fig. 14.16 The illustration (**a**) and corresponding sonoanatomy demonstrate the proximal band (white arrowheads) (**b**) and distal band (black arrowheads) (**c**) of the dorsal intercarpal ligaments in the long-axis views. S scaphoid; L lunate; TRQ triquetrum; TRD trapezoid; C capitate; R radius; U ulna

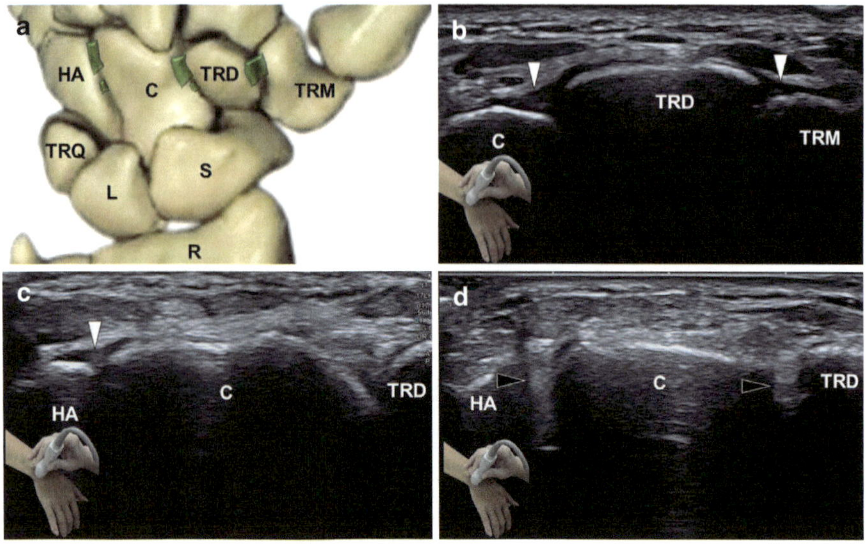

Fig. 14.17 Illustration (**a**) and corresponding sonoanatomy depict the dorsal distal interosseous ligament complexes (white arrowheads) (**b**) between the trapezium, trapezoid, capitate, and hamate (**c**). The deep interosseous portion (black arrowheads) of the dorsal distal interosseous ligament complexes can be observed near the neck or head of the capitate (**d**). TRQ triquetrum; TRM trapezium; TRD trapezoid; C capitate; HA hamate; S scaphoid; L lunate; R radius

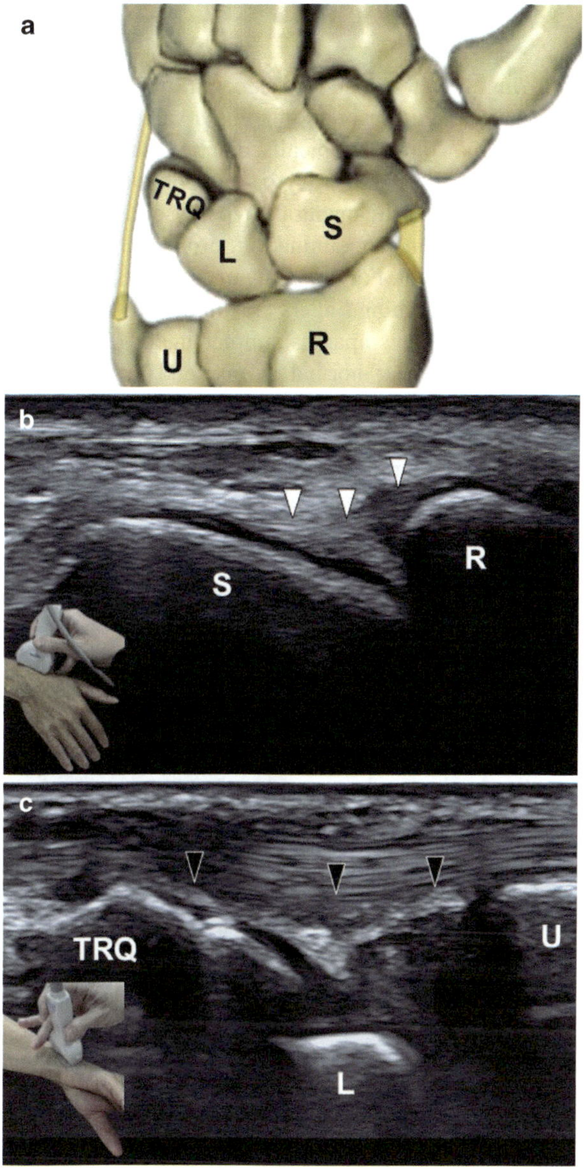

Fig. 14.18 The illustration (**a**) and corresponding sonoanatomy show the radial collateral ligament (white arrowheads) (**b**) and ulnar collateral ligament (black arrowheads) (**c**) in the long-axis views. S scaphoid; L lunate; TRQ triquetrum; R radius; U ulna

14.4 Pathology

Utilizing the ultrasound transducer allows for precise alignment with all wrist ligaments, making ultrasound imaging a valuable tool for exploring wrist pathologies. Wrist sprain injuries typically display thickened, hypoechoic fibers (Fig. 14.19a) with disorganized and wavy patterns on ultrasound images. Power Doppler assists in detecting intra-ligamentous hypervascularity (Fig. 14.19b).

During ligament examination, proper wrist positioning is crucial to tension the targeted ligament. For dorsal ligament inspection, forming a full fist may be beneficial, while stretching fingers aids in palmar ligament scanning. Telling normal and sprained ligaments apart is simpler under tensile stress. Moreover, sprained ligaments may appear normal at one end but abnormal at the other (Fig. 14.20). Traumatic incidents often lead to wrist ligament tears, with complete tears indicated by the absence of ligament fibers and effusion filling the gap (Fig. 14.21a). Conversely, incomplete, or partial-thickness tears present with ligament thinning and intra-ligamentous hypoechogenicity (Fig. 14.21b).

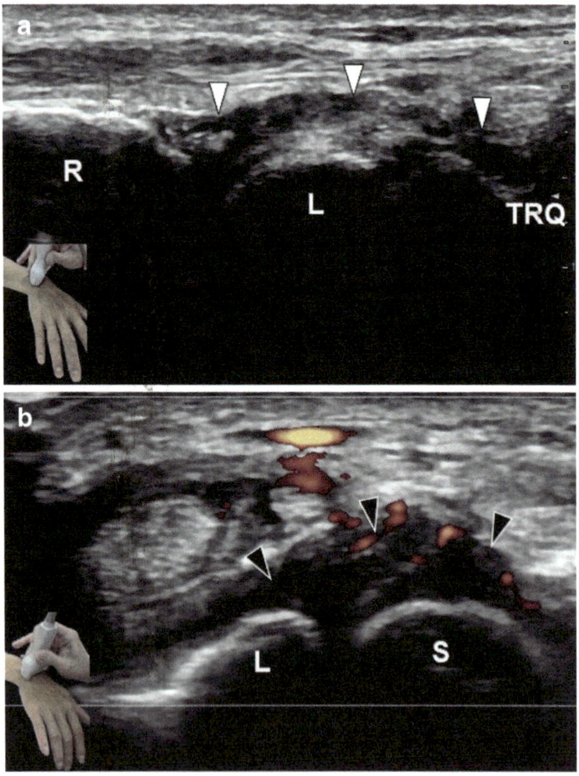

Fig. 14.19 The ultrasound image shows thickening and hypoechoic fibers of the dorsal radiolunotriquetral ligament (white arrowheads) (**a**). In another case (**b**), the ultrasound image demonstrates hypervascularity on power Doppler, indicating inflammation of the dorsal scapholunate ligament (black arrowheads). L lunate; TRQ triquetrum; R radius; S scaphoid

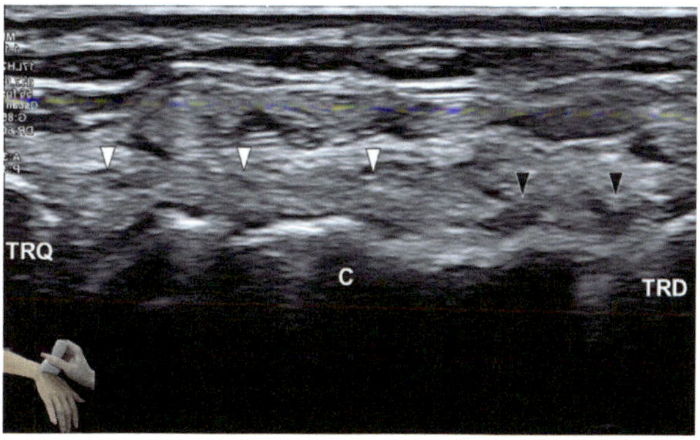

Fig. 14.20 The ultrasound image reveals a normal fibrillar pattern at the triquetral end (white arrowhead), but an abnormal pattern is observed at the trapezoid end (black arrowhead) of the distal band of the dorsal intercarpal ligament. TRQ triquetrum; C capitate, TRD trapezoid

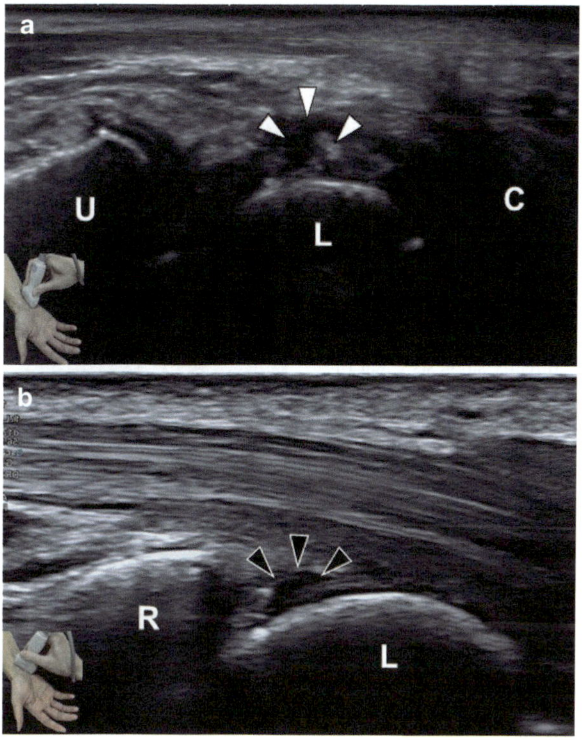

Fig. 14.21 The ultrasound image demonstrates hypoechoic swelling and complete fiber discontinuity with a visible gap, indicating a full-thickness tear (white arrowheads) of the ulnocapitate ligament (**a**). Another image reveals a partial-thickness tear (black arrowheads) of the short radiolunate ligament (**b**). L lunate; C capitate; R radius; U ulna

Presence of bony chips within the joint space suggests a previous avulsion injury (Fig. 14.22). Widening of the joint space during dynamic stress testing indirectly indicates ligament tear (before ulnar deviation, Fig. 14.23a; after ulnar deviation, Fig. 14.23b). Additionally, ganglion cysts (Fig. 14.24), common in wrist pathologies, present as encapsulated anechoic fluid accumulation near wrist carpal ligaments, potentially involving underlying joints. Unlike effusion, ganglion cysts typically are not compressible. The dorsal wrist recess effusion [7], which may arise

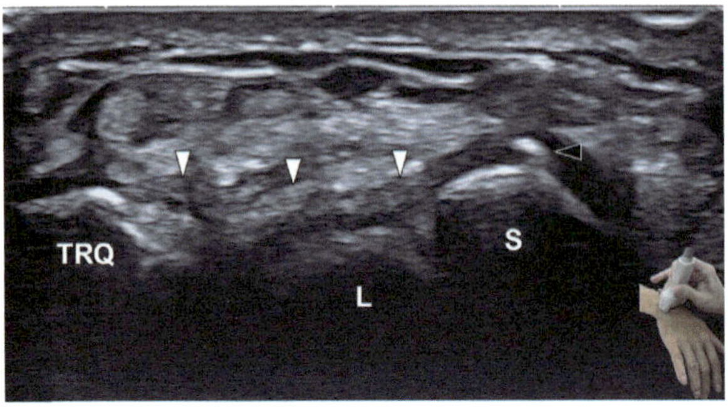

Fig. 14.22 The ultrasound image shows a hyperechoic plaque on the top of the scaphoid (black arrowhead), indicating an avulsion injury of the proximal band of the dorsal intercarpal ligaments. White arrowheads: proximal band of the dorsal intercarpal ligament; S scaphoid; L lunate; TRQ triquetrum

Fig. 14.23 The static ultrasound image of the dorsal scapholunate ligament (**a**) is compared to the dynamic examination image obtained during ulnar deviation (**b**). The widening of the joint space during ulnar deviation indirectly suggests a tear of the ligament. White arrowheads: dorsal scapholunate ligament; S scaphoid; L lunate

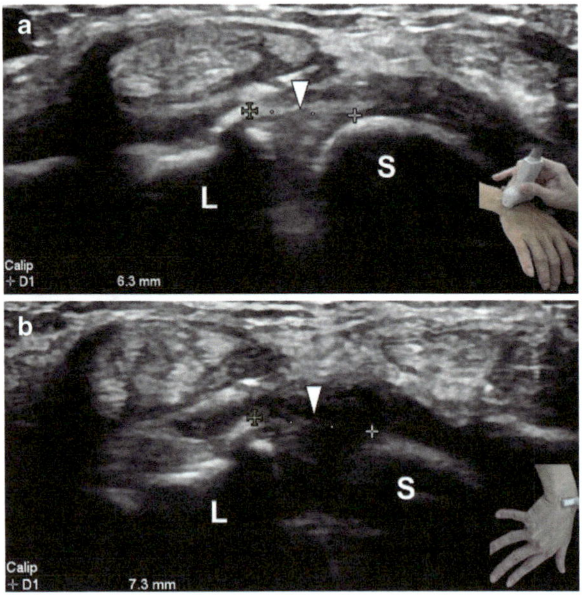

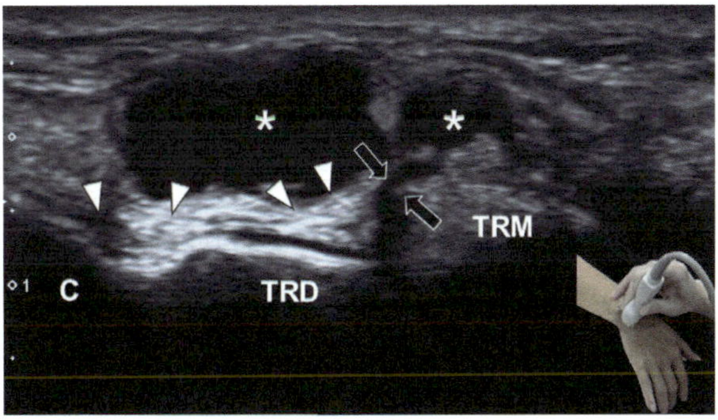

Fig. 14.24 The ultrasound image of the dorsal distal interosseous ligament complex (white arrowheads) reveals an anechoic lesion with a stalk (black arrows) extending to the trapeziotrapezoid joint, indicating the presence of a ganglion cyst (asterisks). TRM trapezium; TRD trapezoid; C capitate

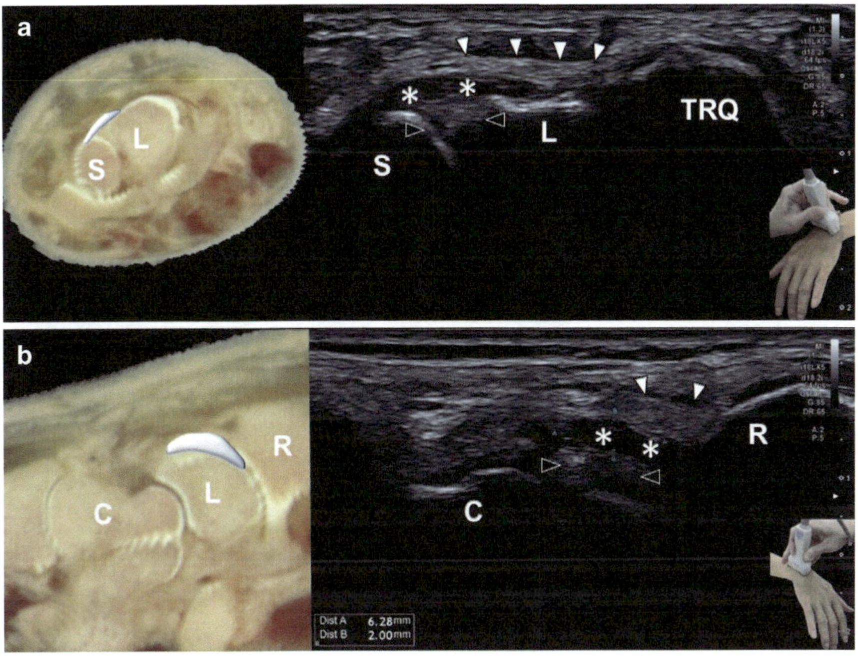

Fig. 14.25 Modified cadaveric illustration and ultrasound images demonstrate the dorsal wrist recess effusion (light blue shade and asterisks) in axial (**a**) and longitudinal (**b**) views. White arrowheads: dorsal radiolunotriquetral ligament; black arrowheads: dorsal scapholunate ligament; S scaphoid; L lunate; C capitate; R radius; TRQ triquetrum

from the joint space between the radiocarpal or midcarpal joints, can mimic a ganglion cyst. However, dorsal wrist recess effusion is significantly more compressible than a ganglion cyst. On a short-axis ultrasound image, the effusion from the radiocarpal joint can be observed dissecting between the dorsal radiocarpal ligament and the proximal row of carpal bones (Fig. 14.25a). On a long-axis ultrasound image, extension of the effusion toward the capitate can be seen (Fig. 14.25b).

14.5 Ultrasound-Guided Injection

For acute sprain injuries, ultrasound imaging may reveal hypervascularity (Fig. 14.26a). In such cases, a low-dose corticosteroid, such as 10 mg triamcinolone, can be injected adjacent to the ligament. Conversely, for partial or full-thickness ligament tears, high-concentration dextrose or platelet-rich plasma can be administered using the peppering injection technique directly into the ligament. A hockey-stick transducer facilitates an in-plane approach for injections in the wrist region (Fig. 14.26b). However, nerve injury is a potential risk during injection. For instance, before injecting the volar wrist ligament and dorsal wrist ligament, it is important to locate the median nerve and its branches [8], as well as the dorsal ulnar cutaneous nerve and superficial radial nerve [9]. On the contrary, the posterior interosseous nerve can be observed over the dorsal intercarpal ligament, serving as a target for nerve blocks in patients experiencing dorsal wrist pain [10].

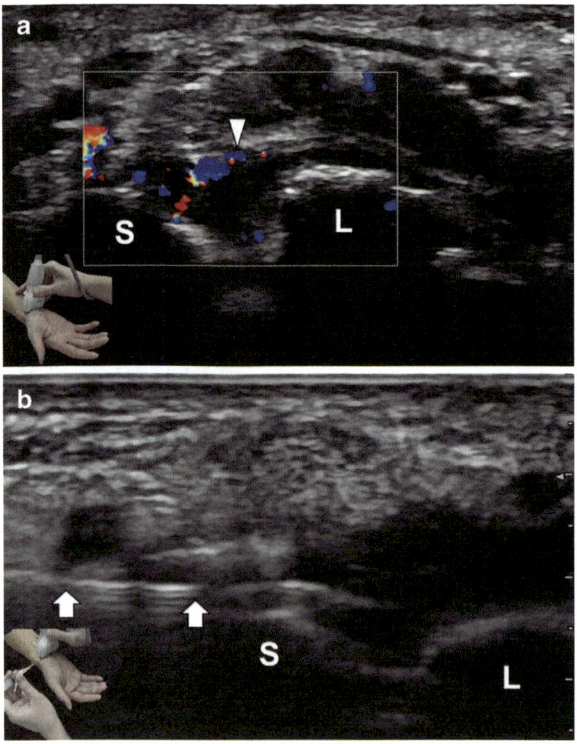

Fig. 14.26 The ultrasound image shows hypervascularity of the palmar scapholunate ligament (white arrowhead) (**a**), along with the guided injection performed using the in-plane approach (**b**). White arrows: needle; S scaphoid; L lunate

14.6 Conclusion

Wrist ligaments are intricate structures, necessitating a systematic approach for thorough examination of their pathology. A crucial step in assessing wrist ligament integrity involves placing the ligament under tension. During ultrasound-guided injections, employing a hockey-stick transducer facilitates the in-plane approach, thereby aiding in the avoidance of inadvertent nerve injury.

Acknowledgments Images and illustrations adapted from cadaveric images provided by the Visible Human Project® of the National Library of Medicine. Excerpts featured in the VH Dissector are used with permission from Touch of Life Technologies Inc.

References

1. Bateni CP, Bartolotta RJ, Richardson ML, Mulcahy H, Allan CH. Imaging key wrist ligaments: what the surgeon needs the radiologist to know. AJR Am J Roentgenol. 2013;200(5):1089–95.
2. Berger RA. The anatomy of the ligaments of the wrist and distal radioulnar joints. Clin Orthop Relat Res. 2001;383:32–40.
3. Özçakar L, Kara M, Chang KV, et al. EURO-MUSCULUS/USPRM basic scanning protocols for wrist and hand. Eur J Phys Rehabil Med. 2015;51(4):479–84.
4. Johnston RB, Seiler JG, Miller EJ, Drvaric DM. The intrinsic and extrinsic ligaments of the wrist. A correlation of collagen typing and histologic appearance. J Hand Surg Br. 1995;20(6):750–4.
5. Falsetti P, Conticini E, Baldi C, et al. Ultrasound evaluation of the scapholunate ligament and scapholunate joint space in patients with wrist complaints in a rheumatologic setting. J Ultrason. 2021;21(85):e105–e11.
6. Wang J-C, Wu W-T, Chang K-V, Chen L-R, Nakashima Y, Özçakar L. Sonoanatomy and step-wise/systematic ultrasound examination of the extrinsic/intrinsic wrist ligaments. Diagnostics. 2021;11(10):1834.
7. Laurell L, Court-Payen M, Nielsen S, Zak M, Fasth A. Ultrasonography and color Doppler in juvenile idiopathic arthritis: diagnosis and follow-up of ultrasound-guided steroid injection in the wrist region. A descriptive interventional study. Pediatr Rheumatol Online J. 2012;10:11.
8. Wu CH, Chang KV, Özçakar L, et al. Sonographic tracking of the upper limb peripheral nerves: a pictorial essay and video demonstration. Am J Phys Med Rehabil. 2015;94(9):740–7.
9. Chang KV, Mezian K, Naňka O, et al. Ultrasound imaging for the cutaneous nerves of the extremities and relevant entrapment syndromes: from anatomy to clinical implications. J Clin Med. 2018;7(11):457.
10. Smith J, Rizzo M, Finnoff JT, Sayeed YA, Michaud J, Martinoli C. Sonographic appearance of the posterior interosseous nerve at the wrist. J Ultrasound Med. 2011;30(9):1233–9.

Chapter 15
Finger Pain Beyond Stenosing Tenosynovitis

Ke-Vin Chang, Wei-Ting Wu, and Shao-Yu Chi

15.1 Introduction

Hand injuries represent a common occurrence, particularly among athletes [1]. Among the myriad of injuries, involvement of the collateral ligaments of the metacarpophalangeal and interphalangeal joints is frequently encountered. Additionally, trigger finger [2], a pathological condition affecting the digital pulleys and flexor tendons, presents a notable challenge. Preceded by pain and joint stiffness, the triggering phenomenon adds complexity to its diagnosis and management. Furthermore, in patients with rheumatoid arthritis, tendon tears can lead to various hand deformities, such as the Boutonniere deformity [3]. Another well-known condition, "Boxer's knuckle" [4], prevalent among boxers, typically results from clenched-fist trauma, primarily affecting the third metacarpal head. Its pathology involves tears of the sagittal bands of the dorsal hood and associated extensor tendon instability. Given the diverse nature of finger disorders, precise imaging diagnosis becomes imperative. Capitalizing on its superior visualization of superficial structures, ultrasound has emerged as a preferred modality for diagnosing finger disorders. This chapter aims to explore the sonoanatomy of the extensor/flexor tendons of the fingers, along with the associated connective tissue structures such as the sagittal band and annular pulley. Additionally, common pathologies like trigger finger will be elucidated through ultrasound findings, along with insights into ultrasound-guided injection techniques for its management.

K.-V. Chang (✉) · W.-T. Wu · S.-Y. Chi
Bei-Hu Branch, National Taiwan University Hospital, Taipei, Taiwan

K.-V. Chang (ed.), *Ultrasonography of Musculoskeletal Pain*,
https://doi.org/10.1007/978-981-96-6787-1_15

15.2 Anatomy

15.2.1 Pulley System

The pulleys, fibrous retinacula found along the volar aspect of the phalanges, play a vital role in stabilizing the flexor tendons of both the thumb and fingers. This system encompasses annular and cruciform pulleys. Annular pulleys secure the flexor tendons onto the volar phalanges, preventing radial or ulnar displacement and volar bowstringing. They are designated sequentially from proximal to distal as A1 to A5 [5] (Fig. 15.1). The cruciform pulleys, situated between neighboring annular pulleys, consist of intersecting fibers that are pliable, facilitating interphalangeal joint flexion. The arrangement of pulleys follows the sequence: A1, A2, C1, A3, C2, A4, C3, and A5, from proximal to distal. In the thumb, the pulley system comprises the A1 and A2 annular pulleys, located at the level of the metacarpophalangeal joint and

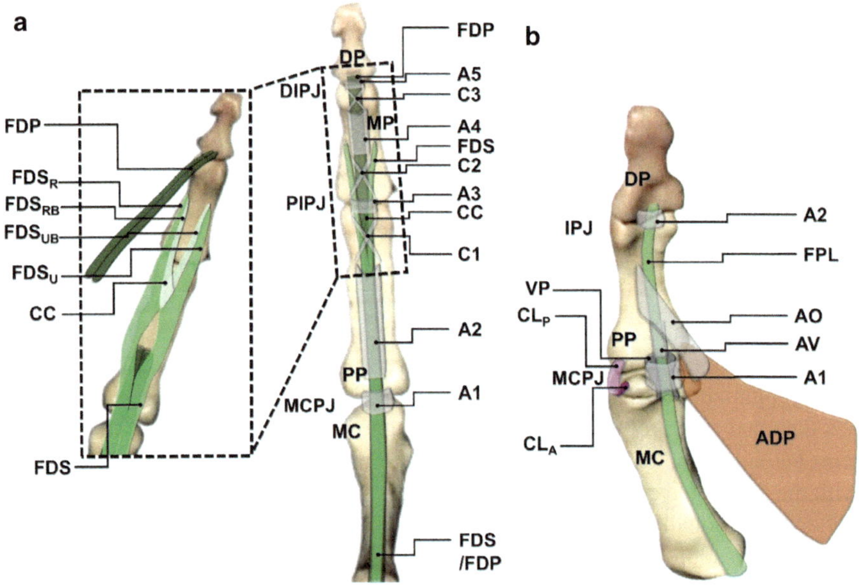

Fig. 15.1 The illustration of the pulley system of the finger (**a**) and the thumb (**b**), along with the nearby flexor tendons and collateral ligaments. A1-A5 the annular pulleys of A1 to A5; C1-C3 the cruciform pulleys of C1 to C3; FDP flexor digitorum profundus tendon; FDS flexor digitorum superficialis tendon; FDS_R radial bundle of the flexor digitorum superficialis tendon; FDS_U ulnar bundle of the flexor digitorum superficialis tendon; FDS_{RB} radial branch of the ulnar bundle of the flexor digitorum superficialis tendon; FDS_{UB} ulnar branch of the radial bundle of the flexor digitorum superficialis tendon; FPL flexor pollicis longus tendon; ADP adductor pollicis; DIPJ distal interphalangeal joint; DP distal phalanx; IPJ interphalangeal joint of the thumb; MC metacarpal bone; MCPJ metacarpophalangeal joint; PP proximal phalanx; PIPJ proximal interphalangeal joint; MP middle phalanx; AO oblique pulley of the thumb; AV variable pulley of the thumb; CC Camper's chiasm; CL_P proper collateral ligament; CL_A accessory collateral ligament; VP volar plate

just proximal to the interphalangeal joint [6]. Additionally, there is an oblique pulley spanning from ulnar proximal to radial distal across the proximal phalanx, positioned between A1 and A2. On the other hand, the variable pulley of the thumb is a pulley structure within the thumb's flexor tendon sheath that can vary in its presence, form, and exact anatomical location. It is often formed by the aponeurosis of the adductor pollicis muscle and serves to stabilize and redirect the flexor pollicis longus tendon, which allows smooth flexion of the thumb.

15.2.2 Finger Flexors and Supporting Systems

At the level of the wrist and hand, the flexor digitorum superficialis tendons lie volar to the flexor digitorum profundus tendons. In the fingers, the flexor digitorum superficialis tendons diverge at the midpoint of the proximal phalanges to allow the flexor digitorum profundus tendons to pass. At the proximal interphalangeal joint, the two slips of each flexor digitorum superficialis tendon merge beneath the flexor digitorum profundus tendon, forming the Camper's chiasm [7]. The flexor digitorum superficialis tendons attach to the middle phalanx, while the flexor digitorum profundus tendons attach to the distal phalanx (Fig. 15.1).

The volar plates are situated on the palmar side of the metacarpophalangeal joint and the interphalangeal joints, serving to strengthen the joint capsule and prevent excessive joint hyperextension [11]. At its wider distal insertion onto the palmar base of the proximal phalanx, the volar plate is fibrocartilaginous, while its proximal attachment to the neck of the metacarpophalangeal joint is membranous. The checkrein ligaments are extensions of the volar plate that attach to the proximal phalanx, reinforcing the volar plate and further limiting hyperextension. Vincula brevia and vincula longa are small bands that anchor the flexor tendons to the phalanges in the fingers. They carry blood vessels that supply the tendons, which otherwise have limited blood flow. Vincula brevia are shorter and closer to the tendon insertions, while vincula longa are longer and located further from the insertions (Fig. 15.2).

15.2.3 Finger Extensors and Supporting Systems

The extensor digitorum communis tendon demonstrates distinct anatomical characteristics proximal to the proximal interphalangeal joint, with its three portions serving specific functions. Close to the proximal interphalangeal joint, the tendon splits into three segments [8] (Fig. 15.3). The central portion forms the central slip, which attaches to the middle phalanx. The lateral portions of the tendon join the intrinsic tendons of the lumbrical muscles and interosseous muscles, contributing to the formation of the lateral bands. These lateral bands converge over the middle phalanx

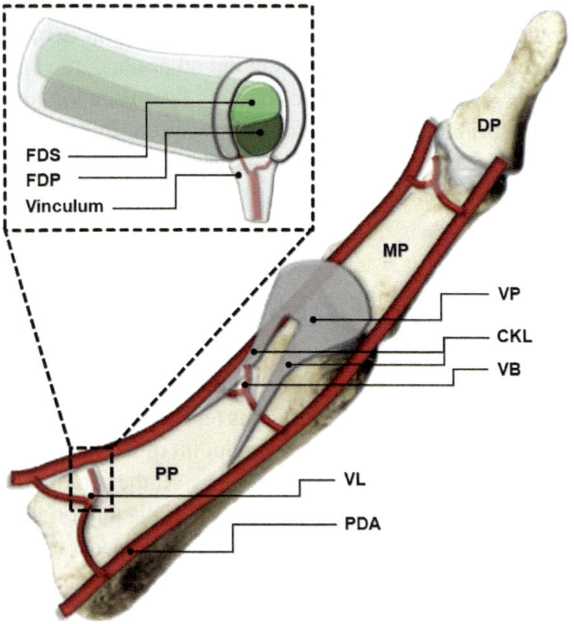

Fig. 15.2 The illustration of the volar plate, checkrein ligaments, vincula longa and vincula brevia. CKL checkrein ligament; DP distal phalanx; FDP flexor digitorum profundus tendon; FDS flexor digitorum superficialis tendon; MP middle phalanx; PP proximal phalanx; VB vincula brevia; VL vincula longa; VP volar plate; PDA proper digital artery

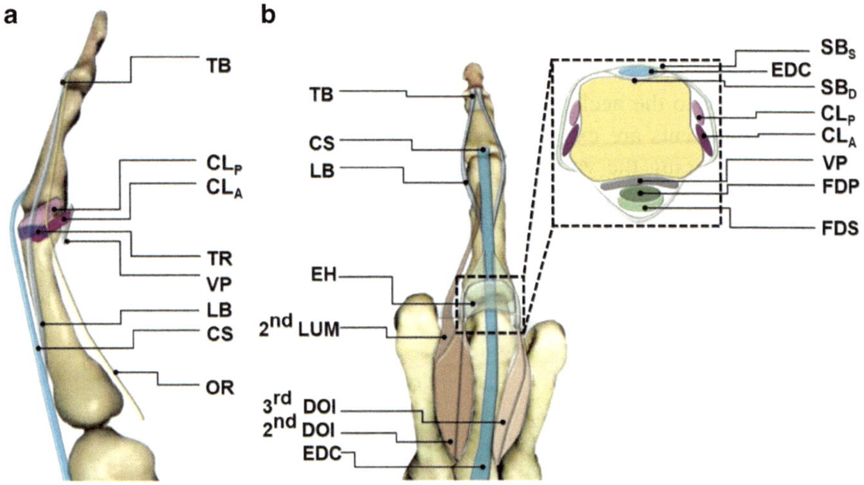

Fig. 15.3 The illustration of the extensor tendons of the fingers and nearby collateral ligaments of the finger (**a**), and the illustration of the extensor hood, nearby muscles, tendons, and associated ligamentous structures (**b**). CL_A accessory collateral ligament; CL_P proper collateral ligament; CS central slip of the extensor tendon; DOI dorsal interosseous muscle; EDC extensor digitorum communis tendon; EH extensor hood; FDP flexor digitorum profundus tendon; FDS flexor digitorum superficialis tendon; LB lateral band; LUM lumbrical muscle; TB terminal band; VP volar plate; SB_D the deep band of the sagittal band; SB_S the superficial band of the sagittal band; TR transverse retinaculum; OR oblique retinaculum

and extend dorsally over the distal interphalangeal joint, ultimately inserting into the distal phalanx, thus forming the terminal band (Fig. 15.3).

The extensor indicis proprius or extensor digiti minimi tendons, located on the dorsal aspect of the 2nd or 5th digit, are situated ulnar to the extensor digitorum communis tendon (Fig. 15.4). Unlike the extensor digitorum communis tendon, both the extensor indicis proprius and the extensor digiti minimi tendons do not attach distally to bone. Instead, they insert with variability onto the ulnar side of the extensor hood of either the 2nd or 5th finger, typically around the level of the proximal phalanx [9]. However, in the case of the 3rd and 4th digits, only a single extensor digitorum communis tendon is present.

The sagittal bands are pivotal components of the dorsal hood, serving to centrally position the extensor digitorum communis tendon at the metacarpophalangeal joint (Fig. 15.3) [10]. This positioning plays a crucial role in preventing excessive excursion, bowstringing, and subluxation of the extensor pollicis longus, extensor digitorum communis, extensor indicis proprius, and extensor digiti minimi tendons during digital extension. Extending from the radial and ulnar margins of the extensor tendon to the volar plate and deep transverse metacarpal ligament, these bands offer indispensable structural support.

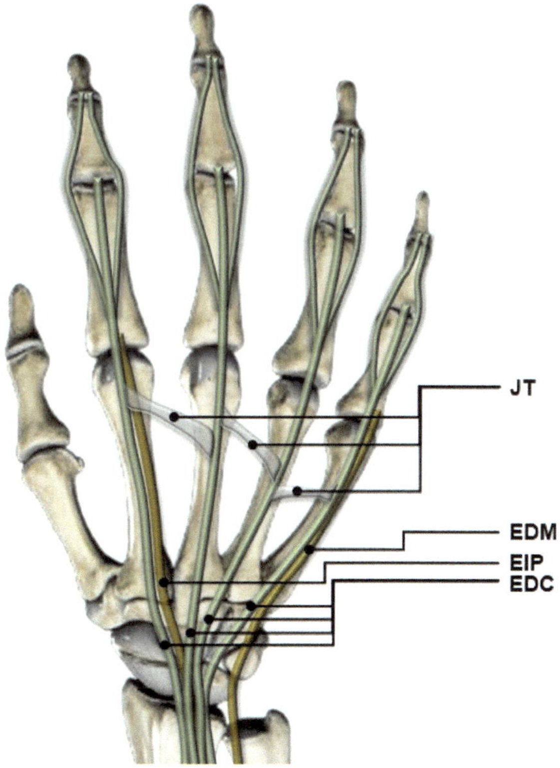

Fig. 15.4 The illustration of the association of extensor indicis proprius, extensor digitorum communis, extensor digiti minimi tendons, and the juncturae tendinae. EDC extensor digitorum communis tendon; EDM extensor digiti minimi tendon; EIP extensor indicis proprius tendon; JT juncturae tendinae

Located just cranial to the 2nd to 5th dorsal metacarpophalangeal joints, the extensor digitorum communis tendons are interconnected by juncturae tendinae [13]. These juncturae tendinae comprise fibrotic bands that extend both horizontally and obliquely between the extensor tendons in the 2nd, 3rd, and 4th dorsal inter-metacarpal spaces. Their function includes realigning the force exerted by the extensor digitorum communis, extensor indicis proprius, and extensor digiti minimi tendons, alleviating undue loads on the sagittal bands, and aiding in the stabilization of the metacarpophalangeal joint.

15.2.4 *Finger Supporting Ligaments*

The deep transverse metacarpal ligament connects the volar plates of the metacarpophalangeal joints of the 2nd to 5th digits horizontally (Fig. 15.5), thereby securing the stability of the transverse metacarpal arch. Its role in preventing the metacarpal heads from separating enhances grip strength. Furthermore, it

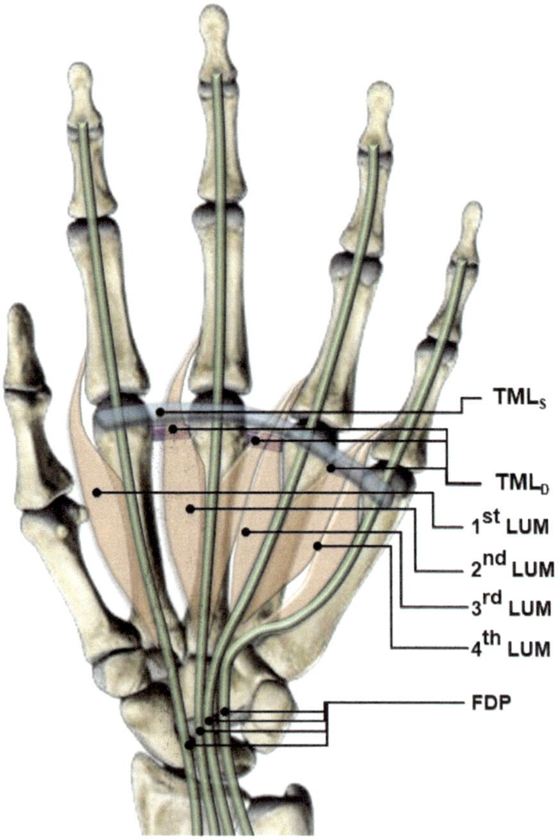

Fig. 15.5 The illustration of the lumbrical muscles and the superficial and deep transverse metacarpal ligaments. TML$_D$ deep transverse metacarpal ligament; TML$_S$ superficial transverse metacarpal ligament; FDP flexor digitorum profundus tendons; LUM lumbrical muscles

synergizes with the accessory collateral ligaments, supporting hand stability and dexterity. By contrast, the superficial transverse metacarpal ligament is a fibrous band located just beneath the palmar skin, connecting the palmar aponeurosis across the heads of the metacarpals and providing stability to the superficial structures of the palm.

On the other hand, for the 2nd to 5th fingers, the ulnar and radial collateral ligaments originate from the medial and lateral tubercles of the metacarpal condyles, respectively. These ligaments are further divided into the proper collateral ligament and the accessory collateral ligament. The proper collateral ligament attaches directly to the proximal phalanx, whereas the accessory collateral ligament extends to the volar plate (Fig. 15.3) [11]. The ulnar (Fig. 15.6) and radial (Fig. 15.7) proper collateral ligaments of the first metacarpophalangeal joint connect the metacarpal bone to the base of the proximal phalanx, while the accessory collateral ligament connects to the sesamoid bone. These ligaments are obliquely covered by the aponeurosis of the abductor pollicis brevis and the adductor pollicis, respectively.

15.2.5 *Intrinsic Hand Muscles*

Regarding the intrinsic hand muscles relating to finger motions, the lumbrical muscles are four muscles that originate from the tendons of the flexor digitorum profundus and insert into the extensor hoods of the index, middle, ring, and little fingers. The 1st and 2nd lumbrical muscles have a unipennate structure, whereas the 3rd and

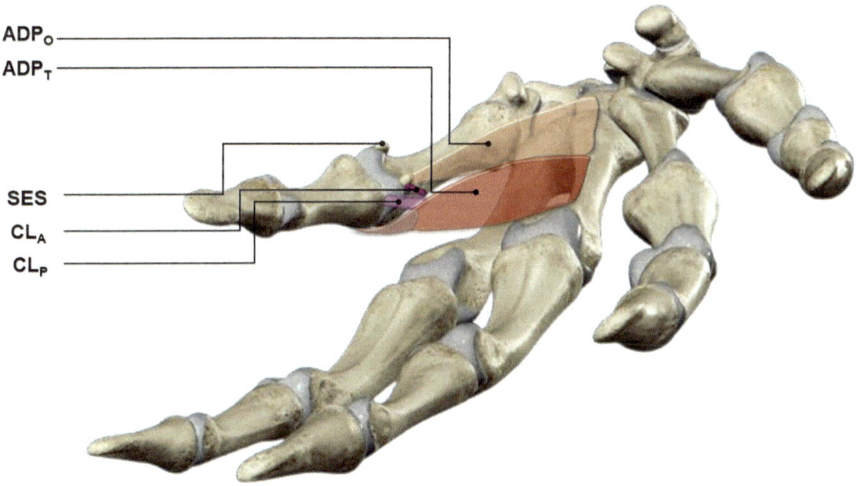

Fig. 15.6 The illustration of the ulnar collateral ligaments of the first metacarpophalangeal joint and their association with the adductor pollicis muscle. ADP$_O$ oblique head of the adductor pollicis muscle; ADP$_T$ transverse head of the adductor pollicis muscle; CL$_A$ accessory collateral ligament; CL$_P$ proper collateral ligament; SES sesamoid

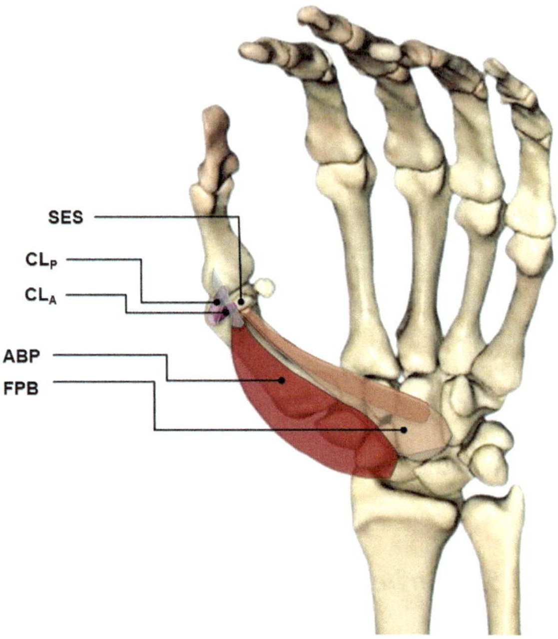

Fig. 15.7 The illustration of the radial collateral ligaments of the first metacarpophalangeal joint and their association with the abductor pollicis brevis. ABP abductor pollicis brevis; FPB flexor pollicis brevis; CL_A accessory collateral ligament; CL_P proper collateral ligament; SES sesamoid

4th are bipennate. These muscles facilitate flexion at the metacarpophalangeal joints while extending the interphalangeal joints (Fig. 15.5).

The adductor pollicis consists of two heads: the transverse and oblique (Fig. 15.6). The transverse head originates from the 3rd metacarpal, while the oblique head originates from the capitate and the bases of the 2nd and 3rd metacarpals. Both heads insert onto the base of the proximal phalanx and the extensor hood of the thumb. This muscle is responsible for thumb adduction.

The dorsal interosseous muscles comprise four muscles that originate from the metacarpals and insert into the extensor hood and the bases of the proximal phalanges of the index, middle, and ring fingers (Fig. 15.8a). They are responsible for abducting the index, middle, and ring fingers at the metacarpophalangeal joints. The palmar interosseous muscles consist of four muscles, originating from the metacarpals and inserting into the extensor hoods of the thumb, index, ring, and little fingers, though the muscle on the thumb is commonly absent (Fig. 15.8b). These muscles facilitate the adduction of the thumb, index, ring, and little fingers at the metacarpophalangeal joints.

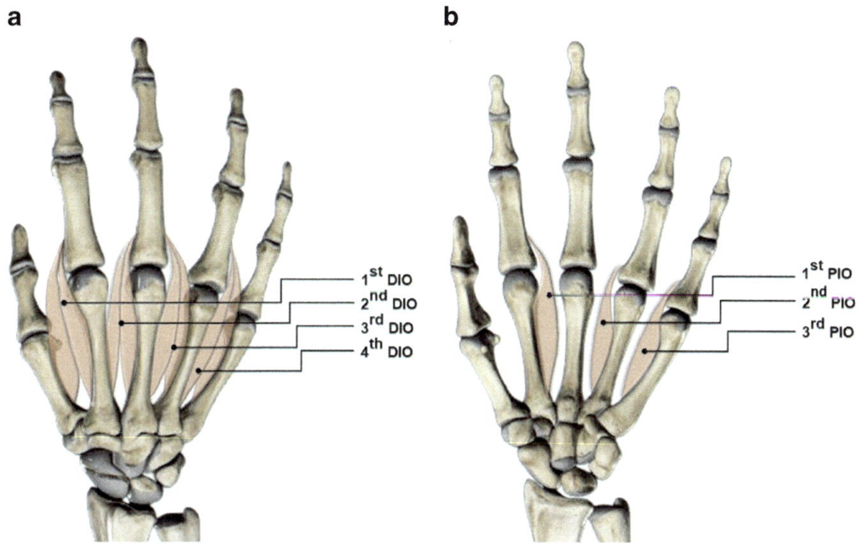

Fig. 15.8 The illustration of the 4 dorsal interosseous (**a**) and 3 palmar interosseous muscles (**b**). Note: The commonly absent palmar interosseous muscle inserting on the thumb is not depicted in the illustration. DIO dorsal interosseous muscle; PIO palmar interosseous muscle

15.3 Sonoanatomy

15.3.1 Volar Aspect

The transducer is positioned horizontally, intersecting the metacarpal heads of the 2nd to 5th digits on the palm side, providing a view of the cross-sections of both the flexor digitorum superficialis and flexor digitorum profundus tendons [12]. Adjacent to the flexor tendons of the 2nd digit, or located between the 2nd and 3rd, 3rd and 4th, and 4th and 5th digits, are the lumbrical muscles. The 1st and 2nd lumbrical muscles exhibit a unipennate arrangement (Fig. 15.9a), while the 3rd and 4th lumbrical muscles demonstrate a bipennate structure (Fig. 15.9b). The transducer is then rotated to align with the long axis of the lumbrical muscle, allowing visualization of its origin alongside the tendons of the flexor digitorum profundus (Fig. 15.9c) and its insertion into the extensor hoods of the fingers (Fig. 15.9d).

The common digital arteries and nerves are superficial to the lumbrical muscles. Beneath the finger flexor tendons lie the volar plates, connected by the deep transverse metacarpal ligaments. Deep to the volar plate lies the metacarpal head, while beneath the deep transverse metacarpal ligaments are the palmar and dorsal interosseous muscles (Fig. 15.10).

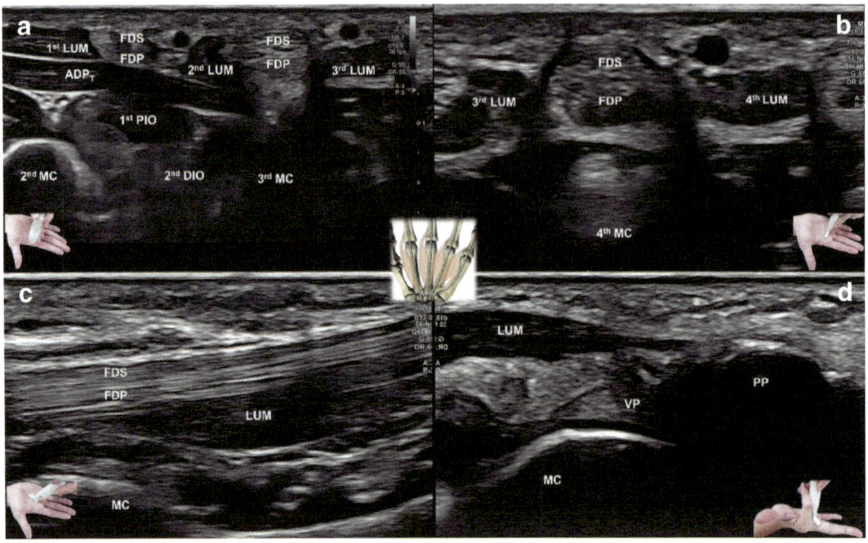

Fig. 15.9 The sonoanatomy of the lumbrical muscles shows a unipennate structure for the 1st and 2nd lumbrical muscles (**a**) and a bipennate structure for the 3rd and 4th lumbrical muscles (**b**) in the short axis. In the long axis, the lumbrical muscles originate adjacent to the tendons of the flexor digitorum profundus (**c**) and insert into the extensor hoods of the fingers (**d**). ADP$_T$ transverse head of the adductor pollicis muscle; PIO palmar interosseous muscle; DIO dorsal interosseous muscle; FDS flexor digitorum superficialis tendon; FDP flexor digitorum profundus tendon; LUM lumbrical muscle; MC metacarpal bone; PP proximal phalanx; VP volar plate

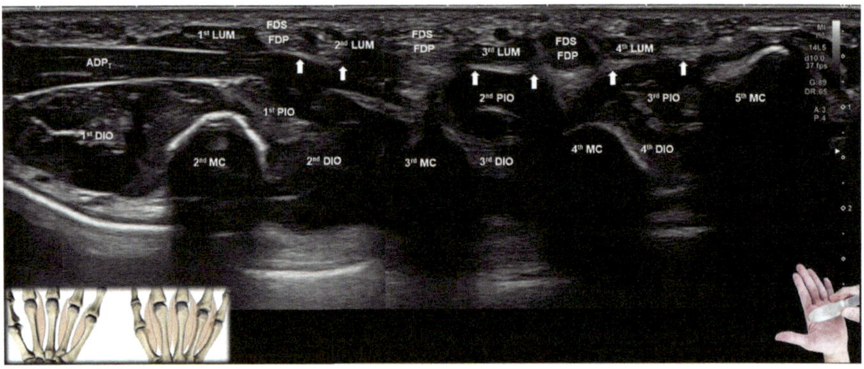

Fig. 15.10 The sonoanatomy of the interosseous muscles in the short axis of the palm, along with the deep transverse metacarpal ligament (white arrows). ADP$_T$ transverse head of the adductor pollicis muscle; PIO palmar interosseous muscle; DIO dorsal interosseous muscle; FDS flexor digitorum superficialis tendon; FDP flexor digitorum profundus tendon; LUM lumbrical muscle; MC metacarpal bone

Distally, the volar plates of the proximal interphalangeal joint are connected by thin bands known as checkrein ligaments, which become more prominent in the presence of joint effusion. These paired, cord-like ligaments contribute to the stability of the proximal interphalangeal joint. They originate from the periosteum of the proximal phalanx at the level of the A2 and C1 pulleys and insert into the volar plate. Dynamic movements, such as extension (Fig. 15.11a) and flexion (Fig. 15.11b), aid in visualizing the checkrein ligaments using ultrasound imaging.

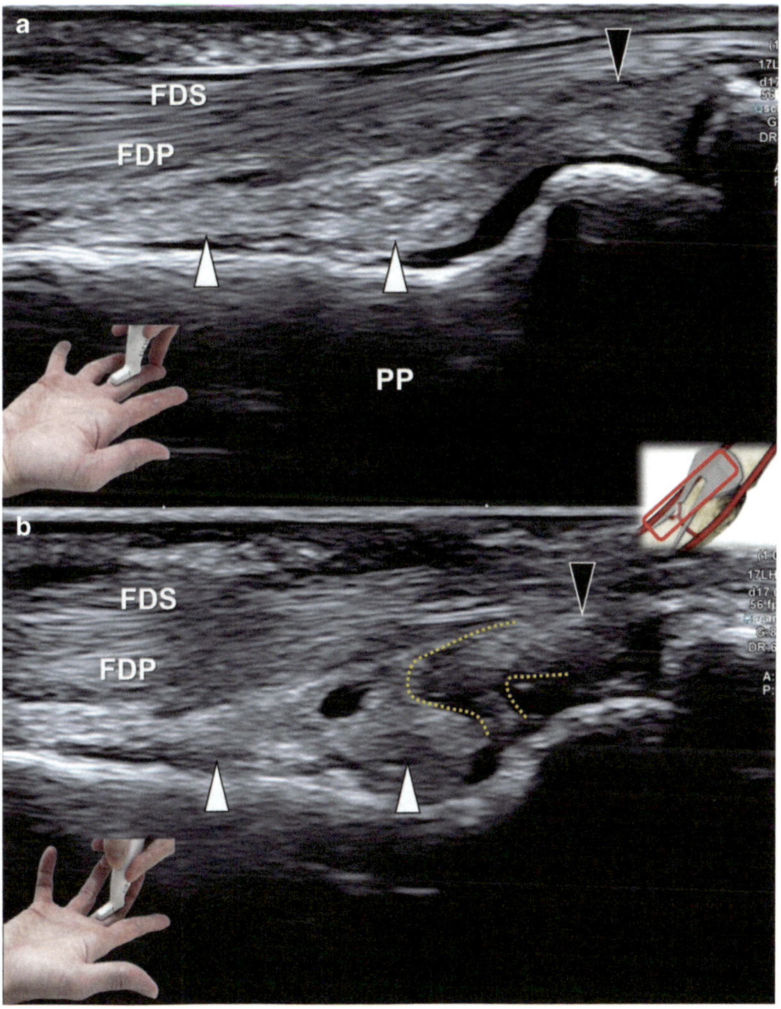

Fig. 15.11 The sonoanatomy of the checkrein ligament (white arrowheads) connecting to the volar plate (black arrowheads) in the long axis of the finger is demonstrated with the proximal interphalangeal joint in extension (**a**) and flexion (**b**). The membranous portion of the volar plate (orange dashed lines) folds during finger flexion to accommodate the movement. FDS flexor digitorum superficialis tendon; FDP flexor digitorum profundus tendon; PP proximal phalanx

Centering the flexor tendon in the middle of the screen and positioning the transducer at the mid-shaft of the proximal phalanx reveals the bifurcation of the flexor digitorum superficialis into two bundles that run alongside the flexor digitorum profundus (Fig. 15.12a). Before reaching the proximal interphalangeal joint, these bundles transition from the lateral sides of the flexor digitorum profundus (Fig. 15.12b) to its undersurface (Fig. 15.12c). At the level of the volar plate, each bundle of the flexor digitorum superficialis tendon splits into radial and ulnar branches. The radial bundle and the radial branch of the ulnar bundle insert on the

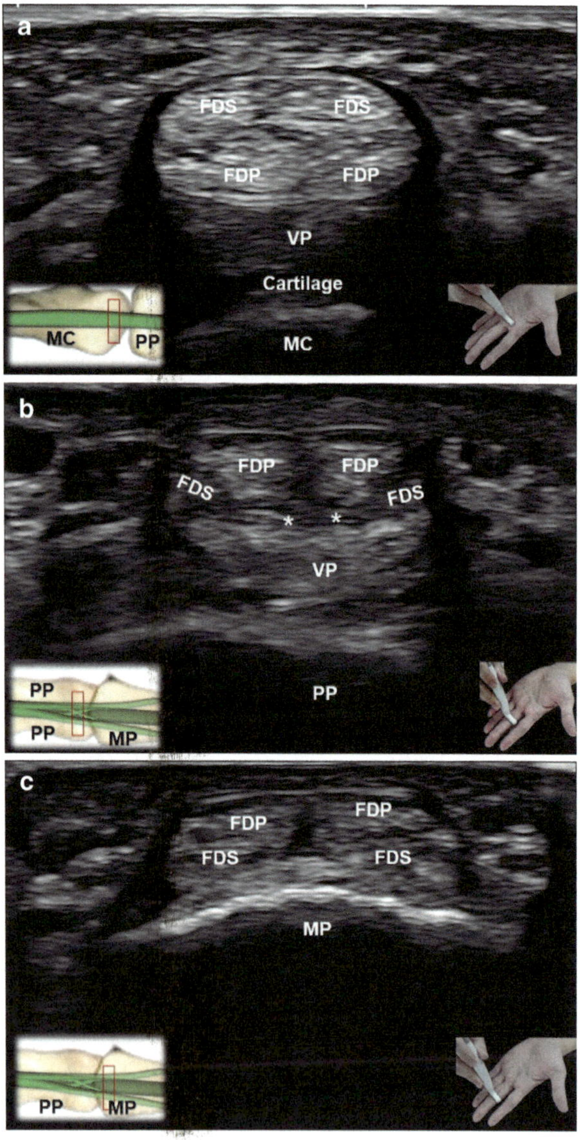

Fig. 15.12 The sonoanatomy of the flexor digitorum superficialis and flexor digitorum profundus tendons in the finger's short axis, imaged at the head of the metacarpal bone (**a**), the head of the proximal phalanx (**b**), and the base of the middle phalanx (**c**). Red squares indicating the transducer's position have been added to the schematic drawing to enhance clarity. Asterisks: Camper's chiasm; FDS flexor digitorum superficialis tendon; FDP flexor digitorum profundus tendon; MC metacarpal bone; PP proximal phalanx; MP middle phalanx; VP volar plate

radial side of the mid-shaft of the middle phalanx (Fig. 15.13a). Meanwhile, the radial branch of the ulnar bundle converges with the ulnar branch of the radial bundle to form the Camper's chiasm, which can be visualized along the long axis of the finger (Fig. 15.13b). Similarly, the ulnar insertion comprises the ulnar bundle and the ulnar branch of the radial bundle. Furthermore, in the short-axis view, the flexor digitorum profundus is observed extending distally to attach to the distal phalanx—at the level of the head of the middle phalanx (Fig. 15.14a) and at the base of the distal phalanx (Fig. 15.14b). Its fibrillar fiber attachments can also be visualized along the long axis of the finger (Fig. 15.14c).

As the transducer moves from the proximal to distal side, the annular pulley appears as a thin band encircling the finger flexor. It can be sequentially identified at the following locations: the metacarpophalangeal joint (A1) (Fig. 15.15a), proximal third of the proximal phalanx (A2) (Fig. 15.15b), distal third of the proximal phalanx (cruciform ligament) (Fig. 15.15c), proximal interphalangeal joint (A3) (Fig. 15.16a), mid-shaft of the middle phalanx (A4) (Fig. 15.16b), and distal interphalangeal joint (A5) (Fig. 15.16c). Finally, the transducer is rotated to align with the long axis of the finger (Fig. 15.17).

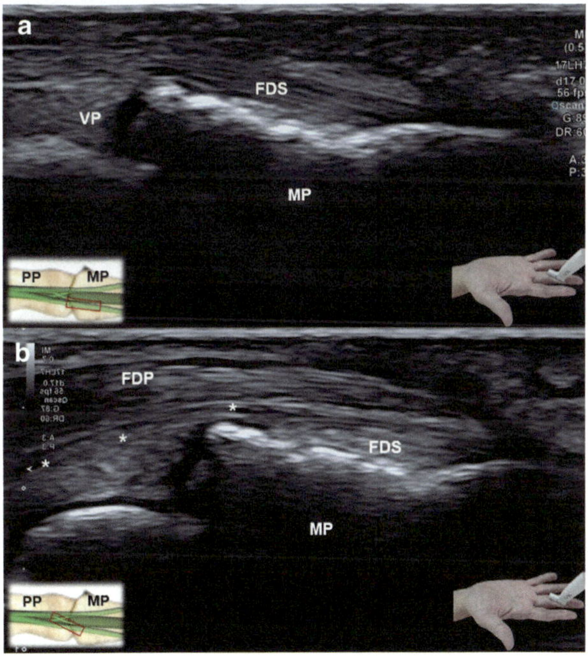

Fig. 15.13 The sonoanatomy of the radial insertion of the flexor digitorum superficialis in the finger's long axis (**a**). When the transducer is moved centrally and the proximal end is rotated toward the ulnar side, the Camper's chiasm (asterisks) and the radial branch of the ulnar bundle of the flexor digitorum superficialis tendon become visible (**b**). Red squares indicating the transducer's position have been added to the schematic drawing to enhance clarity. FDS flexor digitorum superficialis tendon; FDP flexor digitorum profundus tendon; MP middle phalanx; VP volar plate

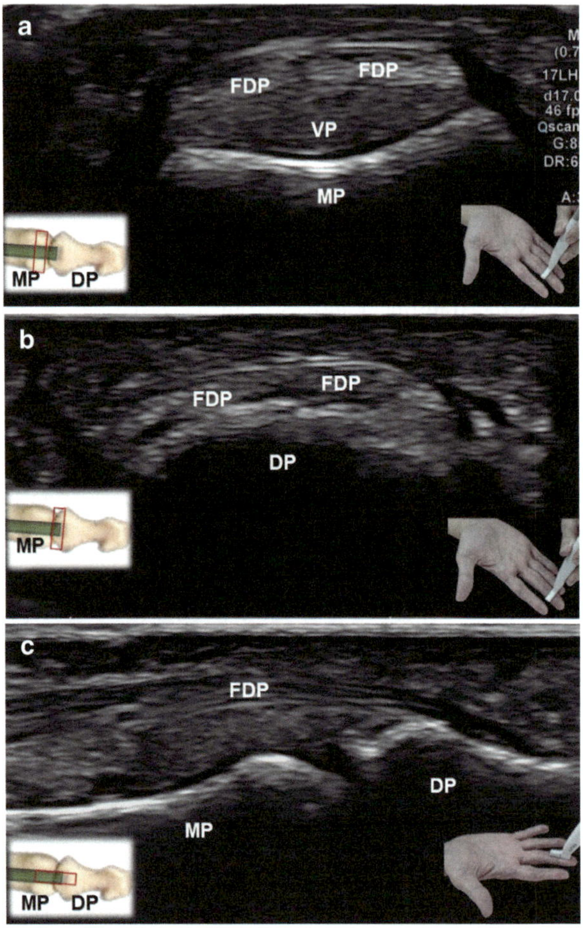

Fig. 15.14 The sonoanatomy of the flexor digitorum profundus: at the level of the head of the middle phalanx in the finger's short axis (**a**), at the base of the distal phalanx in the finger's short axis (**b**), and its insertion in the finger's long axis (**c**). Red squares indicating the transducer's position have been added to the schematic drawing to enhance clarity. FDP flexor digitorum profundus tendon; MP middle phalanx; DP distal phalanx; VP volar plate

For the thumb pulleys, the A1 pulley is positioned between the radial and ulnar sesamoid bones (Fig. 15.18a). As the transducer is moved distally, the variable pulley—formed by the adductor pollicis aponeurosis—comes into view (Fig. 15.18b). Further distal, the oblique pulley appears as a band extending from the ulnar to the radial side (Fig. 15.18c). Finally, the A2 pulley, situated at the interphalangeal joint and superficial to the volar plate, is visualized (Fig. 15.18d).

Tendons surrounded by true synovial sheaths receive their blood supply through vessels that enter via the mesotenon, which is reduced to isolated, cord-like structures called vincula [13]. Each finger contains two types of vincula: the vincula longa and the vincula brevia, positioned similarly across all fingers. The vincula longa connect the flexor digitorum superficialis tendon to the base of the proximal phalanx and link the underside of the flexor digitorum profundus tendons to the flexor digitorum superficialis tendons after the profundus tendons pass through the bifurcation of the superficialis tendons. The vincula brevia are triangular fiber

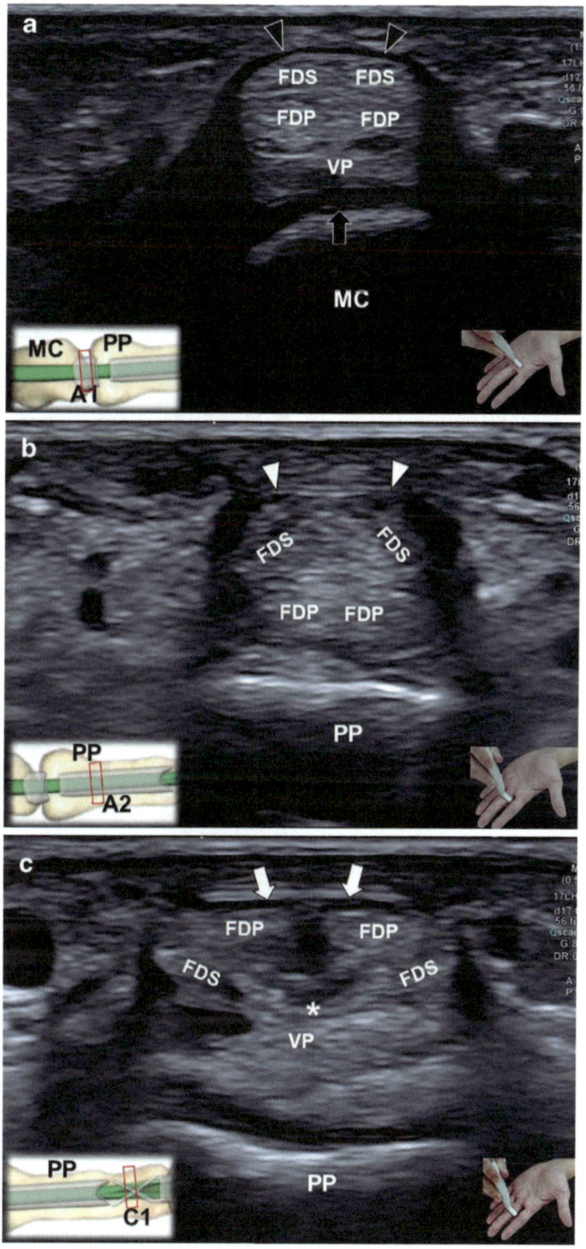

Fig. 15.15 Sonoanatomy of the A1 pulley (black arrowheads) (**a**), A2 pulley (white arrowheads) (**b**), and C1 ligament (white arrows) (**c**) in the short-axis views of the finger. Red squares indicating the transducer's position have been added to the schematic drawing to enhance clarity. Asterisk: Camper's chiasm; black arrow: cartilage; FDS flexor digitorum superficialis tendon; FDP flexor digitorum profundus tendon; MC metacarpal bone; PP proximal phalanx; VP volar plate

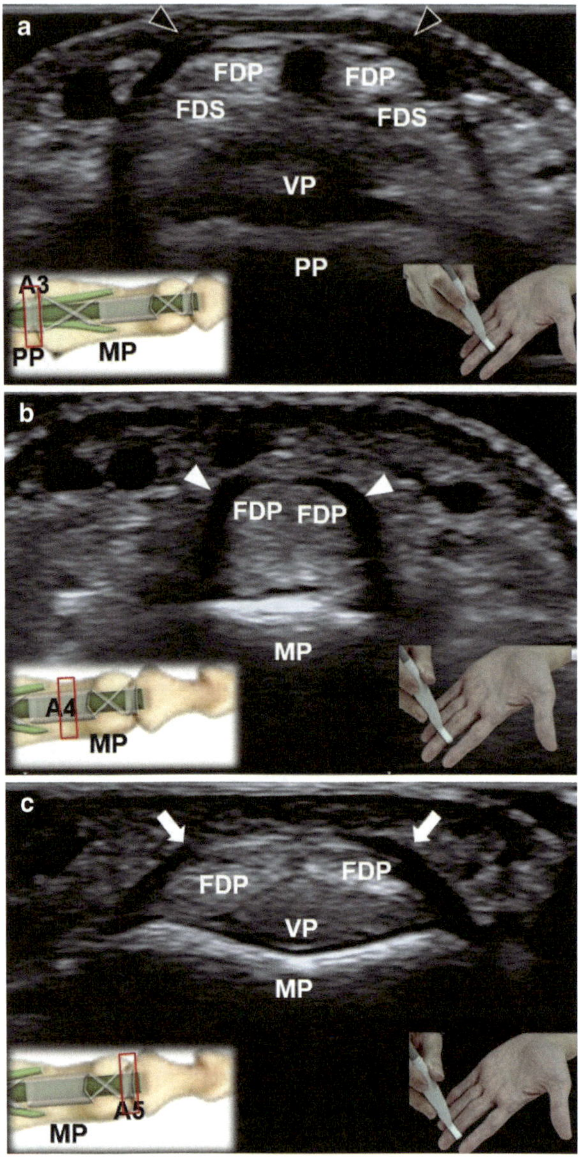

Fig. 15.16 The sonoanatomy of the A3 (black arrowheads) (**a**), A4 (white arrowheads) (**b**), and A5 (white arrows) (**c**) pulleys in the short-axis views of the finger. Red squares indicating the transducer's position have been added to the schematic drawing to enhance clarity. FDS flexor digitorum superficialis tendon; FDP flexor digitorum profundus tendon; PP proximal phalanx; MP middle phalanx; VP volar plate

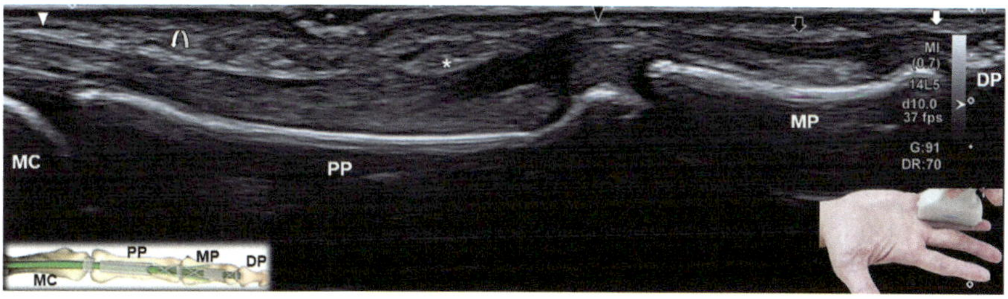

Fig. 15.17 Sonoanatomy of the finger pulley system in the long-axis view of the finger. White arrowhead: A1 pulley; white curve arrowhead: A2 pulley; asterisk: C1 ligament; black arrowhead: A3 pulley; black arrow: A4 pulley; white arrow: A5 pulley; MC metacarpal bone; MP middle phalanx; PP proximal phalanx; DP distal phalanx

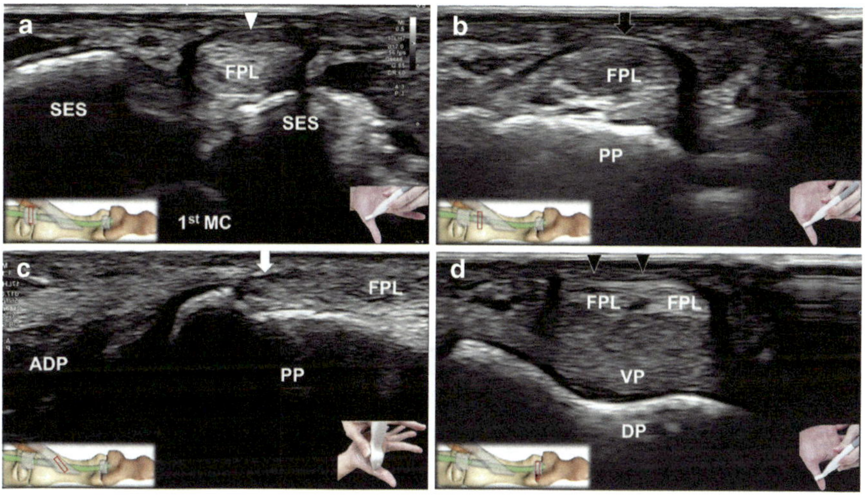

Fig. 15.18 The sonoanatomy of the thumb's pulley system shows the A1 pulley (white arrowhead) (**a**), the variable pulley (black arrow) (**b**), the oblique pulley (white arrow) extending from the ulnar to the radial side (**c**), and the A2 pulley (black arrowheads) (**d**) in the finger's short-axis views. SES sesamoid; 1st MC the first metacarpal bone; FPL flexor pollicis longus tendon; PP proximal phalanx of the thumb; ADP adductor pollicis; DP distal phalanx of the thumb; VP volar plate

bands; one connects the flexor digitorum superficialis tendon to the head of the proximal phalanx, while the other connects the flexor digitorum profundus tendon to the head of the middle phalanx. For simplification, both structures can be easily visualized under power Doppler ultrasound along the finger's long axis: the vincula longa are typically located at the proximal (base) portion of the phalanx shaft (Fig. 15.19a), whereas the vincula brevia are closer to the interphalangeal joint (Fig. 15.19b).

15.3.2 Dorsal Aspect

The transducer should be positioned over the dorsal aspect at the level of the metacarpal head for optimal imaging. To enhance visualization of the finger extensor tendon complex, it is recommended to apply a generous amount of ultrasound jelly on the skin. At the level of the metacarpal head, the extensor digitorum communis tendon, either alone (Fig. 15.20a) or accompanied by the extensor indicis proprius on the 2nd digit (Fig. 15.20b) or the extensor digiti minimi on the 5th digit, is observed encircled by the sagittal band (Fig. 15.20c). Beneath the extensor digitorum communis lies the dorsal plate, situated on the metacarpal head, with the sagittal band extending to the volar side to encircle the proper and accessory collateral ligaments of the fingers (Fig. 15.20d).

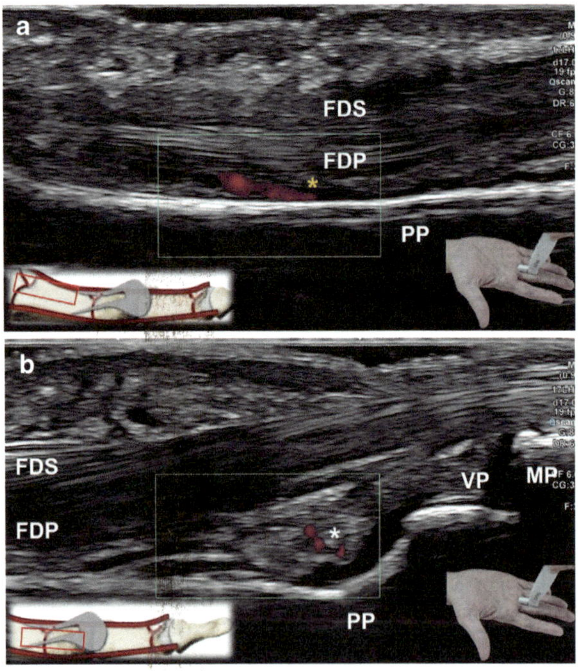

Fig. 15.19 The sonoanatomy of the vincula in the finger's long axis with Doppler mode highlights the arteries within the vincula longa (yellow asterisk) (**a**) and vincula brevia (white asterisk) (**b**). Red squares indicating the transducer's position have been added to the schematic drawing to enhance clarity. FDS flexor digitorum superficialis tendon; FDP flexor digitorum profundus tendon; PP proximal phalanx; MP middle phalanx; VP volar plate

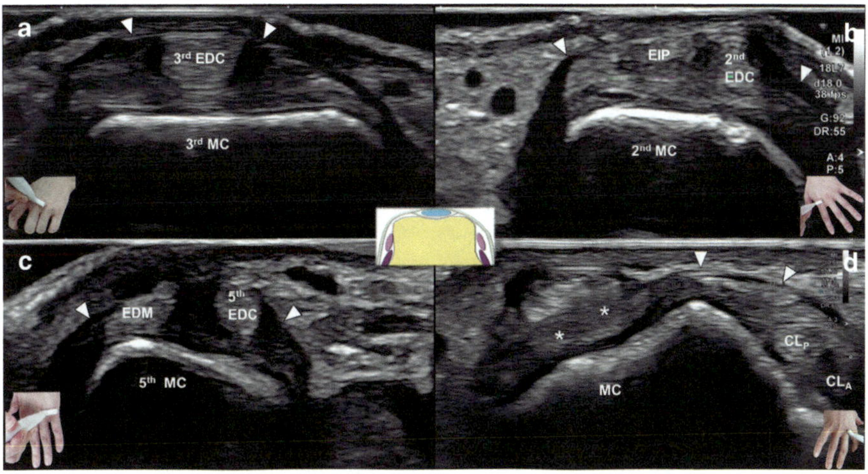

Fig. 15.20 The sonoanatomy of the sagittal band (white arrowheads), extensor tendons, and nearby collateral ligaments at the 3rd metacarpal level (**a**), the 2nd metacarpal level (**b**), the 5th metacarpal level (**c**), and the relationship between the sagittal band and the accessory/proper collateral ligaments (**d**). Asterisks: dorsal plate; EDC extensor digitorum communis tendon; EIP extensor indicis proprius tendon; EDM extensor digiti minimi tendon; MC metacarpal bone; CL_P proper collateral ligament; CL_A accessory collateral ligament

Upon moving the transducer more proximally, the hyperechoic bands crossing over the dorsal interosseous muscles, connecting the finger extensor tendons, are identified as the juncturae tendinae (Fig. 15.21). By pivoting the transducer to align with the long axis of the phalangeal bone, the central slip of the extensor digitorum communis tendon can be visualized, bridging the dorsal plate [14] and attaching to the base of the middle phalanx. (Fig. 15.22a). The transducer can be pivoted back to the axial plane to see the distal attachment of the central slip (Fig. 15.22b). Following the axial plane, the transducer can be moved distally to visualize the bilateral lateral bands at the sides of the middle phalanx (Fig. 15.23a), which converge to form the terminal band that terminates on the distal phalanx (Fig. 15.23b). Similarly, in the long-axis plane, the terminal band of the extensor digitorum communis attaches to the distal phalanx, just proximal to the nail bed (Fig. 15.23c).

15.3.3 Lateral Aspect

To examine the collateral ligaments of the 2nd to 5th fingers, the probe is positioned over either the ulnar or radial side of the metacarpophalangeal, proximal interphalangeal, and distal interphalangeal joints. The proper collateral ligament appears as a fibrillar hyperechoic structure spanning between the metacarpal head and proximal phalanx, as well as between the proximal and middle phalanges, and the middle and distal phalanges (Fig. 15.24a). At the metacarpophalangeal joint, tilting the

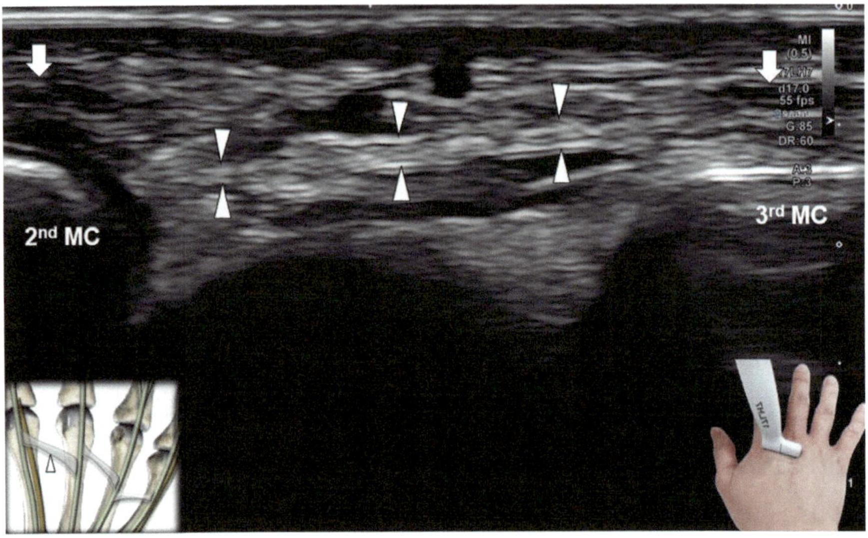

Fig. 15.21 The sonoanatomy of the juncturae tendinae (white arrowheads) in its long axis, connecting the extensor digitorum communis tendons (white arrows) of the 2nd and 3rd fingers. MC metacarpal bone

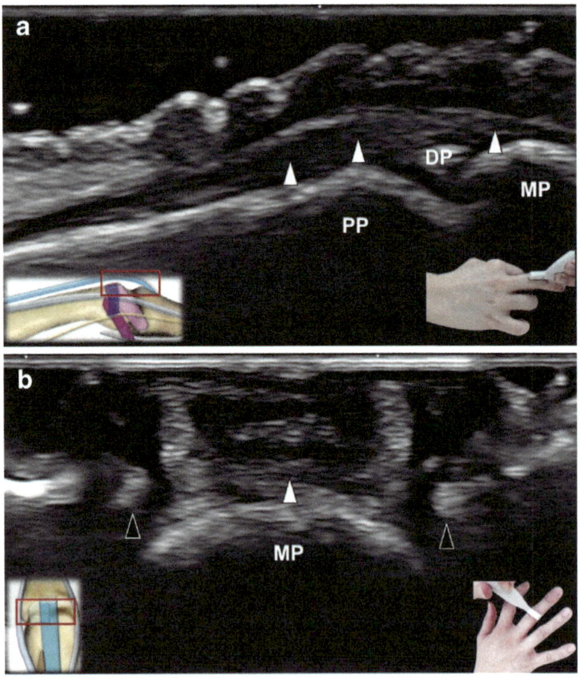

Fig. 15.22 The sonoanatomy of the central slip (white arrowheads) of the extensor digitorum communis tendon shown in the finger's long axis (**a**) and short axis (**b**). Red squares indicating the transducer's position have been added to the schematic drawing to enhance clarity. DP dorsal plate; PP proximal phalanx; MP middle phalanx; black arrowheads: the lateral band of the extensor digitorum communis tendon

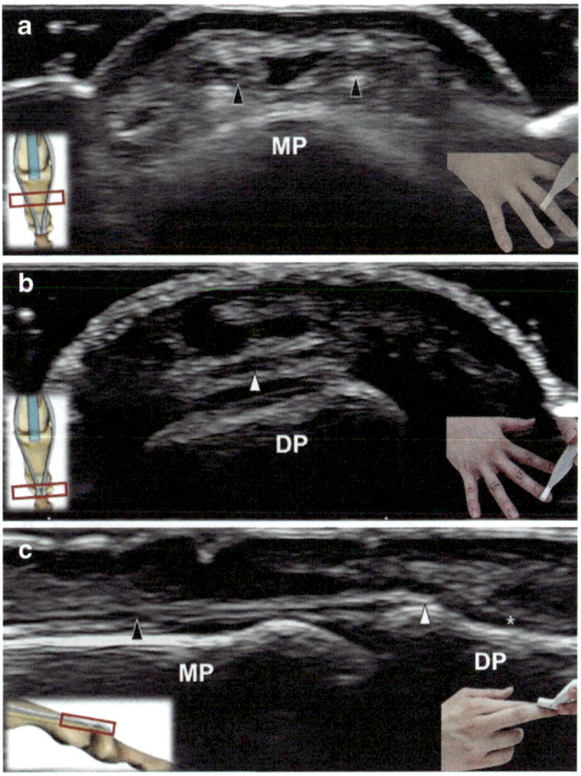

Fig. 15.23 The sonoanatomy of the lateral band (black arrowheads) (**a**) and terminal band (white arrowhead) (**b**) of the extensor digitorum communis tendon in the finger's short-axis view, with the long-axis view of the finger shown in (**c**). Red squares indicating the transducer's position have been added to the schematic drawing to enhance clarity. Asterisk: nail bed; MP middle phalanx; DP distal phalanx

distal end of the transducer toward the volar aspect allows visualization of the accessory collateral ligament, which connects the metacarpal head proximally to the volar plate distally (Fig. 15.24b). The transducer can be rotated to the lateral axial plane of the finger to view both ligaments in the short axis (Fig. 15.24c).

Examination of the ulnar proper collateral ligament of the thumb in the long axis (Fig. 15.25a) follows the same technique used for the other fingers. The proximal edge of the transducer can be slightly rotated toward the dorsal first webspace to visualize the adductor pollicis aponeurosis overlying the ulnar proper collateral ligament (Fig. 15.25b). Similarly, examining the radial proper collateral ligament of the thumb in the long axis follows the same approach as for the other fingers (Fig. 15.26a). Rotating the proximal edge of the transducer slightly toward the volar aspect of the thumb reveals the aponeurosis of the abductor pollicis brevis muscle over the radial proper collateral ligament (Fig. 15.26b). To examine the accessory collateral ligament, the distal end of the transducer should be rotated palmarly to align it toward the sesamoid (Fig. 15.27).

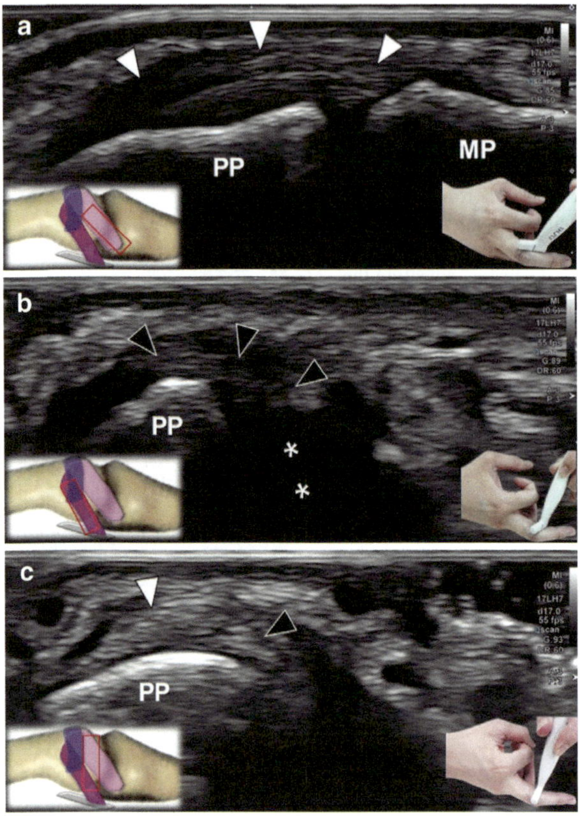

Fig. 15.24 The sonoanatomy of the proper collateral ligament (white arrowheads) (**a**) and accessory collateral ligament (black arrowheads) (**b**) in the long axis, and both ligaments in the short axis (**c**). Red squares indicating the transducer's position have been added to the schematic drawing to enhance clarity. Double asterisks: volar plate; MP middle phalanx; PP proximal phalanx

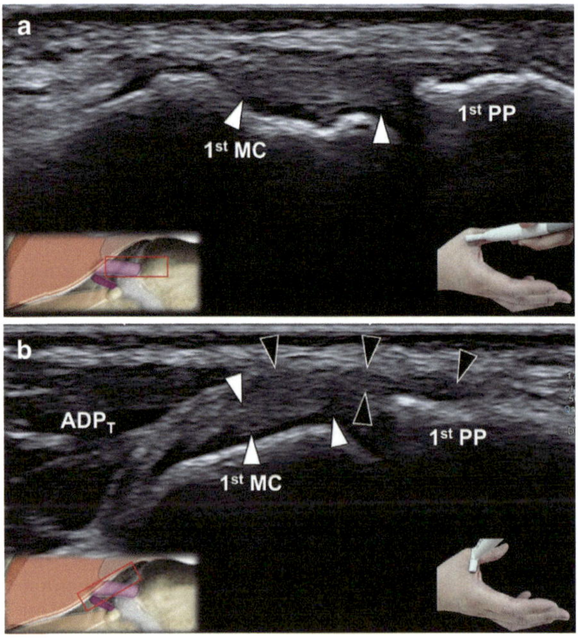

Fig. 15.25 Sonoanatomy of the ulnar proper collateral ligament (white arrowheads) of the thumb in the thumb's long axis (**a**) and in the oblique axis, showing the ligament along with the adductor pollicis aponeurosis (black arrowheads) (**b**). Red squares indicating the transducer's position have been added to the schematic drawing to enhance clarity. ADP_T transverse head of the adductor pollicis muscle; MC metacarpal bone; PP proximal phalanx

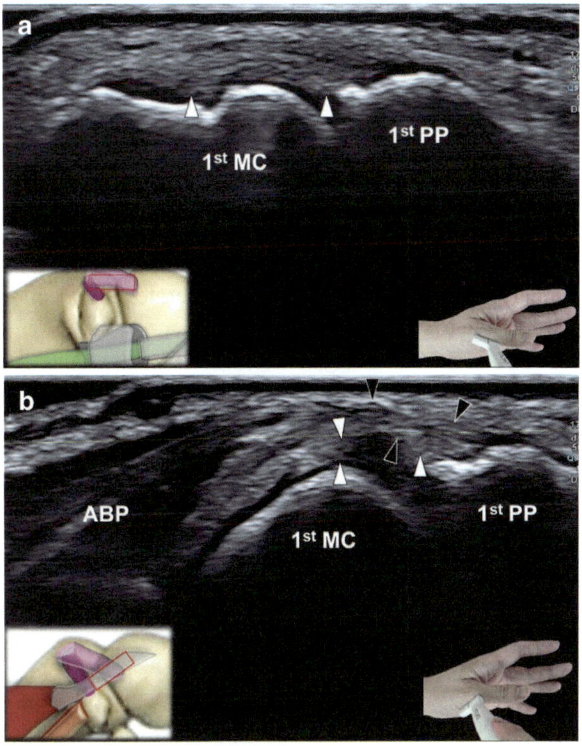

Fig. 15.26 Sonoanatomy of the radial proper collateral ligament (white arrowheads) of the thumb in the thumb's long axis (**a**) and in the oblique axis, showing the ligament along with the abductor pollicis brevis aponeurosis (black arrowheads) (**b**). Red squares indicating the transducer's position have been added to the schematic drawing to enhance clarity. MC metacarpal bone; PP proximal phalanx; ABP abductor pollicis brevis muscle

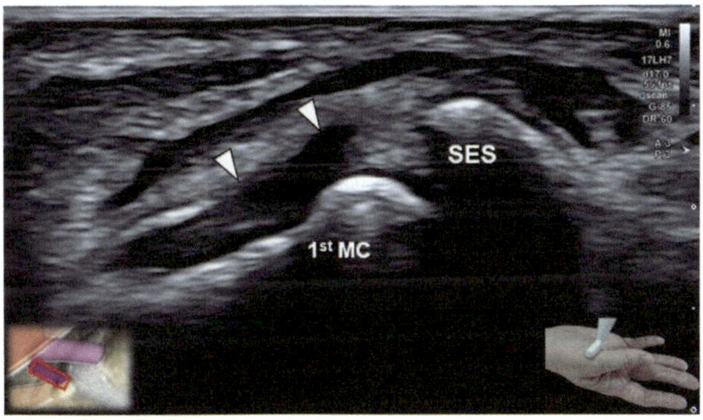

Fig. 15.27 Sonoanatomy of the accessory collateral ligament (white arrowhead) of the thumb in the long axis. Red squares indicating the transducer's position have been added to the schematic drawing to enhance clarity. MC metacarpal bone; SES sesamoid

15.4 Pathology

15.4.1 Volar Finger

The most common pathology affecting the volar finger region is trigger finger, resulting from the thickening of the A1 pulley, which narrows the digital osteofibrous tunnel through which the finger flexor tendons pass, leading to impaired tendon gliding [15]. Typically, axial sonograms over the A1 pulley reveal thickening and hyperemia, alongside tendinosis of the finger flexor tendons (Fig. 15.28a). The long-axis view of the finger is useful for detailing the fibrillar pattern of the flexor digitorum superficialis and profundus tendons, which may be involved in trigger finger (Fig. 15.28b). Progressive nodular thickening of the finger flexor tendon, especially the flexor digitorum superficialis, occurs with repetitive entrapment. During dynamic ultrasound imaging, the thickened segment of the finger flexor tendon may seem locked, hindering gliding into the narrow osteofibrous tunnel while extending the finger. Occasionally, when the flexor tendon becomes stuck inside the tunnel, twisted tendon fibers may generate a hypoechoic vertical shadow within the tendon due to anisotropy.

In patients with trigger fingers, static ultrasound imaging can detect the extosis of the metacarpal head, which may cause secondary trigger finger. Prolonged cases of trigger finger can cause degenerative changes in the annular pulley, leading to pulley tears or the formation of cystic lesions (short axis, Fig. 15.29a; long axis, Fig. 15.29b). Additionally, chronic impingement may result in intratendinous tears in the flexor tendon (Fig. 15.30a), as compared to the normal side (Fig. 15.30b). Moreover, while thickening of the A1 pulley is the most common, the A2 pulley may also thicken, causing symptoms of trigger finger. On the other hand, when the

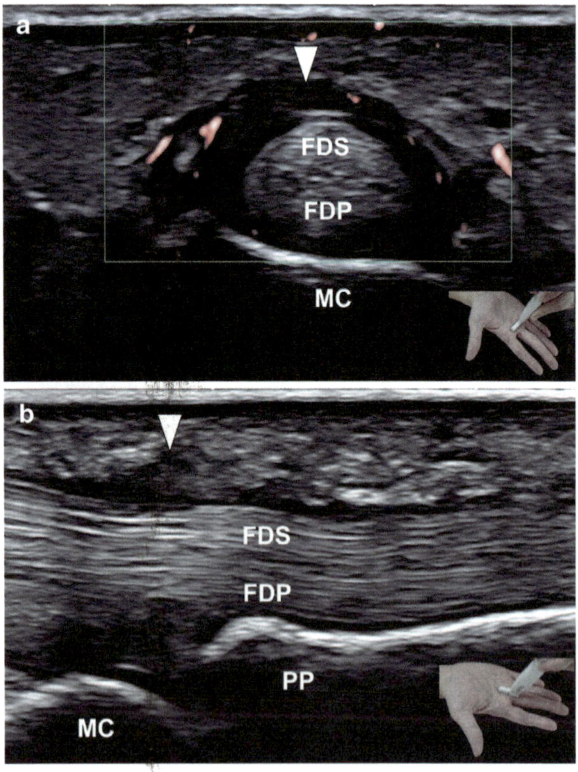

Fig. 15.28 The ultrasound images of trigger finger show A1 pulley thickening (white arrowheads) and hyperemia in the finger's short axis (**a**) and long axis (**b**). FDS flexor digitorum superficialis tendon; FDP flexor digitorum profundus tendon; MC metacarpal bone; PP proximal phalanx

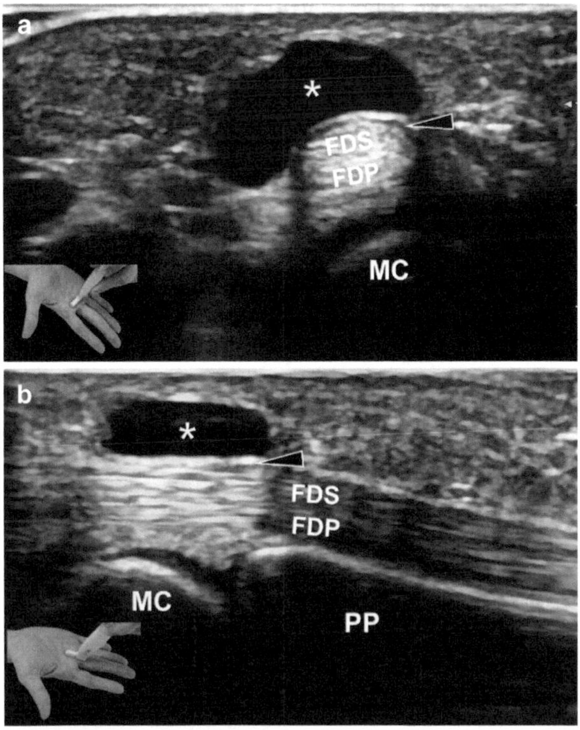

Fig. 15.29 The ultrasound images of a hypoechoic and well-defined ganglion cyst (asterisks) over the A1 pulley (black arrowheads) in the finger's short axis (**a**) and long axis (**b**). FDS flexor digitorum superficialis tendon; FDP flexor digitorum profundus tendon; MC metacarpal bone; PP proximal phalanx

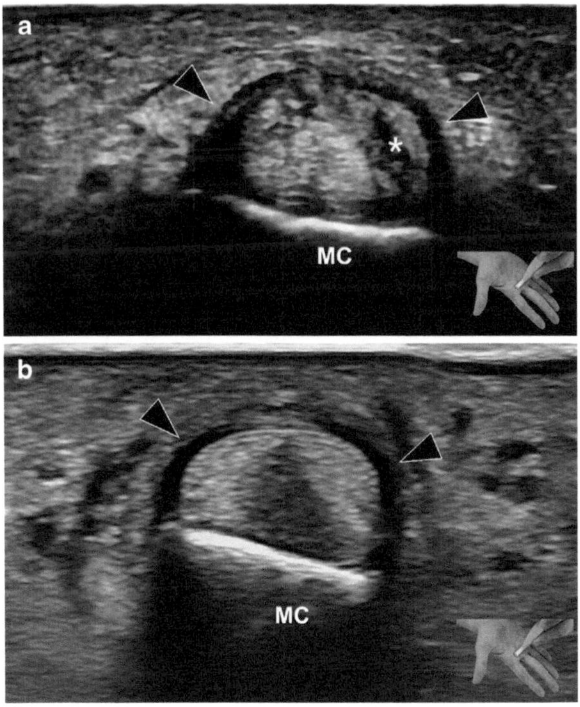

Fig. 15.30 The ultrasound image shows an intratendinous partial tear (asterisk) of the finger flexor tendon (**a**) compared to the contralateral side (**b**) in the short-axis view of the finger. Black arrowheads: A1 pulley; MC metacarpal bone

pulleys are torn (Fig. 15.31a), the finger flexor tendon shifts away from the bone, creating a bowstring sign (Fig. 15.31b). In contrast, on the normal side, the finger flexor tendon remains closely aligned with the phalanx (Fig. 15.31c) [12].

Ultrasound imaging offers valuable insights for patients with flexor tendon injuries [16]. In cases of tendon sprain or tendinitis, increased thickness and reduced echogenicity (Fig. 15.32a), along with a hyperemic pattern (Fig. 15.32b), can be observed without a visible cleft. In partial tears, the finger flexor tendon may exhibit increased thickness, reduced echogenicity, and visible gaps that do not involve the full tendon thickness (Fig. 15.33a), compared to the contralateral unaffected side (Fig. 15.33b).

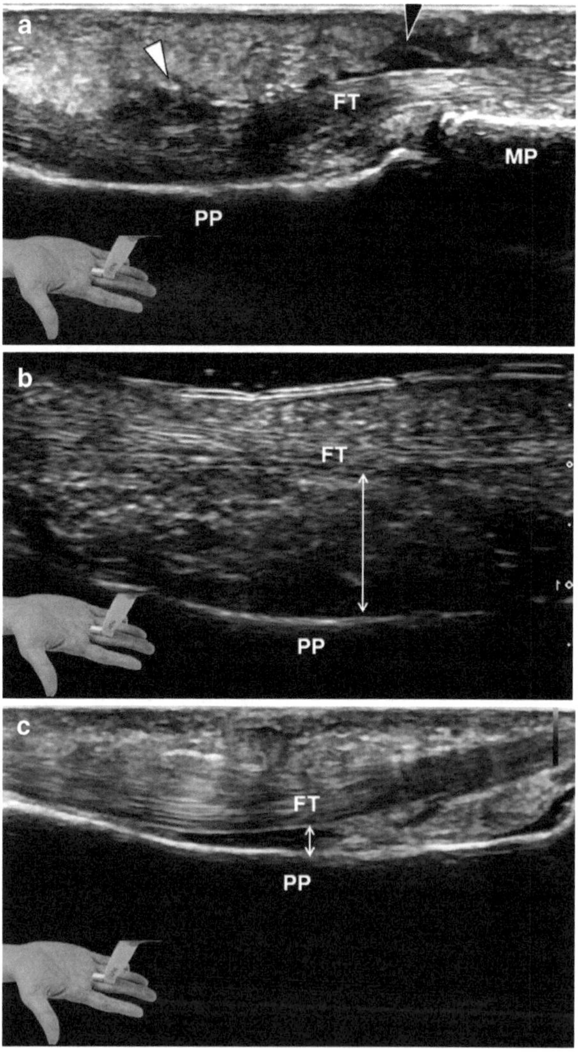

Fig. 15.31 The ultrasound image shows A2 (white arrowhead) and A3 (black arrowhead) pulley ruptures in the finger's long axis (**a**). The bowstring sign (**b**), with the flexor tendon shifting away from the phalanx during flexion, is observed compared to the contralateral side (**c**). FT finger flexor tendon; MP middle phalanx; PP proximal phalanx; double-headed arrows: the distance between the flexor tendon and the phalanx

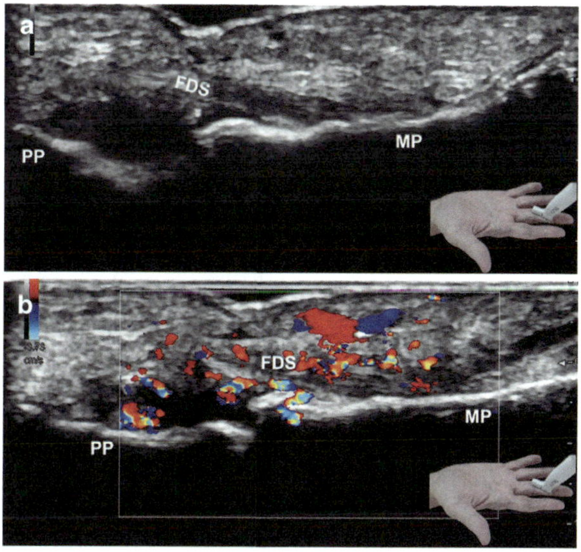

Fig. 15.32 The ultrasound images of flexor digitorum superficialis tendinitis at its distal attachment demonstrate a hypoechoic appearance with loss of the fibrillar pattern (**a**) and hyperemia (**b**) in the long axis of the tendon. FDS flexor digitorum superficialis tendon; MP middle phalanx; PP proximal phalanx

In cases of complete tears, ultrasound images may show an absence of the tendon compared to the adjacent flexor tendon in the short-axis view (Fig. 15.34a). In the long-axis view, no tendon fibers are visible proximal to the distal stump (Fig. 15.34b). In some chronic cases, the distal stump may not be thickened and could adhere to the phalanx (Fig. 15.34c). Although lumbrical muscle injury or inflammation is rare, hyperemic lesions may occasionally be detected between the finger flexor tendons and the superficial and deep metacarpal ligaments (short axis, Fig. 15.35a; long axis, Fig. 15.35b).

Sonographic imaging can differentiate volar plate injuries, categorized into three types: Type A, an avulsion fracture without volar plate rupture (affected side, Fig. 15.36a; normal side, Fig. 15.36b); Type B, a full-thickness tear of the volar plate without fracture (long axis, Fig. 15.37a; short axis, Fig. 15.37b); and Type C, a partial-thickness tear of the volar plate (long axis, Fig. 15.38a; short axis, Fig. 15.38b) [17].

15.4.2 *Dorsal Finger*

Pathologies affecting the dorsal aspect of the fingers commonly result from trauma or are associated with conditions such as rheumatoid arthritis. One such example is a sagittal band injury [4]. During examination of the dorsal aspect of the metacarpophalangeal joint in the short axis, it is important to note that intact sagittal bands exhibit uniform echotexture compared to the radial and ulnar aspects of the finger extensor tendons. It is essential to compare these observations with the corresponding areas in the adjacent asymptomatic metacarpophalangeal joint and the

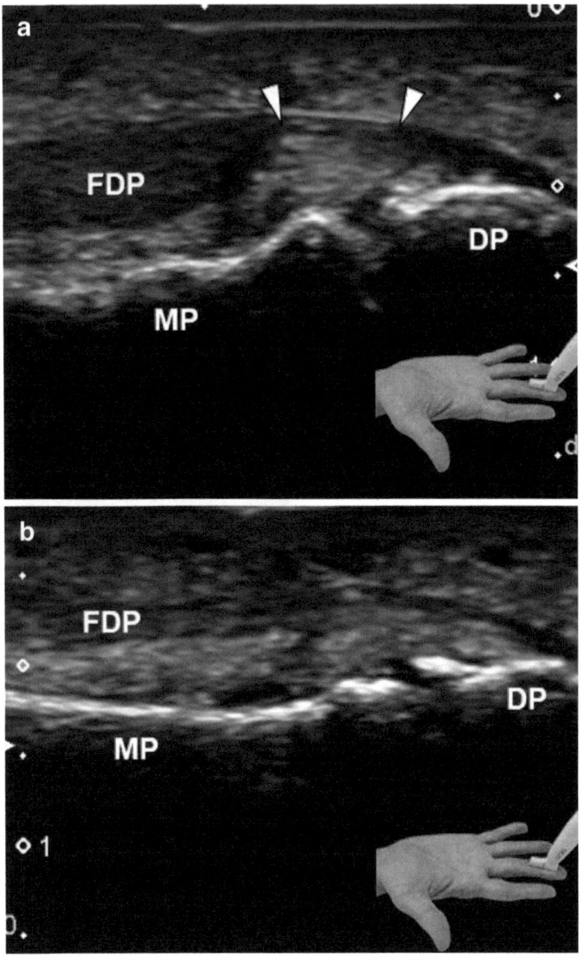

Fig. 15.33 The ultrasound image shows a partial tear of the flexor digitorum profundus tendon, with partial tendon discontinuity (white arrowheads) and proximal thickening (**a**), compared to the healthy side (**b**) in the finger's long axis. FDP flexor digitorum profundus tendon; MP middle phalanx; DP distal phalanx

contralateral limb, particularly when partial sagittal band tears are suspected, as they may cause thickening of the sagittal band.

A comprehensive sonographic evaluation of the sagittal bands is necessary, spanning from the proximal dorsal metacarpophalangeal joint to the mid proximal phalanx level. Dynamic assessment is vital for observing the real-time positioning of the finger extensor tendon relative to the dorsal aspect of the metacarpal head. This dynamic evaluation can help identify potential subluxation or dislocation of the finger extensor tendons towards either the radial or ulnar aspects of the metacarpal head, which are often associated with sagittal band tears.

Partial sagittal band tears typically appear as focal thickening and hypoechoic areas in the sagittal band on the radial or ulnar side (Fig. 15.39a). Complete sagittal band tears, or ruptures, are characterized by a visible discontinuity on the radial or ulnar aspects in short-axis sonographic imaging, with a retracted stump adjacent to

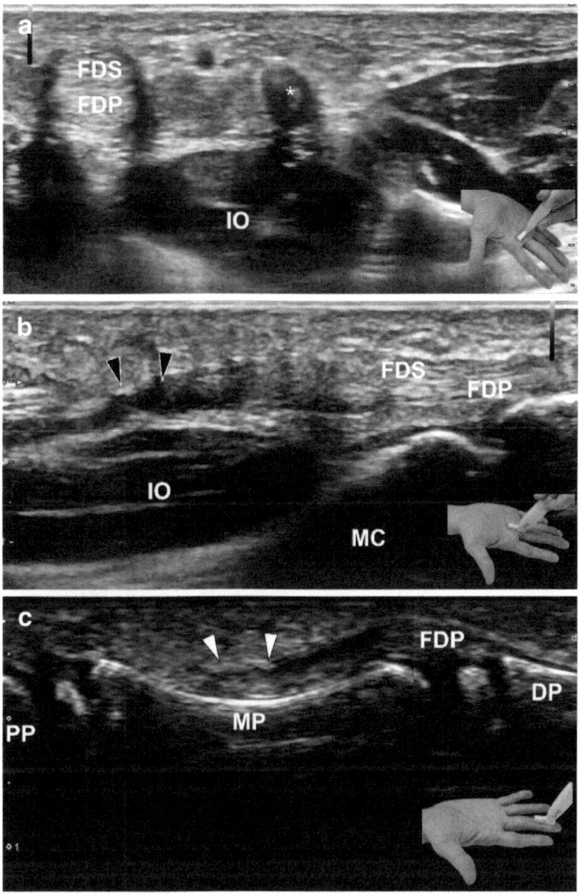

Fig. 15.34 The ultrasound images of a complete finger flexor tendon tear reveal the absence of the tendon (asterisk) compared to the adjacent finger flexor tendon in the short-axis view (**a**). In the long-axis view, no tendon fibers are visualized proximal to the distal stump (black arrowheads) (**b**). In another case, a complete tear of the flexor digitorum profundus tendon is observed, with a visible distal stump (white arrowheads) showing thickness similar to its more distal segment (**c**). FDS flexor digitorum superficialis tendon; FDP flexor digitorum profundus tendon; IO interosseous muscles; MC metacarpal bone; PP proximal phalanx; MP middle phalanx; DP distal phalanx

the finger extensor tendon (Fig. 15.39b). This gap results in the loss of a continuous sagittal band around the finger extensor tendon at the metacarpophalangeal level, which may lead to finger extensor tendon subluxation or dislocation (Fig. 15.39c). In some cases, dorsal plate injury with effusion beside it can also be observed (Fig. 15.39d).

Mallet finger deformity occurs when the tip of a finger or thumb is struck by a rigid object, such as a baseball, causing it to bend [18]. This impact causes a tear in the terminal band and retraction of the lateral band. On longitudinal oblique ultrasound imaging of the phalanx, the lateral band may exhibit a wavy appearance (Fig. 15.40a). In some cases, the terminal band of the extensor digitorum communis is torn (Fig. 15.40b), with or without an associated avulsion fracture. Occasionally, a ganglion cyst with a partial-thickness tear in the terminal band (long axis, Fig. 15.40c; short axis, Fig. 15.40d), potentially associated with osteoarthritic bone spurs, can be observed. This may mimic a solid tumor in the finger.

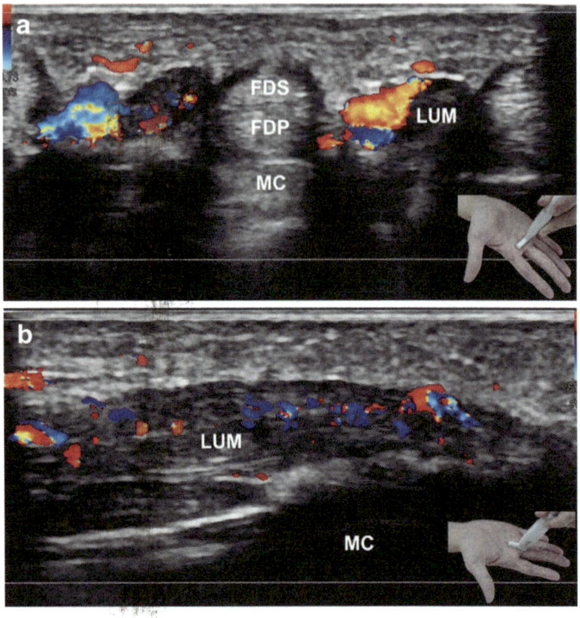

Fig. 15.35 The ultrasound images depict the lumbrical muscle injury with muscle hypervascularity in the finger's short axis (**a**) and long axis (**b**). FDP flexor digitorum profundus tendon; FDS flexor digitorum superficialis tendon; LUM lumbrical muscle; MC metacarpal bone

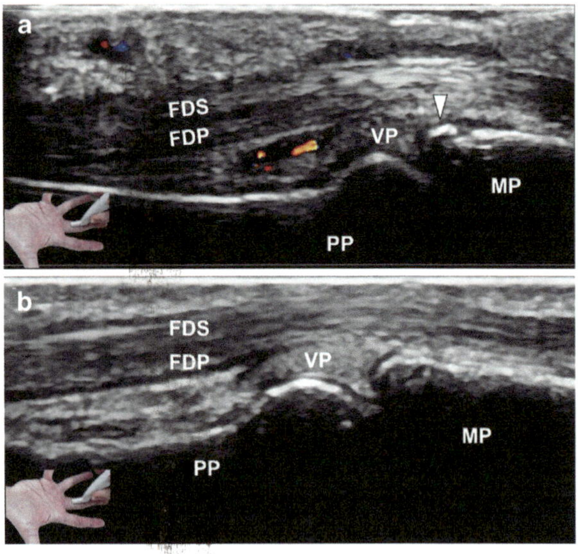

Fig. 15.36 The ultrasound image shows a volar plate avulsion fracture (white arrowhead) (**a**), compared to the contralateral normal side (**b**) in the finger's long axis. FDS flexor digitorum superficialis tendon; FDP flexor digitorum profundus tendon; MP middle phalanx; PP proximal phalanx; VP volar plate

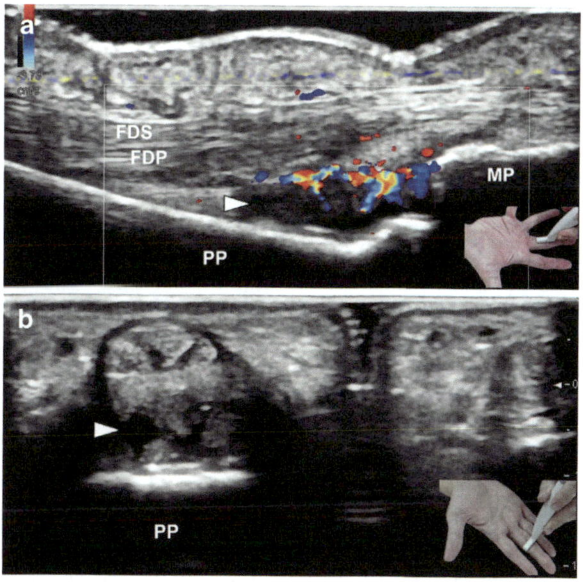

Fig. 15.37 The ultrasound images show a full-thickness tear of the volar plate (white arrowheads) in the finger's long axis (**a**) and short axis (**b**). FDS flexor digitorum superficialis tendon; FDP flexor digitorum profundus tendon; PP proximal phalanx; MP middle phalanx

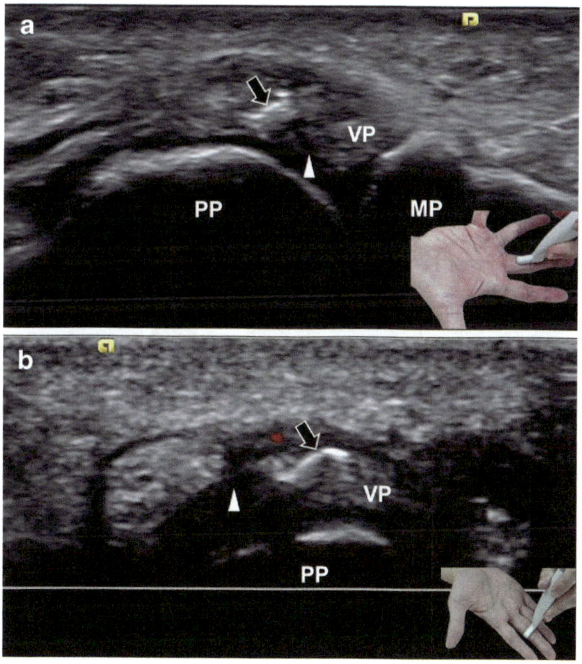

Fig. 15.38 The ultrasound images show a partial tear of the volar plate (white arrowheads) and calcification (black arrows) in the finger's long axis (**a**) and short axis (**b**). PP proximal phalanx; MP middle phalanx; VP volar plate

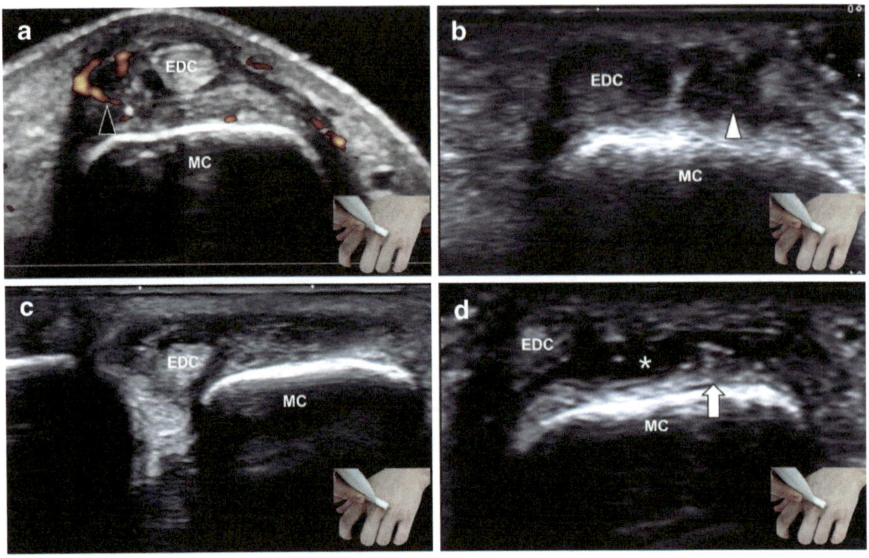

Fig. 15.39 The ultrasound images show various sagittal band injuries: a partial tear with thickening and hypervascularity (black arrowhead) (**a**), a complete tear with a retracted stump (white arrowhead) adjacent to the finger extensor tendon (**b**), a complete tear with extensor tendon subluxation during finger flexion (**c**), and an associated ruptured dorsal plate (white arrow) with effusion (asterisk) (**d**) in the finger's short axis. EDC extensor digitorum communis tendon; MC metacarpal bone

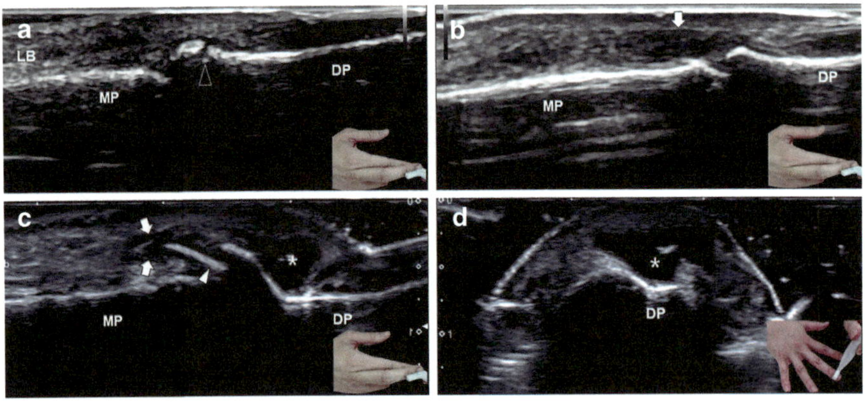

Fig. 15.40 The ultrasound images depict mallet finger deformity, including the avulsion fracture (black arrowhead) of the terminal band with wavy appearance of the lateral band (**a**), partial tear (white arrows) of the terminal band (**b**) in the finger's long axis. In another case, a partial tear of the terminal band with the ganglion cyst (asterisks) along with the spurs (white arrowhead) in the finger's long axis (**c**) and short axis (**d**). DP distal phalanx; MP middle phalanx

Boutonniere deformity presents with flexion at the proximal interphalangeal joint and hyperextension at the distal interphalangeal joint of the finger [19]. Ultrasound imaging reveals a torn central slip of the extensor digitorum communis tendon, with the lateral bands remaining intact. Complete tears of the central slip of the extensor digitorum communis tendon can occur due to blunt trauma, such as forced flexion of the proximal interphalangeal joint, and may be linked to an avulsion fracture of the dorsal base of the middle phalanx (Fig. 15.41a). On the other hand, even with a partial tear of the central slip, ultrasound effectively demonstrates its capability in delineating thickening (Fig. 15.41b), hypoechogenicity, and hypervascularity (Fig. 15.41c) of the tendon fibers.

15.4.3 Lateral Finger

Patients with a sprain of the radial or ulnar collateral ligament of the proximal interphalangeal joint demonstrate characteristic sonographic features, including interstitial hypoechoic areas without fiber disruption and regions of thickening and hypoechogenicity (Fig. 15.42a) [20]. An avulsion fracture may also be present at the distal or proximal attachment of the ligament (Fig. 15.42b). In partial-thickness tears, longitudinal sonography commonly reveals focal hypoechoic areas within the collateral ligament with partial fiber disruption near its insertion (Fig. 15.42c).

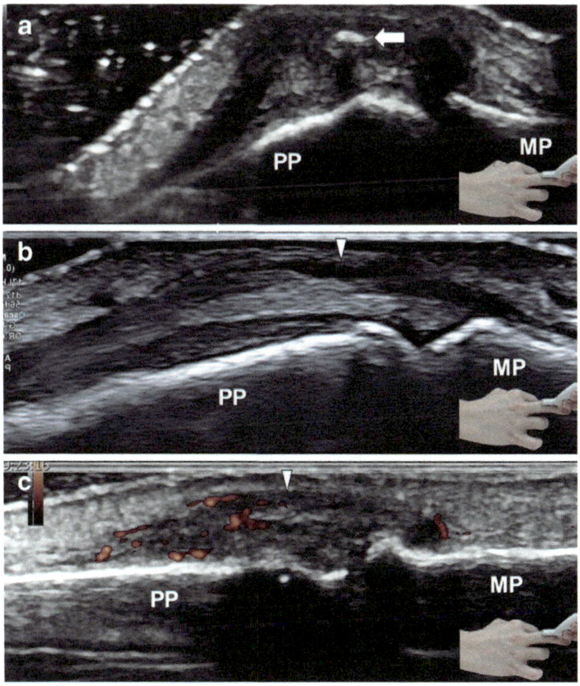

Fig. 15.41 The ultrasound images illustrate central slip injuries, including an avulsion fracture (white arrow) (**a**), a partial tear of the central slip (white arrowheads) (**b**), and a partial tear with swelling and hyperemia (**c**) along the finger's long axis. PP proximal phalanx; MP middle phalanx

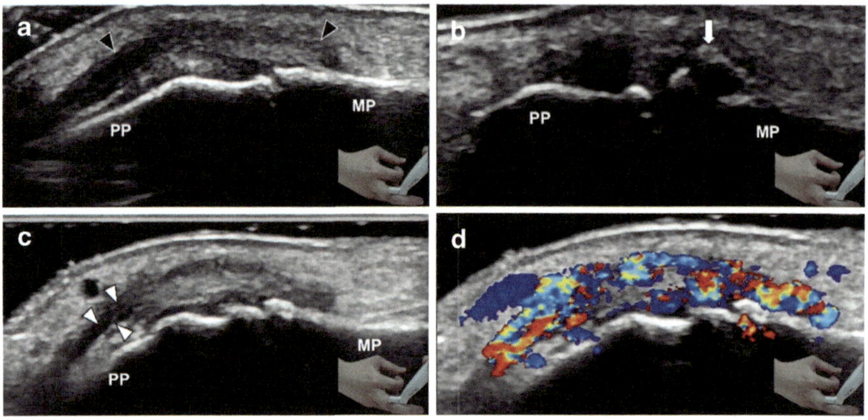

Fig. 15.42 The ultrasound images illustrate different types of collateral ligament injuries, including a ligament sprain with hypoechoic swelling (black arrowheads) (**a**), an avulsion fracture (white arrow) (**b**), a partial-thickness tear (white arrowheads) (**c**), and increased blood flow at the injury site, as shown by Doppler imaging (**d**). PP proximal phalanx; MP middle phalanx

Doppler imaging may show hyperemia near the tear site, indicating increased blood flow associated with the injury (Fig. 15.42d). A full-thickness tear shows a hypoechoic gap extending through the entire thickness of the collateral ligament (Fig. 15.43a), compared to the normal side (Fig. 15.43b). In cases of a complete tear, ultrasound imaging typically depicts ligament swelling and retraction, which appears as a hypoechoic pseudo mass.

An injury to the ulnar collateral ligament of the first metacarpophalangeal joint, often referred to as Gamekeeper's thumb or Skier's thumb [21], is typically associated with abduction injuries. During ultrasound examination, gentle valgus stress applied to the joint may help reveal a ligament tear and retraction, especially if fluid is seen entering the torn ligament gap. Ultrasound imaging may show a stump retracted from the ligament tear (Fig. 15.44a), associated hyperemia (Fig. 15.44b), a tear extending through the full thickness of the ligament (Fig. 15.44c), and an increase in the joint space upon valgus examination (Fig. 15.44d).

In patients with a Stener lesion (migration of the ruptured ulnar collateral ligament superficial to the adductor pollicis aponeurosis), the retracted ligamentous stump appears as a hypoechoic, heterogeneous, mass-like structure located at the juxta-articular region. This type of injury will not heal spontaneously, and surgical intervention is recommended to prevent chronic instability. Conversely, the radial collateral ligaments support the dorsal joint capsule and resist valgus forces on the thumb's metacarpophalangeal joint, providing stability during both flexion and extension, especially during strong pinching motions. Injuries to the radial collateral ligament of the thumb are less common than those on the ulnar side.

Fig. 15.43 The ultrasound image shows a full-thickness tear of the accessory collateral ligament (white arrowhead) (a), compared to the normal ligament (black arrowhead) on the contralateral side (b) at the same joint. PP proximal phalanx

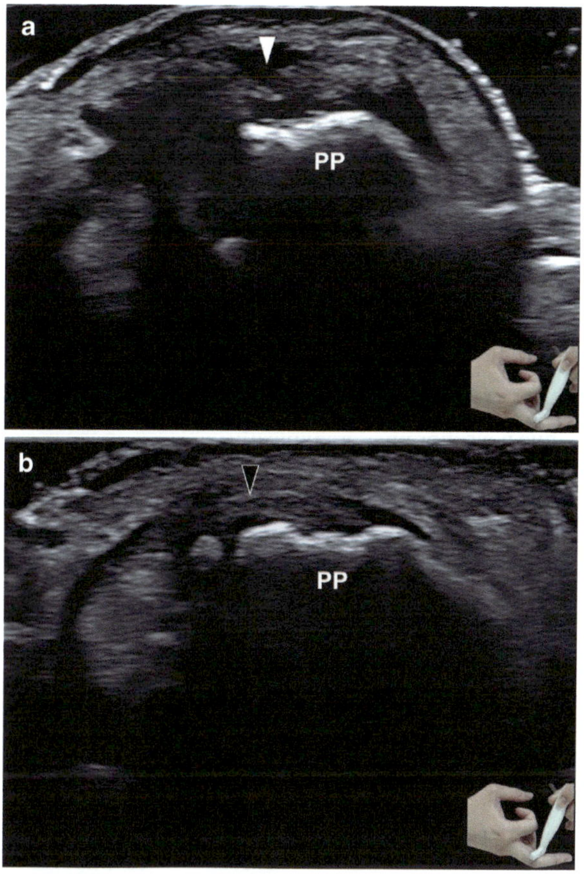

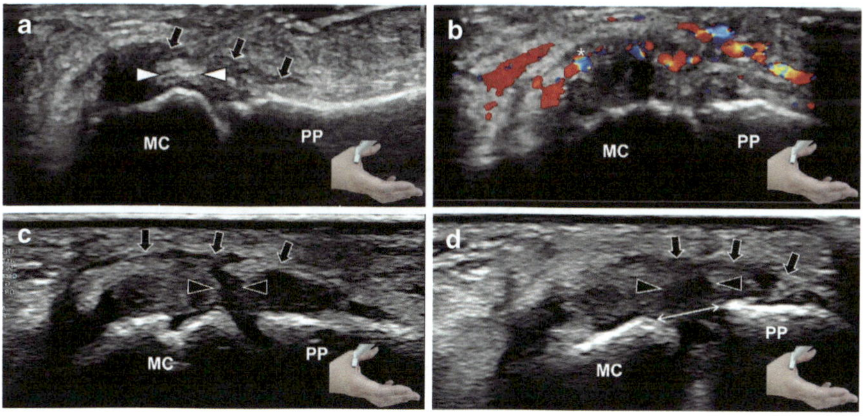

Fig. 15.44 The ultrasound images depict the injury of the ulnar collateral ligament of the first metacarpophalangeal joint. The complete tear is shown with the stump (white arrowheads) retracted from the torn ligament (**a**). Associated hyperemia is observed in another case (**b**). In the third case, a full-thickness tear (black arrowheads) of the ligament is present (**c**), and an increase in the joint space (double-dashed line) is observed upon valgus examination (**d**). Black arrows: adductor pollicis aponeurosis; MC metacarpal bone; PP proximal phalanx

15.4.4 Tumor

Common finger masses include ganglion cysts, glomus tumors, giant cell tumors, neuromas, and Dupuytren's contracture. Glomus tumors (short axis, Fig. 15.45a; long axis, Fig. 15.45b; corresponding magnetic resonance image, Fig. 15.45c) [22], which arise from neuromyoarterial glomus bodies, appear as focal hypoechoic masses with hyperemia and may involve the cortical bone. These tumors most often occur beneath the nail or near the distal digit, presenting with pain and tenderness. The giant cell tumor (short axis, Fig. 15.46a and Fig. 15.46b; long axis, Fig. 15.46c) [23], also known as pigmented villonodular tenosynovitis, presents as a hypoechoic, hyperemic solid mass in contact with the tendon sheath, most commonly affecting the finger flexor tendons. A neuroma that is eccentric to the peripheral nerve is characteristic of a schwannoma (short axis, Fig. 15.47a; long axis, Fig. 15.47b) [24], while neurofibromas are typically centered on the nerve. Both appear as hypoechoic structures, with variable blood flow on Doppler imaging. Dupuytren's contracture presents as a palpable mass or nodularity superficial to the finger flexor tendons of the hand, caused by thickening of the palmar aponeurosis [25], which may lead to contracture. On ultrasound, it appears as nodular or cord-like hypoechoic masses, known as knuckle pads, situated superficial to the finger flexor tendons (short axis, Fig. 15.48a, b; long axis, Fig. 15.48c).

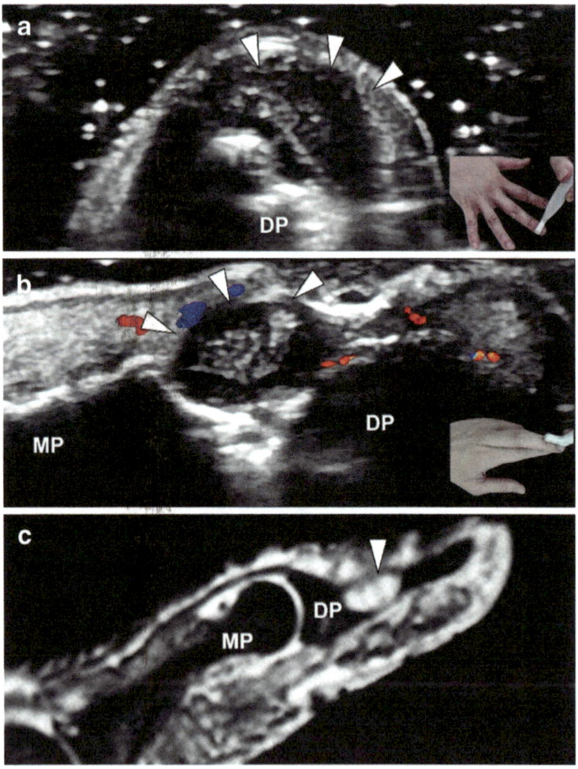

Fig. 15.45 The images show a glomus tumor (white arrowheads) in the finger's short-axis view (**a**), long-axis view (**b**), and the corresponding magnetic resonance image (**c**). MP middle phalanx; DP distal phalanx

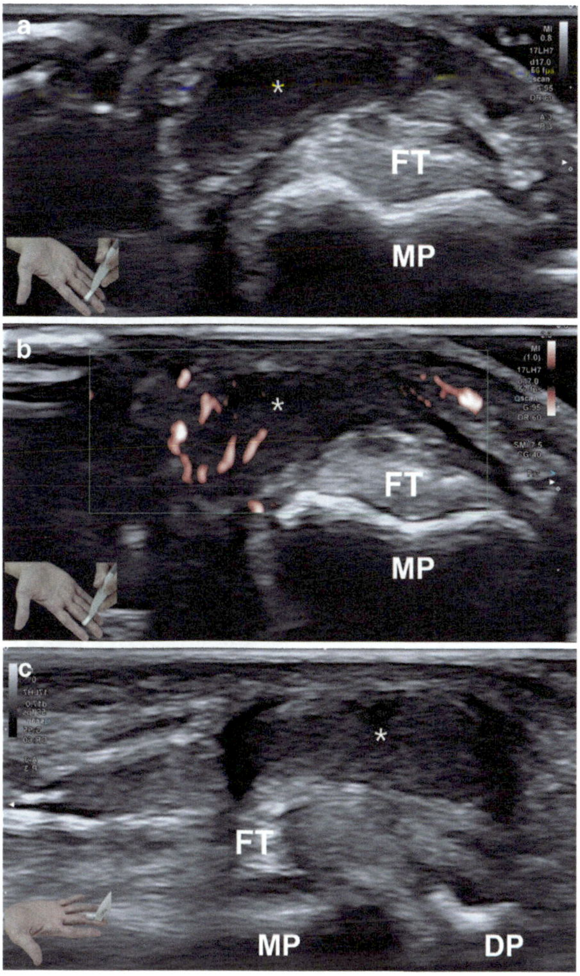

Fig. 15.46 The ultrasound images show a giant cell tumor (asterisks) as a hypoechoic, homogeneous mass (**a**) with a hyperemic pattern (**b**), visualized in both the short-axis and long-axis views of the finger (**c**). FT finger flexor tendon; MP middle phalanx; DP distal phalanx

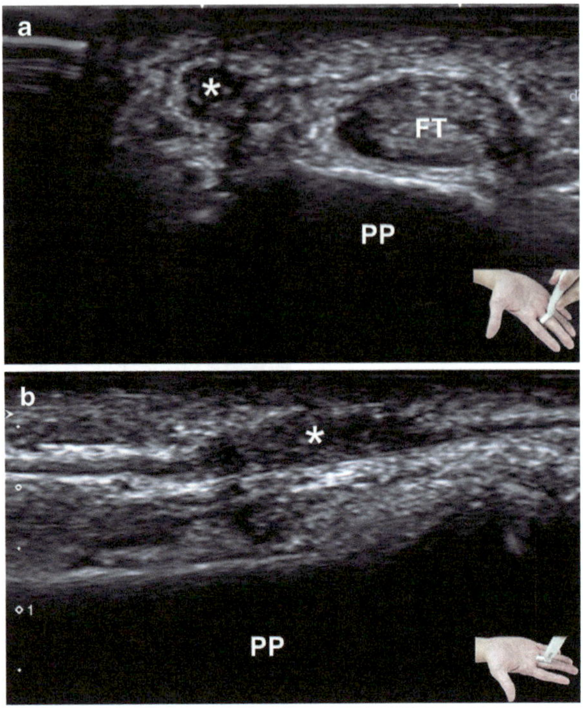

Fig. 15.47 The ultrasound images show a schwannoma of the palmar proper digital nerve (asterisks) in the short-axis (**a**) and long-axis (**b**) views of the finger. PP proximal phalanx; FT finger flexor tendon

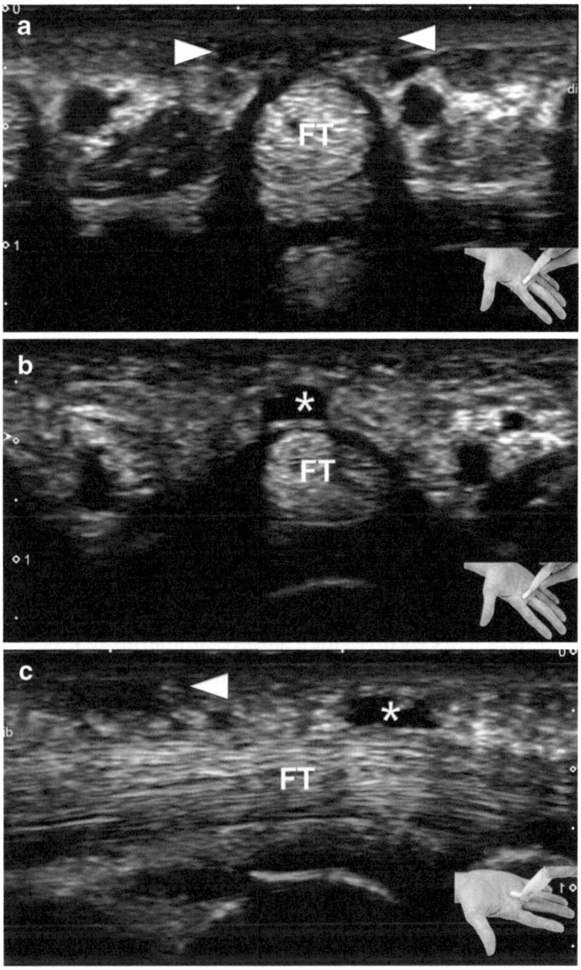

Fig. 15.48 The ultrasound images show Dupuytren's contracture (white arrowheads) (**a**) associated with a ganglion cyst (asterisks) in both finger's short-axis (**b**) and long-axis views (**c**) of the same case. FT finger flexor tendon

15.5 Ultrasound-Guided Intervention

For the management of trigger finger, the transducer can be positioned longitudinally along the long axis of the phalangeal bone. A 1.5-inch, 25-gauge needle is preferred, and the needle shaft can be bent to an angle greater than 60° to facilitate advancement. A local anesthetic ointment can be applied to the puncture site to minimize discomfort. The needle is inserted from the distal to proximal aspect using the in-plane approach, with the injectate consisting of 20 mg of triamcinolone acetonide and 1 mL of lidocaine, targeting the interface between the annular pulley and the finger flexor tendon sheath. If the goal is to thin the annular pulley, a thicker needle, such as a 23-gauge, may be used to scratch and release the pulley (Fig. 15.49a). It is recommended to administer local anesthetics to block the bilateral palmar common digital nerves prior to annular pulley release. An in-plane approach with corticosteroid injection through the finger's short axis, targeting the undersurface of the A1 pulley, is also feasible and carries a lower risk of damaging the finger flexor tendon (Fig. 15.49b).

In cases of chronic sprain of the radial or ulnar collateral ligament, the fingers may exhibit a sausage-shaped appearance and experience difficulty in achieving full flexion. Ultrasound imaging can initially be utilized to confirm the presence of any ligament tears. If no evidence of ligamentous tear is found, a small amount of corticosteroid, such as 10 mg of triamcinolone acetonide, can be administered under

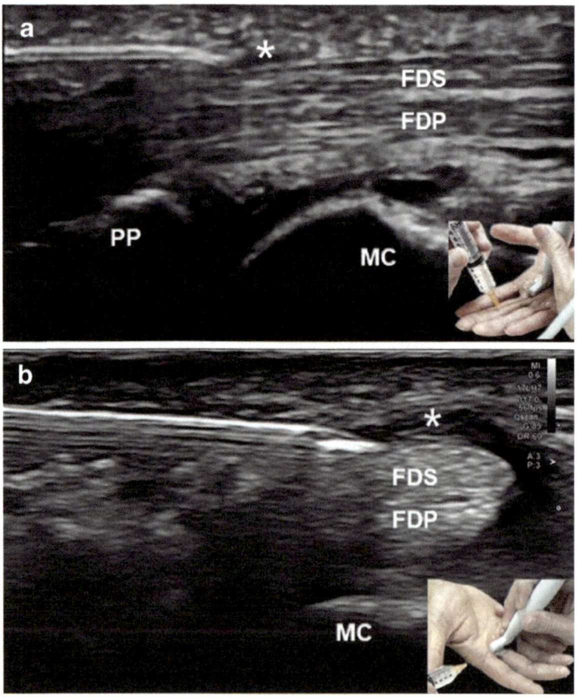

Fig. 15.49 The ultrasound-guided injection for trigger finger using the in-plane technique along the finger's long axis (**a**) and short axis (**b**). Asterisks: A1 pulley; FDS flexor digitorum superficialis tendon; FDP flexor digitorum profundus tendon; MC metacarpal bone; PP proximal phalanx

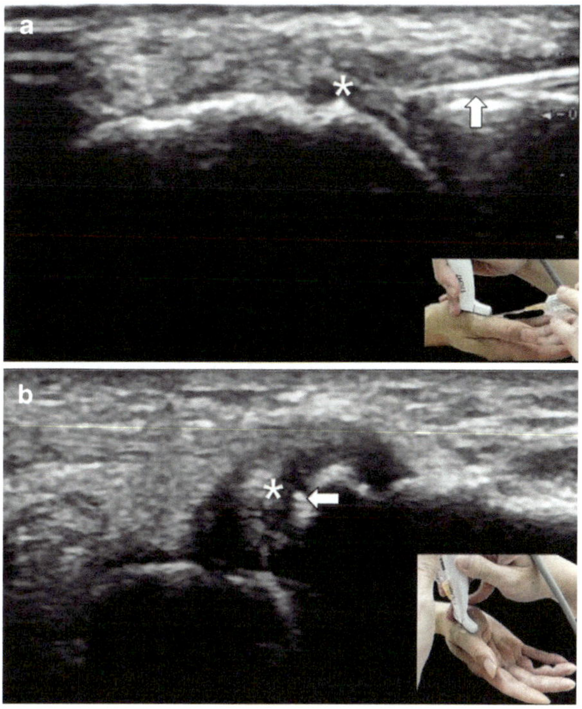

Fig. 15.50 The ultrasound-guided injection of the collateral ligament using the in-plane technique (**a**) or out-of-plane technique (**b**). Asterisks: the injured collateral ligament; white arrows: the needle

ultrasound guidance, either in-plane (Fig. 15.50a) or out-of-plane (Fig. 15.50b). This aims to target the undersurface of the ligament, facilitating its return to a normal appearance.

15.6 Conclusion

The intricate tendinous structures of the fingers are well-documented. Through static and dynamic ultrasound imaging, we have gained valuable insights into the normal and abnormal interactions of tendons and peritendinous connective tissues. Notably, the application of ultrasound-guided curved needle interventions has emerged as a promising approach for addressing common finger pathologies such as stenosing tenosynovitis. This integrated diagnostic and therapeutic approach holds significant potential for enhancing clinical outcomes in managing finger conditions.

Acknowledgments Images and illustrations adapted from cadaveric images provided by the Visible Human Project® of the National Library of Medicine. Excerpts featured in the VH Dissector are used with permission from Touch of Life Technologies Inc.

References

1. Moellhoff N, Throner V, Frank K, et al. Epidemiology of hand injuries that presented to a tertiary care facility in Germany: a study including 435 patients. Arch Orthop Trauma Surg. 2023;143(3):1715–24.
2. Johnson E, Stelzer J, Romero AB, Werntz JR. Recognizing and treating trigger finger. J Fam Pract. 2021;70(7):334–40.
3. Massengill JB. The boutonniere deformity. Hand Clin. 1992;8(4):787–801.
4. Fenech M. Boxer's knuckle: Sonographic anatomy and assessment of sagittal band tears of the dorsal hood. Aust J Ultrasound Med. 2023;26(4):216–29.
5. Doyle JR. Anatomy of the finger flexor tendon sheath and pulley system. J Hand Surg Am. 1988;13(4):473–84.
6. De Las HJ, Simón de Blas C, Salaberri GJ, et al. What is new in flexor tendon pulleys and the gaps between them in triphalangeal fingers of the hand? J Anat. 2024; https://doi.org/10.1111/joa.14031.
7. Faccio D, Montanari S, Maschio N, Bassetto F, Tiengo C, Messana F. The origins of the camper's chiasm asymmetry: a cadaveric study and clinical implications for flexor tendons surgery. J Plast Surg Hand Surg. 2023;57(1–6):471–5.
8. Colzani G, Tos P, Battiston B, Merolla G, Porcellini G, Artiaco S. Traumatic extensor tendon injuries to the hand: clinical anatomy, biomechanics, and surgical procedure review. J Hand Microsurg. 2016;8(1):2–12.
9. Dass P, Prabhu LV, Pai MM, Nayak V, Kumar G, Janardhanan JP. A comprehensive study of the extensor tendons to the medial four digits of the hand. Chang Gung Med J. 2011;34(6):612–9.
10. Young CM, Rayan GM. The sagittal band: anatomic and biomechanical study. J Hand Surg Am. 2000;25(6):1107–13.
11. Allison DM. Anatomy of the collateral ligaments of the proximal interphalangeal joint. J Hand Surg Am. 2005;30(5):1026–31.
12. De Maeseneer M, Meng J, Marcelis S, Jager T, Provyn S, Shahabpour M. Ultrasound anatomy of the fingers: flexor and extensor system with emphasis on variations and anatomical detail. J Ultrason. 2020;20(81):e122–e8.
13. Armenta E, Lehrman A. The vincula to the flexor tendons of the hand. J Hand Surg Am. 1980;5(2):127–34.
14. Slattery PG. The dorsal plate of the proximal interphalangeal joint. J Hand Surg Br. 1990;15(1):68–73.
15. Bianchi S, Gitto S, Draghi F. Ultrasound features of trigger finger: review of the literature. J Ultrasound Med. 2019;38(12):3141–54.
16. Bekhet CNH, Ghaffar MKA, Nassef MA, Khattab RT. Role of ultrasound in flexor tendon injuries of the hand: a new insight. Ultrasound Med Biol. 2021;47(8):2157–66.
17. Wang T, Guo F, Qi H, et al. The role of ultrasonography in diagnosing acute closed volar plate injury of proximal interphalangeal joint. BMC Med Imaging. 2023;23(1):117.
18. Wang T, Qi H, Teng J, Wang Z, Zhao B. The role of high frequency ultrasonography in diagnosis of acute closed mallet finger injury. Sci Rep. 2017;7(1):11049.
19. Westerheide E, Failla JM, van Holsbeeck M, Ceulemans R. Ultrasound visualization of central slip injuries of the finger extensor mechanism1 1No benefits in any form have been received or will be received by a commercial party related directly or indirectly to the subject of this article. J Hand Surg Am. 2003;28(6):1009–13.
20. Draghi F, Gitto S, Bianchi S. Injuries to the collateral ligaments of the Metacarpophalangeal and Interphalangeal joints: Sonographic appearance. J Ultrasound Med. 2018;37(9):2117–33.
21. Melville DM, Jacobson JA, Fessell DP. Ultrasound of the thumb ulnar collateral ligament: technique and pathology. AJR Am J Roentgenol. 2014;202(2):W168.
22. Chiang YP, Hsu CY, Lien WC, Chang YJ. Ultrasonographic appearance of subungual glomus tumors. J Clin Ultrasound. 2014;42(6):336–40.

23. Middleton WD, Patel V, Teefey SA, Boyer MI. Giant cell tumors of the tendon sheath: analysis of sonographic findings. AJR Am J Roentgenol. 2004;183(2):337–9.
24. Lee SJ, Yoon ST. Ultrasonographic and clinical characteristics of Schwannoma of the hand. Clin Orthop Surg. 2017;9(1):91–5.
25. Morris G, Jacobson JA, Kalume Brigido M, Gaetke-Udager K, Yablon CM, Dong Q. Ultrasound features of palmar Fibromatosis or Dupuytren contracture. J Ultrasound Med. 2019;38(2):387–92.

GPSR Compliance

The European Union's (EU) General Product Safety Regulation (GPSR) is a set of rules that requires consumer products to be safe and our obligations to ensure this.

If you have any concerns about our products, you can contact us on ProductSafety@springernature.com

In case Publisher is established outside the EU, the EU authorized representative is:

Springer Nature Customer Service Center GmbH
Europaplatz 3
69115 Heidelberg, Germany

Batch number: 10732076

Printed by Printforce, the Netherlands